HEART DISEASE, CANCER AND STROKE IN CHICAGO

A Geographical Analysis with Facilities, Plans for 1980

Gerald F. Pyle
The University of Akron

THE UNIVERSITY OF CHICAGO
DEPARTMENT OF GEOGRAPHY
RESEARCH PAPER NO. 134

1971

AF691918

Copyright 1971 by Gerald F. Pyle
Published 1971 by The Department of Geography,
The University of Chicago, Printed by The University
of Chicago Printing Department, Chicago, Illinois

Library of Congress Catalog Card Number: 77-167941

Research Papers are available from:
The University of Chicago
Department of Geography
5828 S. University Avenue
Chicago, Illinois 60637
Price: $4.50 list; $4.00 series subscription

ACKNOWLEDGMENTS

This study was made possible through assistance from several agencies. The major basis of support was the Illinois Regional Medical Program grant 7 GO2 RM-00061, operating in cooperation with the Hospital Planning Council for Metropolitan Chicago. At the same time, a fellowship from the Economic Development Administration (OER-019-G-68-2) awarded through the Center for Urban Studies and Department of Geography, University of Chicago, enabled me to do the major portion of the work during the academic year 1969-70.

It would not have been possible to accomplish the study without the thoughtful guidance and assistance of my advisor throughout four years of graduate study, Brian J. L. Berry, Professor of Geography and Director of Training Programs, Center for Urban Studies, University of Chicago. I am also indebted to Chauncy D. Harris, Professor of Geography and Director of the Center for International Studies, University of Chicago, for his interest during the preparation of this study and his valuable suggestions for improvements to the manuscript and the bibliography. Thanks are also due to Jack Meltzer, Director of the Center for Urban Studies, for providing a place to accomplish the processing of data.

Acknowledgments to the assistance of several individuals of the staff of the Hospital Planning Council for Metropolitan Chicago are also in order. Pierre de Vise, Director of the Chicago Regional Hospital Study, carefully reviewed every chapter and drew from his vast knowledge of the practical aspects of health care to make extremely valuable comments and criticisms. Hiram Sibley, Director of the Hospital Planning Council, offered many helpful suggestions about health care facilities research techniques and practical applications. Gerald Falk's keen, perceptive criticisms regarding morbidity and hospital treatment were a great asset. I am particularly grateful for Marian Marshall's record of quietly and efficiently meeting every single typing deadline for the research project. I should also like to thank all other members of the staff of the Hospital Planning Council not specifically mentioned who helped in so many ways.

I am indebted to Brain Lovelace, Assistant Director, Illinois Regional Medical Program, for placing the resources of his agency at my disposal. Particular thanks are due to Robert Rom and Marilyn Voss for making available the results of specialized surveys made by the IRMP staff.

Susan Davies and Marianne Harrison served as research assistants at the Center for Urban Studies by processing and coding morbidity and demographic data. Thanks are also due to Susan and Marianne as well as John Preston Hughes for some of the cartographics drafting in the first four chapters. Larry Finch of the University of Akron assisted with the drafting of the remainder of the maps. Phil Lankford put at my disposal his valuable advice about computer programing, and assisted particularly with Chapter VI.

My wife, Carole, served as a constant inspiration, and, in spite of her own teaching responsibilities, functioned as a research assistant during critical phases of the study. And finally, I am deeply appreciative of golden moments of silence offered by my children, Eric and Frances.

Park Forest, Illinois
1970

PREFACE

This is a study of possible means of improving medical facilities for the treatment of cancer, heart disease, and stroke in Metropolitan Chicago. It would not have been possible if it had not been for a four-year program of research, the Chicago Regional Hospital Study (CRHS), undertaken by the Hospital Planning Council for Metropolitan Chicago in cooperation with the Illinois Department of Public Health, the Center of Health Administration Studies, and the Center for Urban Studies of the University of Chicago.[1] The CRHS undertook extensive in-depth analyses of patient discharge records for all hospitals in the Chicago metropolitan area for the month of February, 1965. The research opportunity was unusual, for the discharge records enabled the complex linkages between patients, doctors, and hospitals to be analyzed and the effects of distance, race, religion, and socio-economic status in hospital use and patients' travel to be described for the first time in a comprehensive manner.

To the findings of this research, supplementary analysis of hospitals[2] determined that apart from two special cases (government hospitals with many long-term beds, and university-related teaching hospitals) the Chicago area is characterized by a hospital hierarchy on the basis of scale of services. Through use of a simple gravity-type model distance-decay relationships between patients and hospitals were revealed. A whole series of these relationships was established for hospitals in the Chicago area.[3] It was thus possible to determine hospital service areas. Not unexpectedly, the large hospitals draw from very large areas. Hospitals of lower levels display substantial overlap in their service areas. In general, service areas in southern Chicago and the south suburbs are more exclusive territorially and they are easier to define. Satellite cities display

---

[1]The Chicago Regional Hospital Study was funded by National Institutes of Health grant HM 00452-01. The study concentrated upon the description and analysis of spatial patterns of use, the prediction of future hospital use, and the measurement of unmet hospital needs.

[2]Richard L. Morrill, "Hierarchy of Hospital Services: Classification of Hospitals," Working Paper I. 8, Chicago Regional Hospital Study, 1966, and "A Principal Components Analysis and Classification of Chicago Area Hospitals," Working Paper I. 9, Chicago Regional Hospital Study, 1967.

[3]Richard L. Morrill, "Relationship Between Transportation and Hospital Location and Utilization," Working Paper I. 14, Chicago Regional Hospital Study, 1967.

distinct areas which overlap little. Overriding each of these is the separation of travel patterns of black and white patients, the former dominated by the service area of Cook County Hospital.

The Morrill-Earickson CRHS Model

Given these study findings, Morrill and Earickson built the CRHS model,[1] the purpose of which was to assign patients to facilities efficiently, given the spatial distribution of patients by broad class of care (medical-surgical, obstetric, pediatric . . .), the spatial distribution and hierarchical position of hospitals, and the interactance parameters linking patients to hospitals via physicians. The model is partly deterministic and partly probabilistic, and has been programmed to account for patient hospital use habits in Chicago on this basis. The model also has a subroutine which redistributes facilities where imabalance exists. It has already been used to evaluate the effects of such proposals as a Southside branch for Cook County Hospital and shows, for example, that whereas at present the black patient has to travel 8 to 12 times farther than the white patient for hospital care (and thus tends to travel less, and only when more seriously ill), either a Southside branch or the requirement that Southside white hospitals admit black patients could do much to eliminate this unwarranted burden.

The CRHS model represents a new approach to hospital planning. The traditional approach had been to allocate N beds to a given population. The new model utilizes as a point of departure the hospital use and hospital service area approach. Initially two kinds of variables are identified:

- I) Patient Variables
  - A) Level and Type of Care
  - B) Ability to Pay
  - C) Race
  - D) Religion
- II) Physician and Hospital Variables
  - A) Physician Locations
  - B) Hospital Locations
  - C) Level and Type of Care
  - D) Policy and Type of Hospital Control

Seven aspects of patient travel are also examined:

- I) To Physicians
- II) Service Areas
- III) Distance
- IV) Level and Type of Care
- V) Economic Variables

---

[1]Richard Morrill and Robert Earickson, "Locational Efficiency of Chicago Hospitals: An Experimental Model," Health Research (Summer, 1969).

VI) Racial Variables
VII) Religious Variables

As explained by Morrill and Earickson:

> The simulation model that has been developed is an interactance model to the extent that probabilities of patients from an area visiting various hospitals are estimated from such a construct, though modified. . . . The model has two additional useful features: a mechanism to achieve replication of the system and one to reallocate hospital capacity in order to improve on the present system.

The first stage allocates patients to physicians or physician clusters:

> If there are large numbers of patients and not too many potential destinations, the probabilities derived from such a modified interactance approach can become deterministic proportions; otherwise a Monte Carlo random number routine allocates the patients in accordance with the probabilities. . . .

Imbalances in clusters are determined rapidly, and as some clusters become saturated, patients are shifted to partially allocated clusters. A second option changes the number of physicians in clusters.

The next operational step of the model is to examine hospital flows:

> The second stage allocates patients to hospitals. The replications of actual patient-to-physician flows are taken as inputs. Using the already identified patient variables of race, religion, and ability to pay, the patient population is divided into six subgroups: paying Negro patients (as above); charity patients (those who did not visit a physician at all but will visit hospitals directly); and four white paying subgroups - Jews, Protestants, Catholics, and the religiously indifferent. Since the capacity of hospitals to care for Negro and charity patients is known, each of these allocations is done separately. All white paying patients are allocated in the same model run, but the religion of the patients is recorded.
>
> Charity patients are allocated to hospitals in the same manner as patients were allocated to physicians above - as a simple function of distance to hospitals and their capacity to treat charity patients. . . . The working hypothesis here, that the choice is a function equally of distance from patient and of distance from physician, seems more reasonable than that the desires of one or the other should be controlling. . . .
>
> White subgroups evaluate distance "religiously" as well as geographically - that is, a mental barrier is erected against a hospital operated under the auspices of a different religion that increases the effective distance to it. Analyses of actual flows and experimental operation of the model suggest that on the average Jews evaluate distance to non-Jewish hospitals as about three times farther; Catholics evaluate distance to non-Catholic hospitals as about twice as far; Protestants evaluate Catholic and Jewish hospitals as about twice as far but evaluate nonreligiously oriented hospitals about the same as Protestant hospitals. These factors, applied to the distances to hospitals, affect the probabilities of visiting various hospitals; otherwise the allocation method is the same as before.

Reiteration of the first option shifts beds from under demanded to over demanded hospitals. This step could also be used to locate new hospitals. The second option shifts the behavioral patterns to fit demand.

Limitations of the CRHS Model

The model, despite its current applicability in other areas, is particularly limited regarding specific morbidity. Since it uses the February, 1965 patient discharge survey as a base, it is also restricted to what that survey reported. Patients were classified by type of care but not by diagnosis. Thus there was no opportunity to link the actual use of hospitals by patients via doctors (revealed demand) with morbidity (disease incidence and need for care, some of which might be unmet), and morbidity in turn with the social, economic and demographic characteristics of health service areas.

Further, since morbidity data were unspecified, it was not possible to link use and need with the availability of special facilities for treatment of specific maladies, for example heart disease, cancer, and stroke, the concern of the Illinois Regional Medical Program (IRMP).

The Regional Medical Model

The purpose of this study is to extend the Morrill-Earickson locational model by (1) building in a morbidity approach so that the need for hospital services can be estimated for small geographic areas, and (2) incorporating the results of analysis of the hierarchy of hospital facilities for the treatment of heart disease, cancer, and stroke, the objects of planning newly instituted in the Illinois Regional Medical Program and the maladies of central concern in the morbidity analysis. It is believed that such an extension will provide an invaluable experimental tool for hospital planners, enabling alternative proposals for improving hospital services to be evaluated in the context of varying patterns of need.

The principal elements of this Regional Medical Program model include:

(1) An explanation of how the planning and operational aspects of the Illinois Regional Medical Program fit into a twenty-five year record of health care facilities planning in the United States (Chapter I).

(2) Analysis of the spatial approach to understanding disease in large cities (Chapter II). The heart disease, cancer, and stroke examples, the three leading killers, account for at least three quarters of all urban deaths. Given this large a sample much can be learned by spatial analysis of these maladies.

(3) In-depth analysis of the incidence of the three diseases in the Chicago SMSA for two time periods, the years 1960 and 1967. Associations are established between disease rates and demographic variables for these two periods. Assuming a similar association in 1980, the demographic variables are forecasted through various means in order to determine 1980 disease patterns (Chapter III).

(4) Analysis of the services provided by hospitals to establish relationships between specialization, scale, service area requirements, and the hierarchy of hospitals (Chapter IV).

(5) A detailed and up-to-date survey of treatment facilities for heart disease, cancer and stroke is accomplished for the Chicago area. The inventory includes capacities for treatment, thus making it possible to add inputs to the planning model (Chapter V).

(6) Replacement of the patient component per se in an allocation model by forecasted morbidity. The treatment facilities are then gradually increased until projected health needs have been met by the supply (Chapter VI).

As with the Morrill-Earickson model, this morbidity-oriented model has applications to geographic locations in addition to Chicago.

TABLE OF CONTENTS

LIST OF TABLES

LIST OF ILLUSTRATIONS

Figure		Page

Figure | Page

CHAPTER I

PLANNING FOR HEALTH CARE FACILITIES AS AN OUTGROWTH OF REGIONAL MEDICAL PROGRAMS

A wide range of interpretations of the history of health planning in the United States is to be found in the literature. To cite a few examples, J. Joel May views the health planning movement in this country as a rather uneven flow of trends which have crested with various highpoints, the most important of which are the Hill-Burton Act of 1946, the report of the Joint Committee of the American Hospital Association and the United States Public Health Service on areawide planning in 1961, and the Comprehensive Health Planning Act of 1966.[1] Hiram Sibley explains health planning as a 3 X 3 matrix with physical, mental, and environmental health planning facets operating as columnar headings and community, metropolitan, and state levels of geographical jurisdiction and/ or operation as rows.[2] Frank Beal explains health planning as an entity which has only recently received anything more than cursory attention by urban planners.[3] According to Beal, planning is new to the health field, which started to use urban planners to any extent only during the 1960's, and it is even newer to urban planning agencies, many of which are just now starting to consider planning of health care facilities as part of their responsibility. That a significant shift may have taken place in the 1960's is echoed by Odin W. Anderson and Joanna Kravits in the introduction to a recent publication:[4]

---

[1] J. Joel May, Health Planning: Its Past and Potential, Health Administration Perspectives No. A5 (Chicago: Center for Health Administration, 1967). The various highpoints suggested by May are discussed in detail later in this text along with other important events and contributions.

[2] Hiram Sibley, "The Hierarchy of Health Planning" (unpublished manuscript, Hospital Planning Council for Metropolitan Chicago).

[3] Frank Beal, The Urban Planner in Health Planning (Washington, D.C.: U.S. Department of Health, Education, and Welfare, Public Health Service, 1968). This report was prepared through the American Society of Planning Officials.

[4] Odin W. Anderson and Joanna Kravits, Health Services in the Chicago Area--A Framework for Use of Data, Research Series No. 26 (Chicago: Center for Health Administration Studies, 1968), p. 3. For a similar analogy dealing with policy and urban planning see Ashley A. Foard and Hilbert Fefferman, "Federal Urban Renewal Legislation,"

Recently Congress passed three laws which may have incalculable effects on the prevailing structure of delivering personal health services in this country. They portend a new era because personal health services are experiencing the end of a free-wheeling development of the prevailing structure and financing of the health care system. The structure and financing of personal health services in the United States have been determined largely by the providers of services with few, and noncontroversial, government restraints such as licensure.

In contrast to these views, the approach of this study is to view the complex process of change toward more and more planning on the part of health care interests as a part of a longer continuum in which many external elements have forced the changes. Although obviously not all change is forced by the changes in our social structure, in many instances the choice for health care establishments is one of either planning or not surviving. In other instances cooperation in a plan can mean maximizing use of facilities and hence "profits." In many respects, whether trends are viewed as a series of policy implications or as a group of highpoints, the emphasis in health planning since its real beginnings on a national level with the Hill-Burton Act of 1946 have shifted in emphasis with changes in the degree and type of urbanization in the United States.

In other words, changes in health planning would appear to be aligned strongly with urban change. At the end of World War II, the greatest emphasis was on small towns and rural areas. Here was the area of concentration most likely to welcome hospital planning--Main Street U. S. A. As both the state administered Hill-Burton programs and metropolitan areas grew, regional planning emerged in the development and proliferation of "area-wide" health planning agencies in the early 1960's. Meanwhile the problems of the central cities were brought swiftly to the attention of the American population. Ghetto riots were followed by several types of inner city health planning in the late 1960's. Also, the population of the country had started to spread out and disperse apace. Concurrent with this movement are to be found state and federally controlled health care payment procedures which perhaps herald an American version of "universal" health care.

Developmental Trends in Health Care Facilities System prior to 1946

By 1946 there had developed in this country a wide array of health care facilities.[1] But the system which had developed by the middle of the twentieth century was described

---

in Urban Renewal, The Record and the Controversy, ed. James Q. Wilson (Cambridge: M. I. T. Press, 1967), pp. 71-125.

[1]During the early 1940's, when it was apparent to the health care community that the United States would embark upon a new era of hospital growth after World War II, the American Hospital Association established for planning purposes a Commission on Hospital Care. The Commission was financed by the Commonwealth Fund, the Kellogg Founda-

by its critics as "disorganized," "unrelated," "overlapping" in terms of patterns of care, "uneconomic," "ineffective," and "haphazard in development." The Commission on Hospital Care described the general lack of coordinated planning in the country in the following manner:[1]

> In most states, anyone can establish the most meager facility for the bed care of the sick and call it a hospital. There is little supervision of the establishment, the organization, or the quality of care in our hospitals. A few states have passed legislation designed to raise the quality of care. Professional organizations have established standards with which hospitals may voluntarily conform. These efforts at improving the quality of service have had a wholesome influence. But the supervision of hospitals has been very largely extra legal in that each institution has been permitted to rest its case with the public it serves. For the most part, the current program of supervision has not resulted in effective controls, particularly in the case of the many small institutions, because public judgments usually are based upon incomplete information or misunderstanding of the elements which contribute to a high quality of hospital care.

The above paragraph represents a realistic and yet pessimistic appraisal of the situation in 1946. First, by that time planning, albeit uncoordinated, was determined by type of control, and the actual implementation of plans was further determined by revenues and sources of revenues. There had developed, and this situation still holds true, three broad types of general hospital in accordance with type of ownership. These groups are (1) Government (Federal, State, Local, --) facilities depending upon taxes for operating revenues, (2) Voluntary (Community Organization, Church, Fraternal, --) hospitals operating with fees and gifts as sources of revenue, and (3) Proprietary (Private) units operating on profits. In addition, there were "plans" developed from 1920 to 1946. The plans had either a local or statewide orientation, and there were perhaps only a half dozen of any real significance.[2] However, the major plans lend impetus to a thrust which in fact became the basis for post-World War II planning. This thrust consisted of two elements posed in the form of the following questions: Is there adequacy of facilities to serve target populations? and, How can coordination among facilities be accomplished? These questions and the other problems already mentioned were in fact based upon a long series of developmental trends which can be examined within two eras, and knowledge of related health care trends hence serves as an asset in understanding the present structure.

---

tion, and the National Foundation for Infantile Paralysis. The primary purpose of the Commission was to conduct a survey of existing health care facilities and make recommendations for planning which would avoid mistakes of the past. The major outcome of the two-year study which was produced in conjunction with the United States Public Health Service was the following publication: Commission on Hospital Care, Hospital Care in the United States (New York: The Commonwealth Fund, 1947).

[1] Ibid., p. x.

[2] May, Health Planning.

The Hospital as a Health and Social Welfare Agency: The Eighteenth and Nineteenth Centuries

Several European traditions regarding health care facilities were transferred to the New World. The needs for collective treatment centers were of course most clearly manifested during the great epidemic plagues.[1] When existing treatment facilities and personnel were taxed beyond all human limits, the structure became the most crystal clear. Those who could afford treatment (when available) received it privately at home. Those who could not relied upon charity. Initially, charity treatment was in the hands of the Church. After the Reformation, pesthouses developed in Protestant countries and the Church continued its function in Catholic regions (it should be pointed out here that during periods of extreme political power the Church largely ignored this obligation but many religious orders continued to care for the indigent ill population). Spanish Catholics carried the notion of the chapel-mission to the New World, and the Portuguese took care of the sick as a part of the less well-known *Misericordia*.

In pre-revolutionary colonial North America, the Protestant traditions were largely reflected. Almshouses were developed in the early eighteenth century for public charity cases, including the sick-poor, the poverty-stricken, the orphaned, the blind and the deaf, the mentally ill, and any other persons considered derelicts.[2] William Penn established the first of these places in Philadelphia in 1713. By 1750 most of the larger urban places and/or seaports had almshouses (the latter functioned for quarantine purposes in an attempt to ward off pending epidemics). Eventually many of the long-term inhabitants of almshouses were sent to special asylums.

Another trend was developing, and for those who could afford to pay voluntary hospitals came into being. The first successful such venture has been attributed to the efforts and influence of Benjamin Franklin in conjunction with Dr. Thomas Bond.[3] In 1751 Franklin solicited £2000 from the Assembly of Pennsylvania with the stipulation that he could match the amount from private contributions. The latter was accomplished and Pennsylvania Hospital was formed. This trend continued as New York Hospital was formed in 1773, Massachusetts General Hospital in 1810, and New Haven Hospital in 1826.

---

[1] For what is perhaps an account of some of the earliest efforts to control and isolate large groups of sick-poor and otherwise infirm populations see Philip Ziegler, *The Black Death* (New York: The John Day Company, 1969).

[2] Commission on Hospital Care, *Hospital Care in the United States*.

[3] *Ibid.*, pp. 432-53.

The tradition of voluntary hospitals continued, and the initiation of this type of institution constituted the first real break with the European ways.[1]

In comparison with other periods of time, the nineteenth century was not represented by very rapid growth in the number of hospitals; important biomedical advances, however, were to herald an era of rapid hospital growth. As voluntary (including religious) hospitals continued to grow slowly they eventually gave up their treatment of mental patients to governmental (mostly state) institutions. In addition, many hospitals developed medical schools. Biomedical advances included the discovery of many causative agents by researchers such as Koch and Pasteur; the beginning of modern nursing partly as a result of treatment of war wounded and dying; social and economic pressures for better treatment and more facilities related to the progressive labor movement; and the development of effective public health agencies which in turn led to control of epidemics.[2]

Still, by 1873 there were only 178 hospitals of all types in the United States with a total capacity of 34,453 beds.[3] In addition, one-third of the beds were for mental patients in custodial care. Two things happened between 1873 and 1909, the date of the first reliable American Medical Association census of hospitals. First the number of hospitals grew rapidly. Second the number of hospital beds increased even more rapidly. As public confidence in hospitals grew the death-house stigma was removed, and public demands led to unprecedented growth.

The Era of "Free-Wheeling" Development: 1900 to 1945

The period from the turn of this century to 1946 was one not only of rapid growth; it was also the time when the infrastructure for our present system of health care facilities became firmly implanted. The voluntary short-term hospital dominated a system which was characterized nationally by uneven geographical distribution and general uncoordination, at least in terms of planning on any sort of comprehensive scale. These hospitals were largely the result of local initiative or private philanthropy. Large medical schools provided health care of the very best type in some urban centers. The attitude in

---

[1] Leslie Morgan Abbe and Anna Mae Baney, The Nation's Health Facilities: Ten Years of the Hill-Burton Hospital and Medical Facilities Program, 1946-1956 (Washington, D.C.: U.S. Department of Health, Education, and Welfare, Public Health Service, 1958), p. 11.

[2] For the story of the development of the New York Board of Health in relation to cholera epidemics see Charles Rosenburg, The Cholera Years (Chicago: University of Chicago Press, 1962).

[3] Commission on Hospital Care, Hospital Care in the United States, Chapter III.

many rural areas of regarding the hospital as the last possible resort combined with a lack of financial resources to inhibit the construction of hospitals and the formulation of other health care plans in these places. Near the end of this period, efforts toward planning were developing in several places, and some of these plans were previews to an era of extensive planning and national coordination. However, some facets of the system were so firmly entrenched that it became necessary either to incorporate many of these traits of the system into new plans or simply not plan at all.

This period can further be divided into two very different subperiods. The first of these dates to 1929. When the Depression hit the United States it marked the end of fifty years of some of the most rapid progress in hospital construction the country had ever witnessed. Already by 1909 the A. M. A. census showed 4,359 hospitals, and by 1928 there were 6,852 hospitals.[1] However, conditions during the Depression forced some 700 hospitals to close by 1938. There was little construction activity during the Depression, and government hospitals were able to survive at a somewhat better rate than others. World War II further halted voluntary and proprietary hospital growth. By 1945, there were 6,098 hospitals in operation. These comparisons in figures must also be tempered by the knowledge that there was attrition among the hospitals all the while; thus the more recent figures represent hospitals which were either built or continued to survive during the entire period 1909 to 1945.

Furthermore, the number of beds available to the population actually showed a gradual increase during this period in spite of a leveling off in the number of hospitals (Fig. 1). While the number of hospitals decreased 6.4 per cent from 1927 to 1941, the number of beds increased 55.2 per cent. Governmental beds increased at the most rapid rate (70 per cent).

Hospitals in 1945 showed the following types of sponsorship: voluntary hospitals made up 50 per cent of the total; governmental, 29 per cent; and proprietary, 21 per cent. Figure 2 shows how, from 1846 to 1946, the various types compared. Most of the supply of voluntary hospitals in 1946 was made of general short-term ones.

During the first half of this century other health care facilities were also changing in orientation. Public health departments grew slowly until after World War I, and by 1935 there were 561 county and multicounty health departments representing some 762

---

[1] Ibid., Chapter IV. Also, see Monroe Lerner and Odin W. Anderson, Health Progress in the United States, 1900-1960 (Chicago: University of Chicago Press, 1963), Chapter XXIII. It should be pointed out that governmental hospitals were not included in 1909, but they were in 1928; however, there were not nearly the number of governmental hospitals in 1909 that there were in 1928.

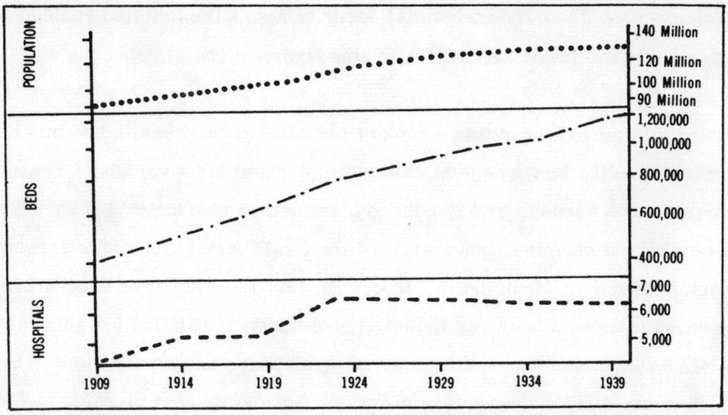

Fig. 1.--A comparison of the growth of hospitals and hospital beds, 1909 to 1939

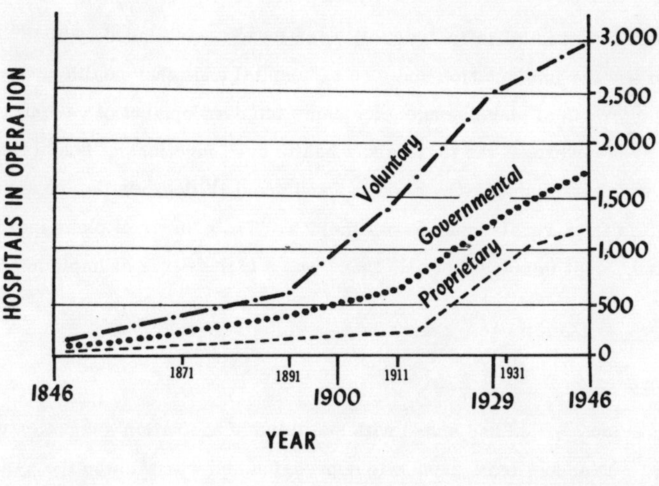

Fig. 2.--The growth of various hospitals by type of sponsorship

counties.[1] By 1946 both the number of counties covered and the number of departments had nearly doubled, and many had assumed some responsibility in taking care of health needs of charity patients. Much of this increase took place during the Depression under Title VI provisions of the 1935 Federal Social Security Act. The act also enabled care of medically indigent through increased aid to nursing homes. The almshouses were being replaced.

All during this period there was a lack of planning to meet health needs. Hospitals were built either where the land was available (often donated for a variety of reasons), near good transportation access, or adjacent to high income residential areas. Some interests had considered planning, however, and the first formal effort was accomplished by the New York Academy of Medicine in 1920.[2] By 1927 the American Hospital Association officially recommended 5 beds per thousand community population for general hospitals. The A. H. A. suggestion was followed by other similar recommendations. In 1931 the Bingham Associate Fund made recommendations for coordinated planning in New England. The Michigan Hospital Survey Committee developed a plan in 1942, and the city of Rochester developed one in 1946. The concept of planning was thus known by the end of World War II, and the Hill-Burton Act added the long overdue impetus to the movement.

Changes, Trends, and Advances from 1945 to 1970

Although the hospital infrastructure was already established by 1946, the next 25 years were to see the implantation and rise of hospital and other health care planning agencies. With the growth of planning agencies came the development of various notions about geographical area coverage; the ideas about health care functions of hospitals having already been well established. Over the two and one-half decades the focus of attention gradually shifted from rural-small town America. The number of plans increased at a rapid rate, and, most important of all, there was a high degree of implementation of these plans.

Hill-Burton programs

The previous period had ended with one third of the nation's counties not having any hospital beds.[3] Freedom from economic depression and war allowed the nation to gather

---

[1]Joseph W. Mountin, Emily K. Hankla, and Georgie B. Druzina, "Ten Years of Federal Grants-in-Aid for Public Health, 1936-1946," Public Health Service Bulletin No. 300, Washington, D. C., 1946.

[2]May, Health Planning, pp. 13-18. [3]Ibid., pp. 24-33.

its resources and attempt to start correcting the shortcomings of the existing system. In January, 1945, Senators Lister Hill and Harold Burton introduced a bill, which was enacted in August 1946 as the Hospital Survey and Construction Act (Title VI of the Public Health Service Act: P. L. 79-725). The initial intent of the bill was simply to supply aid in constructing hospitals in particular parts of the country. The expanded law actually took the idea several steps further, and the purpose of the Hill-Burton Act was stated in two parts:

(1) The various states were to survey their existing supply of hospitals in order to determine needs.

(2) Funds would be supplied to help in new construction.

States were to be given funds through agencies which they established. In order to get the monies each state had to develop a state plan. One of the requirements was that one or more regions had to be established for planning purposes. Service areas were to be determined on the basis of travel habits of the population to hospitals. There were several categories of service area in accordance with hospital size, but the ultimate goal was to supply from 2.5 beds per thousand population in sparse rural areas to at least 4.5 beds per thousand in more settled areas. The actual funding of projects which were approved was accomplished on a variable matching fund basis depending upon each state's per capita income. In 1949, a similar option was added for local communities. Furthermore the nature of the voluntary system was such that these and many other types of hospitals serving the public were included so long as they were "nonprofit."

Much progress could be viewed after ten years.[1] The Act had been amended twice. The first of these amendments was the 1949 one, mentioned above, which authorized the Public Health Service to supply research grants (P. L. 81-380). The second amendment, commonly referred to as the Wolverton Amendment of 1954 (P. L. 83-482), greatly broadened the Hill-Burton program. This amendment provided specific grants for the construction of public and voluntary nonprofit nursing homes, diagnostic and treatment centers, rehabilitation facilities, and facilities for chronic disease. Also funds were appropriated to support the 1949 authorization for grants. Figure 3 shows the national distribution by state of dollars per capita allocated by June 1956. The national average was \$4.8 per capita while the highest (Mississippi) amount was \$10.8 and the lowest (New York) was \$2.1.

By the end of the 1950's Hill-Burton trends and accomplishments could be fairly well evaluated.[2] More than one half of the new hospital beds were in areas which had had

---

[1] Abbe and Baney, Nation's Health Facilities.

[2] For example, see: Alan E. Treloar and Don Chill, Patient Care Facilities: Construction Needs and Hill-Burton Accomplishments, Hospital Monograph Series No. 10 (Chicago: American Hospital Association, 1961), Chapter II.

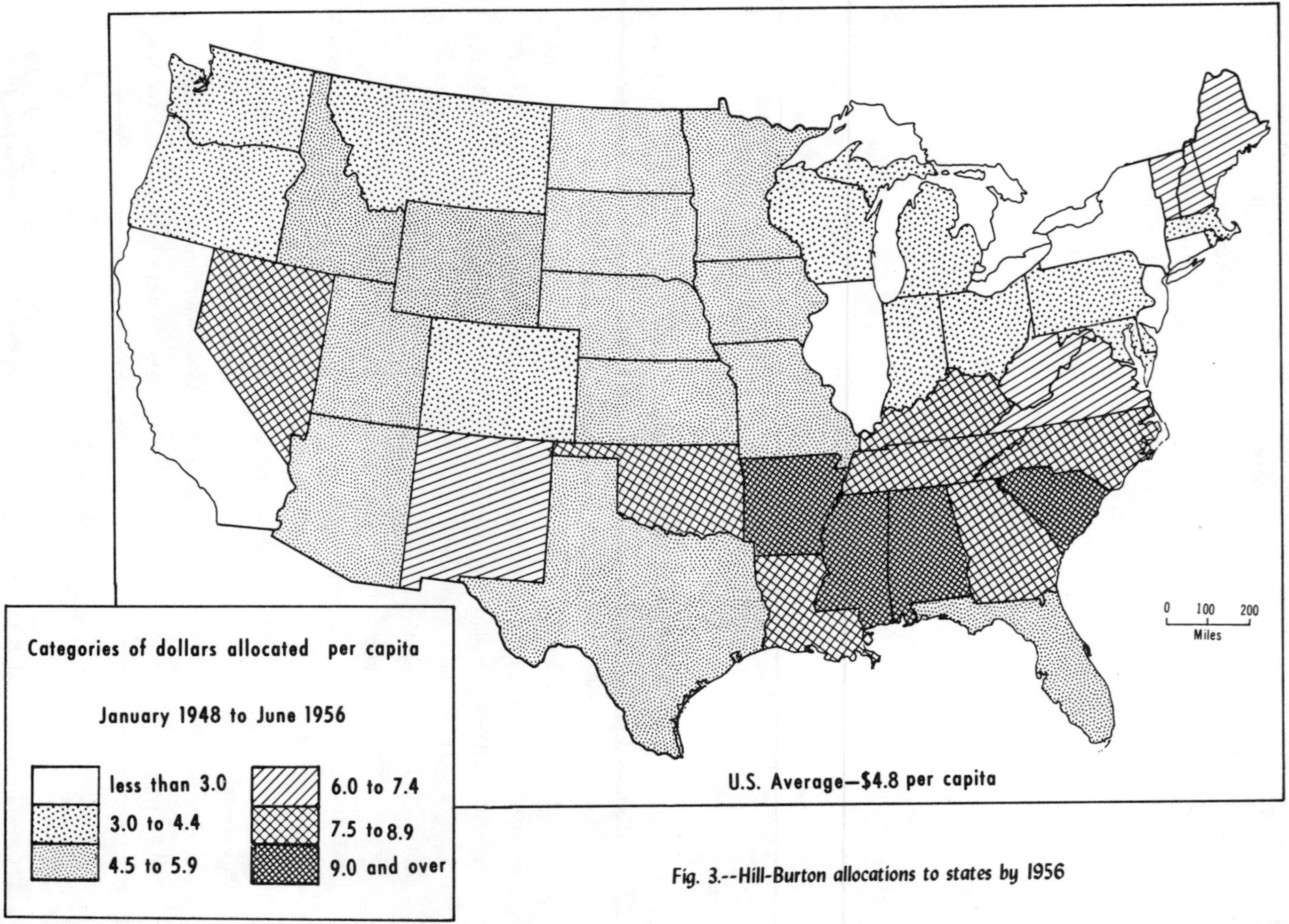

Fig. 3.--Hill-Burton allocations to states by 1956

no hospitals. About 25 per cent were in areas where previous facilities were unacceptable. Medical education was greatly aided by the construction of teaching hospitals. Of necessity surveys and plans had become more systematic. However, the Hill-Burton program became bogged down due to several reasons: (1) many facilities had become obsolete; (2) the population of the United States showed a tremendous increase; (3) people were living longer; (4) hospitals were universally being used more; and (5) construction costs had started to skyrocket.[1] One additional amendment (P. L. 85-589) was passed in 1958 which enabled eligible sponsors to take out long-term loans in lieu of grants.

Many writers have been perhaps too quick to say that the Hill-Burton programs had essentially accomplished their goals by the early 1960's. For in addition to providing new hospitals, beds, and health centers there were many initially unexpected and rewarding results. A 1965 publication lists the following nine important accomplishments:[2]

(1) Systematic statewide planning for hospital facilities.

(2) Development of standards of need.

(3) Development of standards for evaluating the condition of the physical plant.

(4) Achievement of better distribution of facilities.

(5) Improvement of hospital design.

(6) Improvement in hospital operation.

(7) Effective cooperation between government and voluntary health agencies.

(8) Improvement of medical care in low income states and rural areas.

(9) Aid to teaching centers for training physicians and nurses.

The implications regarding planning became more and more obvious. Two Hill-Burton Amendments in the early 1960's related directly to planning. The first of these was the Community Health Services Act of 1961 (P. L. 87-395) which authorized $10 million worth of research funds as well as increased appropriations for nursing homes. The law demonstrated the organizational framework for planners.[3] It encouraged local participation in planning and stimulated community-wide planning. The second amendment was the Hospital and Medical Facilities Amendment of 1964 (P. L. 88-443), commonly known as the Hill-Harris program. It revitalized the survey and construction programs for an

---

[1] Ibid., p. 20.

[2] U. S. Department of Health, Education, and Welfare, "Hill-Burton Program Progress Report, July 1, 1947-June 30, 1965," Public Health Service Publication No. 930-F-3, Washington, D. C., 1965. In an earlier work, Cavanaugh lists the first seven of these items. See James H. Cavanaugh, "Areawide Planning for Hospitals and Related Health Facilities: A National Survey," Ph. D. dissertation, State University of Iowa, 1964 (Ann Arbor: University Microfilms, Inc.).

[3] Cavanaugh, "Areawide Planning . . . ," p. 89.

additional five years, but now much more attention would be given to urban regions. Equally important was the fact that the law authorized additional research and planning funds. After nearly two decades, the importance of planning had become clearly apparent.

Funds from the federal government continued to be appropriated hence maintaining the notion that construction is still important. Table 1 shows how much money was appropriated to June 30, 1965. Of the money 74.6 per cent went to general hospital facilities, 10.2 per cent went to long-term care facilities, 3.1 per cent went to mental hospitals, 1.1 per cent went to tuberculosis care facilities, and 11.0 per cent went to other health care facilities.[1] During this period all the above categories and several others had become incorporated under the general umbrella of comprehensive health care. The comprehensive definition also developed implications of regional and areal coverage, and these notions became part of another "school" of health planning which had developed.

Areawide planning

Improvements in handling and the increased expansion of scope of Hill-Burton programs led to increased amounts of social capital, both from private and public sources, inputs into the hospital system. In addition, newer health care legislation was geared to a metropolitan power base. The natural outcome of such change was the establishment and proliferation of planning agencies, the most common of which were voluntary in nature. Near the end of the 1950's there were nearly a dozen voluntary agencies engaged in metropolitan, or as the term became precisely known, areawide, planning. They were generally one of three types:[2]

(1) Traditional hospital membership organizations.

(2) Community-centered agencies.

(3) Agencies integrating the above two notions.

The subsequent release of large amounts of federal funds intended to help organize further planning in many cities called for closer governmental control, and in order to accomplish this some guidelines had to be developed.

Headed by George Bugbee, the Joint Committee of the American Hospital Association and the United States Public Health Service formulated a viable set of guidelines for the establishment of areawide planning agencies.[3] The idea of establishing such agencies

---

[1] U. S. Department of Health, Education, and Welfare, "Hill-Burton Program Progress Report."

[2] May, Health Planning, p. 37.

[3] "Areawide Planning for Hospitals and Related Health Facilities," A Report of the Joint Committee of the American Hospital Association and the Public Health Service, U. S.

TABLE 1

THE FIRST TWO DECADES OF HILL-BURTON APPROPRIATIONS[a]

Fiscal Year	Number of Projects	Facilities Provided		Total Cost	Federal Funds Obligated
		Inpatient Beds	Other Health Facilities		
Total	7,850	333,280	2,259	$7,470,108,546	$2,351,758,830
1948	448	22.019	74	283,137,023	74,404,235
1949	366	18,354	59	283,190,888	74,869,859
1950	536	27,235	101	459,286,727	149,722,023
1951	266	12,849	62	250,002,856	84,722,023
1952	250	12,281	67	271,003,456	82,184,988
1953	263	11,555	76	244,942,643	74,912,105
1954	215	8,761	72	179,835,760	64,915,444
1955	458	13,858	187	367,671,691	95,529,871
1956	428	17,301	136	376,315,203	109,424,927
1957	501	18,801	165	414,015,132	122,671,582
1958	448	18,375	139	441,588,728	119,025,688
1959	636	23,731	215	585,277,821	184,295,889
1960	558	23,337	165	554,184,539	183,904,768
1961	538	23,296	149	549,111,514	183,948,495
1962	562	25,455	158	655,368,526	209,161,029
1963	600	24,233	186	652,801,706	217,186,663
1964	538	22,254	171	638,888,658	216,714,864
1965[b]	239	9,585	77	263,485,675	104,181,406

Source: U. S. Department of Health, Education and Welfare, "Hill-Burton Program Progress Report."

[a]Available for the fiscal year under appropriation and for the succeeding fiscal year, or a two-year period.

[b]One fiscal year.

had already started to spread rapidly, and, as pointed out by J. Joel May, the "joint report" incentive and justification for more formal organizational procedures. The report was amplified two years later by a U. S. Public Health Service manual on organizational procedures.[1]

Department of Health, Education, and Welfare, Public Health Service Publication No. 885 (Washington, D. C.: U. S. Government Printing Office, 1961).

[1]"Procedures for Areawide Health Facility Planning," U. S. Department of Health, Education, and Welfare, Public Health Service, Division of Hospital and Medical Facilities, Washington, D. C., September, 1963.

On actually establishing a local planning agency the following principles were suggested:[1]

(1) Key public or private agencies should take the initiative to establish planning units in localities where there are particular problems.

(2) Governing bodies of agencies should be comprised of community leaders in general and not include full-time health workers.

(3) The agency should be established on a permanent basis.

(4) The agency should have official Hill-Burton recognition as the authorized planning agency for the region, and the two agencies should work closely together.

(5) A geographic region, normally centered upon one or more cities and incorporating the SMSA, should be delimited. The area should be consistent with the Hill-Burton area. State lines may be crossed.

(6) Liaison with related community organizations should be established.

It was further recommended that several types of data be collected:

(1) Profiles of all health care facilities within the geographic region should be maintained.

(2) Other types of related community data, e.g., demographic, socioeconomic, and topographic, should be procured.

(3) Health facilities data should include:

(a) Obsolescence information.

(b) Distribution of available services.

(c) Patient origins.

(d) Educational programs.

(e) Use of clinics and other specialized services.

(f) Distribution of physicians and other health facility personnel.

(g) Length of stay.

Other suggested activities included projections of future need, planning for an orderly distribution of facilities, projections of financial resources, scheduling construction work, and devising means to carry out plans. All these goals plus the points listed above helped to place a high value on coordinated planning efforts. It was becoming increasingly difficult for individual hospitals to develop plans without consulting with surrounding units. In addition, areawide planning agencies were to discourage the duplication and a variety of other possible results which might develop from the unwise construction of new facilities.

These guidelines were to assist the Public Health Service in actually granting funds. According to Jack C. Haldeman, grants were in fact to serve three purposes:[2]

---

[1] "Areawide Planning for Hospitals and Related Health Facilities."

[2] Cavanaugh, "Areawide Planning . . . ."

(1) To demonstrate to various community settings the organizational framework required by planning agencies in order to effectively carry out their function.

(2) To stimulate area-wide planning in the communities where demonstrations are being carried out as well as in other communities which will be able to benefit from the results of the demonstration.

(3) To reduce the time lag between the development and adoption of improved planning methods.

Thus, according to Haldeman the accomplishment of Hill-Burton objectives in metropolitan areas could be facilitated through such agencies.

Fortunately, a very early study of the effectiveness of the joint committee guidelines is offered in the work of Cavanaugh. By 1963, 38 of the agencies were under discussion in the United States. Cavanaugh sent questionnaires to these agencies, and in a 78.9 per cent (30 agencies) response he was able to determine how, along with many other things, the agencies were following the guidelines. An elaborate checklist of 36 points was developed by Cavanaugh. The most salient conclusion reached was that there was a great deal of variation in many areas among the agencies, and the variation was due to the following points:[1]

(1) Few state boundaries were crossed in determining planning areas.

(2) There was in actuality a general lack of cooperation from state Hill-Burton agencies.

(3) There was also reluctance on the part of many hospitals to supply data.

(4) Some new agencies were not getting cooperation from the more traditional medical and hospital associations.

(5) There appeared to be a lack of representation on the new governing boards from both organized labor and Hill-Burton advisory councils.

(6) Some agencies were receiving all their support from the federal government.

(7) Few agencies had started to receive and disburse capital funds.

Since the Cavanaugh study, the number of agencies has increased about threefold. It would appear that some but not all the problems spelled out have been solved; however, only a national survey would really tell the story. Meanwhile, areawide planning has become entrenched to the point where the term has lost its early and very explicit meaning. For example, the traditionally strong powers which individual hospitals exercised regarding planning could by no means be completely ignored.[2] Conversely, opposition to

---

[1] Ibid., pp. 270-71.

[2] See C. Rufus Rorem, "Areawide Planning Is Here to Stay, Auspices and Areas," The Modern Hospital, August, 1964.

areawide planning agencies has lessened considerably. Charles I. Stone spells out planning progress in the following manner:[1]

> Inherent in areawide planning is the fundamental advantage that viewing the community as whole results in the consideration of each individual hospital's role in perspective. It is thus possible to develop an overall program designed to bring hospital care to the community on an organized coordinated basis. The situation is one where in the past competition has been the byword. The future bespeaks a more integrated system for the provision of health facilities care with cooperation and coordination the guiding principles.

Obviously many but not all of the above goals have been accomplished, and somewhat belated efforts toward bringing increased health care to this country's urban poor were greatly accelerated in the 1960's.

Focus on the central city

As more national attention is given to the health problems of the ghettos, changes are starting to take place in the method of delivery of health care. Universities, some of which have long operated ghetto mental and other health clinics, are starting to open the doors of their medical school clinic more and more. The OEO has opened a number of general health clinics in the nation's ghettos, but these are still limited in number and in ability to provide for the needs of large numbers of people. Part of the answer to the problem of improving ghetto health care facilities lies in the future of two programs, Medicaid and "Model Cities."

Described as a "potentially large program of medical assistance" in 1966, Medicaid (more specifically Title XIX, the Medical Assistance Programs of P. L. 89-97) is in fact a part of the trend toward increasing social welfare activity under the aegis of the Social Security Act. Although critically important, Medicaid is in fact an extension of earlier post-World War II legislation. In 1950 the Bureau of Family Services of the Welfare Administration of the U. S. Department of Health, Education, and Welfare started to provide direct payments for medical care to public assistance recipients.[2] The passage of the Kerr-Mills Act (P. L. 86-778) caused the program to be broadened in 1960. Title XIX programs have now replaced the previous (MAA) programs in most states.

The Medicaid programs are joint Federal-State operations which provide medical care to public assistance recipients and others who do not qualify for public aid but are unable to pay for medical care. Programs are administered by state agencies and the

---

[1] Charles I. Stone, "Areawide Planning for Health Facilities," Hospitals, XLI (April 1, 1967), 51-53.

[2] Dennis E. Stump, Jr., "The Major Aspects of Medical Assistance under Title XIX," Public Health Reports, LXXXI (October, 1966), 867-69.

national government provides from 50 to 83 per cent of the costs, depending upon state average per capita income.[1] Some states, New York and California for example, have utilized this federal incentive to provide extremely progressive medical assistance programs. Other states have moved more slowly.

The Title XIX provisions expressly spell out that any state participating in Medicaid shall provide five minimum services to participants:[2]

(1) Inpatient hospital services.

(2) Outpatient hospital services.

(3) Physicians services (include physicians offices).

(4) Nursing home services for those over 21.

(5) X-ray and other laboratory services.

Furthermore, the legislation specifies that these services be of high quality.

By 1970 many critics of Title XIX stated that, along with other programs, Medicaid has greatly contributed to unnecessary increases in hospital services. The American Hospital Association released as a service to hospitals some interpretive questions and answers about Medicaid reimbursement in 1967.[3] These guidelines include the following key points. A health care recipient is generally free to select a vendor, but some states have amended that option. The major element regarding cost is that it should be "reasonable." Procedures on admission vary greatly from state to state. The administration of proper standard is up to the state office.

Although Illinois was one of the first states to start a Medicaid program, it has lagged behind other states in actually offering health care to the needy.[4] For example, if a family of four makes more than $3,600, it is not eligible. The program is also bogged down in administrative red tape and inefficiency. Many potential recipients of Medicaid in Chicago's ghettos are not aware of the program.[5] The best possible methods of track-

---

[1] See U. S. Department of Health, Education, and Welfare, "Questions and Answers on Medical Assistance," Welfare Administration, Bureau of Family Services Publication 13-29, Washington, D. C., May, 1967.

[2] Ellen Winston, "The New Medical Assistance Program," Public Health Reports, LXXXI (October, 1966), 863-66.

[3] "Title 19 Questions and Answers," Special Bulletin, Medicare No. 31, October, 1967.

[4] Lawrence Bloom, Joyce Lashof, and Pierre de Vise, "Toward Comprehensive Health Care for All Chicagoans," in Slum Medicine: Chicago's Apartheid Health System, by Pierre de Vise et al. (Chicago: University of Chicago Community and Family Study Center, 1969), pp. 71-91.

[5] Lawrence S. Bloom, Peter R. Bonavich, and Daniel Sudran, "Medicaid in Cook County," Inquiry, V (June, 1968), 1-12.

ing medically indigent is through persons receiving general or categorical assistance. Little has been done by either the Cook County Department of Public Aid or the Illinois Department of Public Aid to make the public aware of the programs. Some hospitals have been reluctant to take on Medicaid recipients, and many hospitals have a poor record in seeing this type of patient. Among hospitals that see Medicaid patients, one had unpaid accounts of $1.5 million and five others had unpaid claims of from $250,000 to $750,000.[1] In terms of the growth and development of health care planning much must be accomplished before Medicaid is a working reality.

Another recent program important to health care facilities planning is the Demonstration Cities and Metropolitan Development Act of 1966 (P. L. 89-754), or the Model Cities Act. The Model Cities Act actually represents a major thrust in urban planning for at least two reasons important to this study. The first of these is that the emphasis has shifted from the earlier redevelopment/renewal approach to urban planning to one of changing the "total environment."[2] The second reason is that much attention is given to the health problems of cities. Many studies have shown that some of the unhealthiest areas of cities are the same areas involved in Model Cities programs.[3]

The Model Cities Act can develop into one of the bright new stars in health planning provided the individual cities administering the programs allow this to happen. Title I of the program is primarily concerned with correcting certain existing deficiencies, and Title II, the comprehensive metropolitan development part, is where health planners are looking for future improvements. However, the program is primarily one of urban planning, and the hope of many is that it be linked to an additional program for comprehensive areawide planning.

The integration of health planning and urban planning

The most promise yet in health planning progress appears to be the legislative and financial basis for the establishment of a new kind of planning agency: the Comprehensive Health Planning Act of 1966 (P. L. 89-749) and the Partnership for Health Amendments of 1967 (P. L. 90-174). For the first time in health planning the term comprehensive takes on a very specific meaning. The major purpose of this program is to bring some sort of

---

[1] Bloom, Lashof, and Vise, "Toward Comprehensive Health Care for All Chicagoans," pp. 71-91.

[2] Ellis D. Sox, "New Resources for Urban Health Programs," American Journal of Public Health, LVIII (June, 1968), 1030-35.

[3] Bloom, Lashof, and Vise, "Toward Comprehensive Health Care for All Chicagoans."

organized coordination to health planning.[1] The most important result thus far appears to be the increased cooperation of urban planners and health planners.

The purpose of these laws is generally stated as promoting and assuring the highest level of health care to the entire population. As stated by Cavanaugh, the Act is in fact "a natural extension and restructuring of previous federal commitments to aid the states and localities in protecting and improving the health of their citizens."[2] Before this Act, the Public Health Service provided grants, including those for planning, by means of many of the programs already mentioned in the study. The approach showed results but as the programs became more complex, it became increasingly difficult for federal funds to achieve the desired health improvement goals.

Simply stated, the Act is structured around the premise that there are basically two types of health interest, the provider and the consumer. And in spite of the fact that there are about 80 areawide or regional planning councils in this country, many are perhaps too closely tied to voluntary hospitals to truly represent consumer interests. Membership must be from both state and areawide agencies. It must include organized medicine, hospital associations, and consumer groups. In some cities it has become necessary to establish new agencies with the approval of the designated state agency.

The real foundations of the Act are with a state office of comprehensive planning.[3] Two kinds of grants can be approved from a state office. One is for initial organizational development projects and the other is for actual support in organizing an agency locally. Under most circumstances the federal share will be 50 per cent, but that share may go as high as 75 per cent.

Beal points out that while there is considerable optimism regarding comprehensive health planning, there are several severe limitations which must be overcome. These include:

(1) In spite of widespread support, the basis for the support is quite variable. Some view this type of planning as "self-policing," others would use it to gain control of a system, and still others see it as "inevitable" and would prefer to be part of it rather than oppose it.

(2) There is a lack of consensus regarding the purpose of the Act. The purpose must be more clearly defined.

(3) There is some confusion about method. As health and urban planners start to work together the differences in traditions becomes obvious. Also there are wide spectrums of approach amongst urban planners.

---

[1] James H. Cavanaugh, "Past, Present, and Future Goals and Philosophy in Comprehensive Health Planning" (paper presented at the American Hospital Association's Invitational Conference on Comprehensive Health Planning, October 24-25, 1968).

[2] Beal, "Urban Planner in Health Planning."

[3] _Ibid._, pp. 28-31.

(4) There aren't enough qualified health planners to go around.

(5) The program is supposed to move quickly, but it has neither the capacity nor the authority to do so.

The program has not yet been fairly tested. Only time will tell if this is the answer to coordination in planning and the provision of health care where it is needed. One importnat aspect largely neglected is the capability of this program to become the health planning arm of Model Cities.

Broad Programs for the 1970's

Two similar and yet very different programs will have an effect upon health planning in the 1970's and beyond. These developments are Medicare and the Regional Medical Programs. The programs are similar in that they offer means for providing medical care for the aged. Medicare does so directly by means of insurance programs and the Regional Medical Program in a more subtle way by providing alternate plans for establishing treatment for the leading killers of the elderly (and the entire population). Although the Regional Medical Programs actually do much more, they are also similar to Medicare in that they provide for health care in a broad way for a general class of need on a nationwide basis.

Medicare

Public Law 89-97 is the basis for Medicare under Title XVIII, Health Insurance for the Aged. The law establishes two health insurance programs for persons 65 or over.[1] The major portion of Medicare is a hospital insurance program designed to help pay bills when eligible persons are hospitalized. The second part is an optional additional medical insurance service geared to help pay physicians costs. The federal government matches a modest fee paid out monthly for the latter benefit.

The major provisions of Medicare are as follows:[2]

Part A, Basic Hospital Plan

(1) Up to 90 days of inpatient hospital service for each illness on a deductible basis.

(2) Up to 100 days of posthospital extended care.

---

[1] See U. S. Department of Health, Education, and Welfare, "A Brief Explanation of 'Medicare' Health Insurance for the Aged," OASI-1965-2, Washington, D. C., August, 1965, and *idem*, "Your Medicare Handbook," SSI-50, Washington, D. C., May, 1968.

[2] "Medicare, What It Is, What It Means," *Trustee, Journal of Hospital Governing Boards,* Special Issue, XVIII (September, 1965).

(3) Outpatient diagnostic services.

(4) Posthospital home health services.

(5) Inpatient psychiatric hospital services to 190 days.

Part B, Physicians' Services

(1) Physicians' and surgeons' services.

(2) Home health service.

(3) X-ray, laboratory, and other tests.

(4) X-ray, radium, and radioactive isotope therapy.

(5) Ambulatory service.

(6) Surgical dressings and splints.

The coverage provided by Medicare was bound to have an impact on the hospital system in many ways. Although there were often examples of unoccupied beds in hospitals, many of these were geared to obstetrical and pediatric uses.[1] Furthermore, very careful standards had to be developed for nursing homes due to the extended care aspects of Medicare. Already suffering from a shortage of qualified personnel, the hospitals were faced with the challenge of finding more of the required specialized type in order to conform with the legislation which helped provide the kind of care requirements of aged people. One 1967 study of 100 hospitals alone showed a 19 per cent increase during the third quarter of 1966 for persons 65 and older.[2] This increase, which was in patient days, also was augmented by longer average stays. Since 1966 many hospitals have started to make adjustments necessary for Medicare.

Regional Medical Programs (RMP's)

The other general program, the Regional Medical Program, was created by P. L. 89-239 (1965). The primary purpose of this program is to find methods to improve the provision of services for cancer, stroke, and heart disease. It is strongly tied to medical centers and medical schools and unlike Medicare it is not restricted to any age group. Unlike many other health planning programs, the Regional Medical Program (RMP) structure is also more closely tied to the traditional "establishment." It has not received the publicity most of the other programs have and not nearly so much of the federal monies have been spent on RMP activities.

---

[1]Charles U. Letoureau, "Medicare, Its Effects upon Hospitals and Health Facilities," Hospital Management, August, 1966, pp. 31-33.

[2]Richard P. Ament, "Medicare Boosts Bed Usage by Elderly," The Modern Hospital, CVIII (February, 1967).

The RMP program was a creation and responsibility of the medical profession. As stated by one physician:

> The RMP program has stimulated widely favorable reaction from the medical profession. As a whole, the medical profession at the beginning of 1968 is probably more deeply involved in the planning process to determine the nature of the RMP's than it has been in the planning of any previous federal program. Many of our most distinguished medical leaders are participating full or part-time in the regional programs. Many state and county medical societies are cooperating actively or in an advisory capacity and have expressed their enthusiastic support.[1]

The program was started when President Lyndon B. Johnson's Commission on Heart Disease, Cancer, and Stroke presented its two-volume study in late 1964.[2] The Commission's research and final reports were coordinated by a physician, Michael De Bakey. The Commission made very specific recommendations pertaining to the establishment of a hierarchy of centers for the treatment of the diseases. Congressional hearings preceded the passage of P. L. 89-239. While many of the Commission's recommendations were significantly altered by the Congress in the legislative process, the Act reflects a response to the need for planning.

In its present form, P. L. 89-239 relies heavily upon local initiative. Rather than a federally sponsored network of regional centers, the program offers a framework for the development of "regional cooperative arrangements." The basic concepts behind this philosophy include:[3]

(1) The best in modern diagnostic and treatment methods is not readily accessible to many Americans suffering from or threatened by heart disease, cancer, stroke, and related diseases.

(2) There should be more cooperation within major medical centers regarding diagnostic and therapeutic capability.

(3) If medical innovations are to be made available in an efficient manner, medical and health planning efforts must be combined.

(4) The diversity of local resources calls for a coordinated variety of efforts.

Local initiative, then, is the key to a successful Regional Medical Program. The Act provides a system of grants as the vehicle for the establishment of a Regional Medical Program, and the needs of heart disease, cancer, and stroke facilities planning are then left to the devices of local "creative partnership."

---

[1]Dwight L. Wilbur, "Quality and Availability of Care under Regional Medical Programs," Journal of the American Medical Association, CCIII (March 11, 1968), 143-47.

[2]The President's Commission on Heart Disease, Cancer and Stroke, Report to the President: A National Program to Conquer Heart Disease, Cancer and Stroke (2 vols.; Washington, D.C., December, 1964).

[3]William H. Stewart, Surgeon General, Public Health Service, "Report on Regional Medical Programs to the President and Congress," U. S. Department of Health, Education, and Welfare, Washington, D. C., June, 1967.

Regionalization for RMP's

The urban planner functioning as a regional scientist would no doubt question the use of the term "regionalization" as defined by the RMP planners. However, as with other health care facilities planning programs, the term has a very specific meaning. According to the RMP Guidelines, regionalization means regional cooperative arrangement.[1] The arrangements are not officially sponsored by governmental agencies; they are voluntary agreements to plan for improved treatment of the diseases which in turn are defined as a categorical approach to planning.

The RMP regionalization process has several important facets. It is geographical in that nearly all the RMP's have defined boundaries in spite of the fact that the guidelines specify that for most purposes the boundaries should be flexible (see Fig. 4). The programs provide a means of sharing health manpower, which is in short supply, and includes the involvement of physicians. The programs have to offer their morbidity-centered approach as one important element in overall comprehensive planning. This morbidity facet is a new approach to health planning that will no doubt increase in importance as more and more public attention is given to the everyday health hazards of our urban environment.

In addition to the general characteristics above, the cooperative regional arrangements are expected to reflect the following elements:[2]

(1) There should be maximum involvement of available health care practitioners within each RMP. This can be accomplished through the mandatory Regional Advisory Group where the many public and health care interests can maintain communication.

(2) A RMP must identify the needs regarding heart disease, cancer, and stroke for the entire Region. Furthermore, these needs must be identified in terms which offer opportunities for solution.

(3) An inventory of available treatment resources should be accomplished in order to determine gaps in the supply.

(4) Objectives of each RMP should be spelled out.

(5) Due to manpower and other limitations, priorities should be scheduled.

(6) Plans should be implemented within the constraint of RMP programs. The major problem with this element rests with the fact that no new facilities can be constructed.

(7) Programs will be periodically evaluated.

It is important to note that not all funds are awarded at once. After sufficient local initiative has generated an arrangement, a first phase planning grant is possible.

---

[1]Division of Regional Medical Programs, "Guidelines, Regional Medical Programs" (rev.; Washington, D.C.: U.S. Department of Health, Education, and Welfare, May, 1968).

[2]*Ibid.*

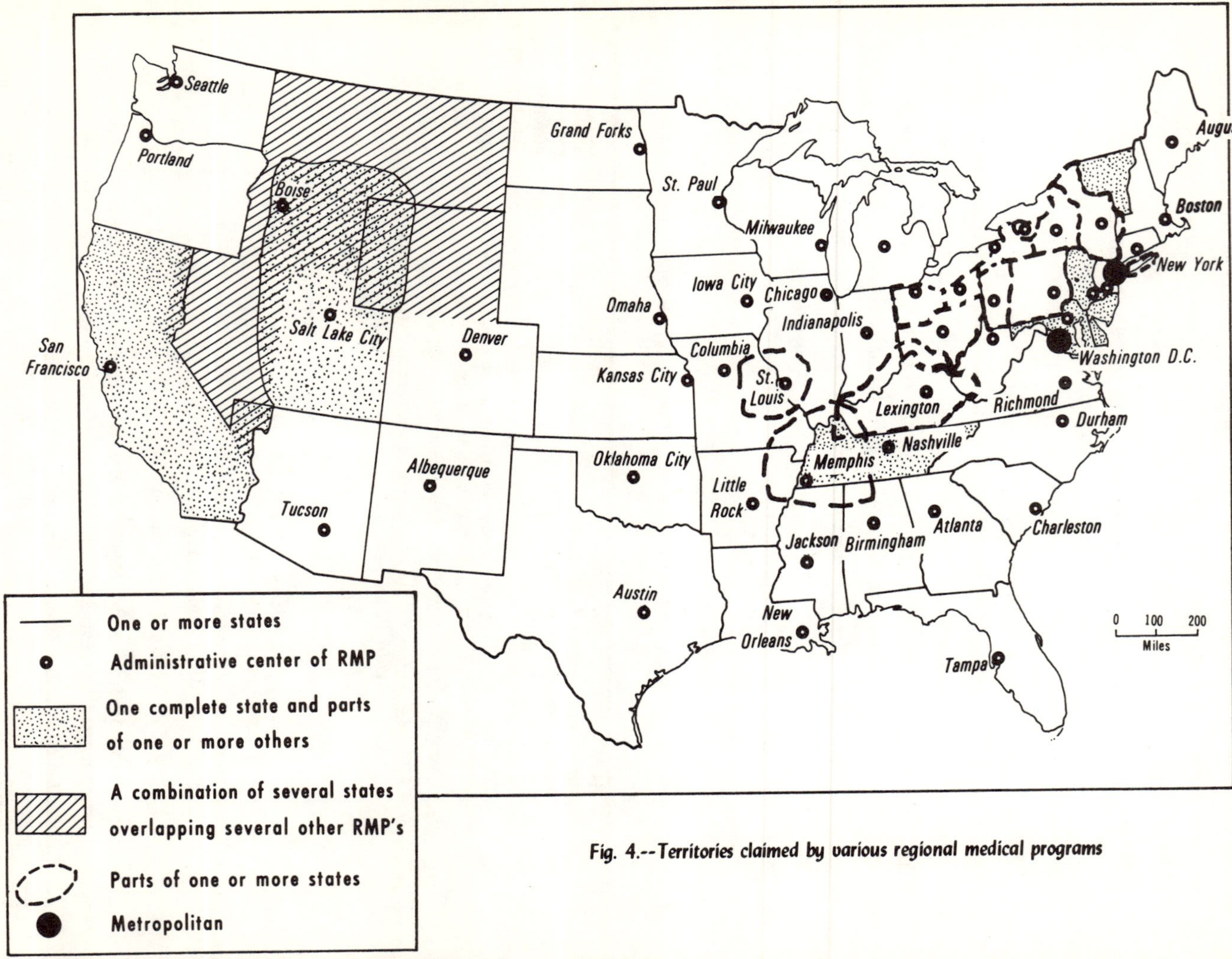

Fig. 4.--Territories claimed by various regional medical programs

This is a very basic grant geared to assist in the development of a program. After sufficient of the elements spelled out have been accomplished a second phase operational grant can be acquired. By the first of 1970, 55 RMP's claiming combined coverage of all parts of the United States had been awarded planning grants. Of these, 44 had been awarded operational grants.

Spatial organization

In spite of the fact that geographical boundaries neither have to be clearly specified nor strictly adhered to, most RMP's have their territories fairly well carved out.[1] Figure 4 shows the various types of spatial arrangement which has resulted. There are essentially five kinds of territory claimed:

(1) One or More States. These RMP's make up most of the number, and with the exception of some Western and Mountain States, they usually consist of one State.

(2) One Complete State and Parts of One or More Others. There are six RMP's in this category.

(3) A Combination of Several States Overlapping Several Other RMP's. There is one RMP in this category, the Mountain States program occupying the States shown on Figure 4.

(4) Parts of One or More States. These RMP's are to be found in the Northeast and the Ohio and Mississippi Valley areas. Some of these areas simply center about one city and overlap other RMP's. Conversely some are mutually exclusive parts of States, e.g., Ohio and Pennsylvania. New York has 6 such nearly initially exclusive areas.

(5) Metropolitan. In spite of the fact that many RMP's have major urban programs only two cities, New York and Washington, D.C., have distinctly separate programs.

It is clear from the spatial organization of the programs that there is a degree of overlap. Western Wyoming, for example, is part of three programs. Southwestern Kentucky is part of three programs, also. The Bi-State Program centered in St. Louis includes parts of the Illinois and Missouri areas, but metropolitan St. Louis is excluded from the Missouri RMP. The Ohio State Program includes the southern and central portions of that State except metropolitan Cincinnati, and the Ohio Valley Program centered in Lexington picks up Cincinnati along with additional parts of Southwestern Ohio. Two programs in category 2 overlap to include southern Delaware, and Southern New Jersey is included in two RMP's. Given the nature of the RMP Guidelines it is surprising there are not more overlapping areas. In addition, when compared to various federal planning subunits, the RMP's are well organized spatially.

---

[1] News Information Data (Director of Regional Medical Programs), III, Nos. 23 and 29 (July 15 and October 14, 1969) (Washington, D.C.: U.S. Department of Health, Education, and Welfare, Division of Regional Programs).

The administrative centers reflect the strong university medical center ties of the RMP organization. Centers appear to be either university towns, state capitals, large metropolitan centers, or any combination of the above types.

Functional organization of RMP's: a sample

The "regionalization" process of the RMP's is also functional, and the activities of the 55 programs are well documented.[1] Much understanding of the programs and the variety of efforts can be gained by viewing a selected sample of RMP accomplishments. The sample includes a Black ghetto, a Midwestern State, a Western Mountain area, a program in Upper New York State, and a Southern State.

Watts[2]

The most populous in the nation, California RMP has subdivided its territory into 8 subdivisions centered about a medical school. Until recently, the Watts-Willowbrook ghetto area was split between the program administered by UCLA and the one administered by USC. A special RMP has now been organized in the ghetto for many reasons; the most obvious one being the fact that there is little immediate access for care, and the nearest hospital willing to treat black and charity patients is the outpatient department of Los Angeles County General Hospital 9 miles from the area. The joint program is working closely with planners of the new Charles R. Drew Post-Graduate Medical School to be built in the area in order to formulate methods for meeting RMP diagnosis and treatment goals. Meanwhile, Paul Ward has suggested that as a short-term program a mobile multiphasic unit similar to areas used in industry be established in the Watts-Willowbrook Area.

Iowa[3]

While health planning between physicians and hospitals is not new to the State of Iowa, the aspect of coordinated health planning and urban planning is. The Iowa RMP has

---

[1]News Information Data, III, Nos. 23 and 29 (July 15 and October 14, 1969); Stewart, "Report on Regional Medical Programs to the President and Congress"; and Regional Medical Programs, Proceedings: Conference Workshop on Regional Medical Programs (2 vols.; Washington, D.C.: U.S. Department of Health, Education, and Welfare, 1968).

[2]For a detailed discussion of the Watts-Willowbrook RMP see Donald J. Brayton, "Watts-Willowbrook Regional Medical Program," and Paul D. Ward, "The Impact of RMP on Hard Core Poverty Areas," in Proceedings of Regional Medical Programs.

[3]John C. Bartlett, "Complementary Relationship Between Iowa Regional Medical Program, Comprehensive Health Planning and Voluntary Health Planning: A Necessary Accomplishment," in Proceedings of Regional Medical Programs; and News Information Data, III, No. 29 (October 14, 1969), 74-76.

chosen an avenue whereby it will become directly involved with the Comprehensive Health Planning Agency (P. L. 89-749) and the more established voluntary Health Planning Council of Iowa in a "super cooperative arrangement." Planning arrangements, including some contracting of work, appears to be the present state of the program. Objectives eventually include the establishment of stroke management teams, developing method of training and retraining new personnel in cardiopulmonary resuscitation, and developing several courses for intensive coronary care units (ICCU's).

The Intermountain program

There are several major approaches for this RMP centered in Salt Lake City. The first of these objectives is the establishment of a tight information services and communications network centered about a Salt Lake City data bank. The second, and certainly no less important, is the further development of education and training programs in all phases of categorical RMP treatment. Other aspects include the establishment of several 89-239 related laboratories. One important program is geared to the establishment of coronary care units for small hospitals. The sparse population of the area cannot support urban-sized hospitals, and yet the RMP goal is to create enough cooperative arrangements so that the population has access to care within 2 hours of onset of symptoms.[1]

Albany

Centered at Albany Medical College of Union University the Albany RMP was one of the first of these programs to become operational. A two-way radio communications system has been established between 57 hospitals, 24 high schools and numerous other key locations. A post-graduate program in categorical care has been organized for physicians. Several subregional coronary care units for demonstration have been established at Poughkeepsie, Pittsfield, Massachusetts, and Herkimer, New York. In addition, a cancer coordinator has been established in Albany.

Alabama

The Alabama RMP is unique in that very careful arrangements had to be made in the planning stages of the program. According to a law dating to 1875 the Medical Association of Alabama is also the State Board of Health. Ten elected members from the association serve simultaneously as the State Board of Censors, State Board of Medical Examiners, and the State Committee on Public Health. According to J. O. Finney,

---

[1]News Information Data, III, No. 29 (October 14, 1969), 67-73.

Associate Director of the Alabama RMP, "Without initial support of the State Association the program would have been doomed to utter failure."[1] As finally established, the Alabama RMP works through a network of county or multicounty offices reporting to a central office which works very closely with the Medical Association of the State of Alabama. The program has been operational since 1969. No specific details regarding activities are listed in RMP News Information Data.

Health Planning Trends and Responsibilities in the Chicago Region

Although various agencies in the Chicago region have been engaged in degrees of health care facilities planning for a greater part of this century, most of the formal planning as explained in the previous discussions has been accomplished since World War II.[2] The following discussion, although hardly exhaustive in terms of all Chicago area health care interests, summarizes the planning activities of several agencies during the last 25 years.

Hill-Burton programs

Illinois was one of the first states to develop a survey and plan in accordance with Hill-Burton requirements.[3] The survey section of the early plan included some 700 hospitals considered in the following categories:

(1) General and Allied Special

(2) Tuberculosis

(3) Neuro-Mental

(4) Chronic and Convalescent

(5) Public Health Facilities

Of the hospitals surveyed 38.8 per cent were in the first category, general, and three-fourths of these were voluntary hospitals containing 78 per cent of all general hospital beds. Most of the first category hospitals, had a capacity of 50 or more beds, and only

---

[1] J. O. Finney, "Development of the Relationship Between the Medical Association of the State of Alabama and the Alabama Regional Medical Program," in Proceedings of Regional Medical Programs, pp. 52-56.

[2] For a review of studies of the growth of Chicago area hospitals prior to World War II, see Gerald F. Pyle, "Methods of Analyzing Chicago's Hospital Hierarchy," Chicago Regional Hospital Study, Working Paper VI.4, October, 1969.

[3] See State of Illinois, "The Illinois Hospital Survey and Plan," Illinois Department of Public Health, July, 1947.

36 per cent had more than a 100-bed capacity. The other categories were divided up in the following manner: (2) Tuberculosis, 3.7 per cent of all institutions; (3) Neuro-Mental, 4.4 per cent; (4) Chronic and Convalescent, 53.1 per cent.

After the inventory it was possible to analyze the seriousness of the situation. As had been indicated by the initial rationale for the Hill-Burton legislation, there were strong deficiencies in rural areas. There were 26 counties with no hospital, 16 had less than 25 beds in the county, and another 16 had only from 25 to 50 hospital beds. These counties totaled to more than half the area of the state.

The State of Illinois then set out to do something about these deficiencies. Within ten years, substantial growth was stimulated by Hill-Burton. For example, general hospital beds had increased from 28,447 in 1945 to 36,309 in 1956, mental hospitals increased from 21,911 to 28,439 beds for the same period, and, also for that period, nursing home beds went from 11,521 to 15,873.[1]

Illinois continued to catch up on the backlog of rural hospital requirement for the next decade and a half, but the programs for metropolitan areas were somewhat less than dynamic. By the early 1960's the Hill-Harris Amendment combined with the growth of voluntary areawide planning agencies in Illinois to augment metropolitan hospital growth. By 1964 the State Hill-Burton Agency had started to develop joint programs with the Hospital Planning Council for Metropolitan Chicago. One of the studies was the establishment of service areas in the Chicago area for Hill-Burton planning.[2]

Areawide planning: the Hospital Planning Council for metropolitan Chicago

The major thrust in recent times for hospital planning in the Chicago metropolitan area has been spearheaded by Chicago's version of an areawide planning agency, the Hospital Planning Council for Metropolitan Chicago. This agency was formed early within the context of the areawide movement. Incorporated in 1957 and staffed late in 1958, it started releasing published materials to the public in 1959. Interests supporting the formation of the organization included the Chicago Association of Commerce and Industry, the Welfare Council for Metropolitan Chicago (an agency that already had a 40-year record of health care facilities planning), the American Hospital Association, organized labor, and various medical schools. As was spelled out in the guidelines for areawide agencies, the board of directors was made up of many top leaders in industry and business.

---

[1] U.S. Department of Health, Education, and Welfare, "Hill-Burton Program Progress Report."

[2] See Pierre de Vise, "Hospital Study Districts for Metropolitan Chicago," Hospital Planning Council for Metropolitan Chicago, Technical Report No. 2, 1966.

Authority for operation has been provided by a variety of sources.[1] Initially, the agency was financed from private contributions. The second major assist came from Blue Cross. During the first and second phases of Hill-Burton, the Hospital Planning Council worked on reviewing permits for new hospitals. Another facet came to include helping hospitals arrange financial support. As stated in 1966, the major objectives of the agency were:[2]

(1) To plan the development of health treatment facilities in the area and to render economic advice to agencies executing the development of such facilities,

(2) To function as a coordinator for agencies and establishments rendering health services,

(3) To be concerned with standards and methods of improvement, including cost,

(4) To coordinate community, hospital and medical interests,

(5) To promote public awareness of health treatment needs and fund raising for appropriate agencies, and

(6) To make the general public aware of available treatment facilities.

Over the past dozen years, these objectives have been furthered through the publication of various bulletins, technical reports, and research papers and through special consultations with health care facility supporters.

The Research Bulletins have functioned in a variety of ways to describe and analyze the supply of facilities in the area. Descriptions include measures of sponsorship, types of service offered, bed components, and obsolescence in places. The methods of analysis deal with the hospital supply in a more dynamic way in that they offer procedures for expansion and construction. In addition, the Hospital Planning Council has applied a step-by-step procedure to determine the viability of establishing a new hospital. The primary considerations which contribute to the request-generating agency's evaluation included determination of overlap in area with existing hospitals through use of a bed ratio measure (the Hill-Burton 2.5/1000 minimum to 4.5/1000 maximum), and an evaluation of community needs for the type of service suggested.[3] A similar procedure has been utilized for the evaluation of planned expansion of new facilities but in this instance cost considerations are much more heavily weighted.

---

[1]Interview with Hiram Sibley, Executive Director, Hospital Planning Council for Metropolitan Chicago, December, 1969.

[2]Hospital Planning Council for Metropolitan Chicago, 'Eighth Annual Report, July 1, 1965-June 30, 1966," pp. 2-11.

[3]Hospital Planning Council for Metropolitan Chicago, Research Bulletins No. 3, "The Evaluation of Proposed New Hospitals" (May, 1960), and No. 4, 'Evaluation of Proposed Changes in Existing Hospitals" (January, 1961).

The Technical Reports are much more detailed than the Research Bulletins. One Report, for example, spells out the methods utilized in establishing subdivisions in accordance with Hill-Burton provisions.[1] Many factors, including access to hospitals, size, urban ecological constraints, age of structures and "trade areas," were utilized to develop these districts. Use data for 1965 were utilized to construct the areas, and they were still in use in 1969. In fact, the areas were used as "building blocks" for a series of facilities use reports. Some recent reports show the use of short-term, general, special, and nursing home facilities by district.[2] Also, the agency is now in the process of developing sets of socioeconomic and demographic profiles for these districts.

The Chicago Regional Hospital Study is another example of hospital planning research in which the Council has participated. Co-sponsored by the Council and the Illinois Department of Public Health and properly titled, "Computer Simulation Model--Metropolitan Hospital Use," the study was financed by Public Health Service grant HM00452-01A1. The first phase of the project lasted for 3 years (1966-69), and the second "planning" phase is now under way. (Two additional agencies, the Center for Urban Studies and the Center for Health Administration Studies, both of the University of Chicago, participate in the project.)

Early in the project, three broad goals were outlined,

(1) To describe and analyze spatial patterns of hospital use,

(2) To predict future use, and

(3) To measure unmet hospital needs.

At the outset it proved useful to utilize as a foundation many of the measures, standards, study areas, and other criteria previously established by the Council. This was especially true of the bed population ratio. Other factors, behavioral, transportation, cost, and morbidity were eventually analyzed. The findings of the study have been released as a series of research papers classified under four general topics.

Series I The Health Care System
Series II The Urban System
Series III Methods and Concepts
Series IV The Planning Component

The Hospital Planning Council has also played an important role in local applications of recent health planning legislation (P. L. 89-97, P. L. 89-239, and P. L. 89-749).

---

[1]Vise, "Hospital Study Districts for Metropolitan Chicago."

[2]Hospital Planning Council for Metropolitan Chicago, "Utilization and Status of Nursing Homes and Nursing Care Units in Homes for the Aged in the Chicago Metropolitan Area for Calendar Years January 1, 1964-December 31, 1966," Report No. 8, June, 1968, and "Utilization of Short-Term General and Special Hospitals in the Chicago Metropolitan Area Calendar Year 1968," Report No. 9, April, 1969.

In a study of Oak Forest Hospital, the agency (Hospital Planning Council) made a dozen recommendations necessary for this facility for chronically ill and geriatric patients to comply with Medicare. In terms of P. L. 89-749, the Hospital Planning Council has taken an active role in working with other Chicago area agencies to develop a separate comprehensive health planning agency. The agency's P. L. 89-239 activities include the undertaking central to this study.

The Welfare Council of Metropolitan Chicago

This organization, now in operation for 50 years, is the major Chicago social welfare agency engaged in aspects of health planning. Before the formation of the Hospital Planning Council, the Welfare Council made contributions to informal planning. The Welfare Council was, as stated before, one of the agencies which helped establish the Hospital Planning Council. By the mid-1960's the Welfare Council shifted its emphasis even more to a community orientation, and this orientation included an examination of health conditions in various Chicago area neighborhoods.[1]

Some of the Welfare Council's more recent activities and research publication include:

(1) The Maternal, Infant, and Preschool Health Survey in Chicago and Suburban Cook County. This study lasted 3 years, and its primary purpose was to assess the health states of expectant mothers and children in the Chicago area. A program to implement improvements recommended in this study will soon be undertaken as part of a comprehensive health effort.

(2) Home Delivered Meals. This program which ended July 31, 1968, was a demonstration of how meals could be delivered to aged, chronically ill and convalescent persons. The Welfare Council is now in the process of attempting to extend this program in three Model Cities areas.

(3) Development of Criteria for Comprehensive Planning for Services to the Handicapped. The purpose of this effort is to coordinate planning efforts for the future provision of many unmet needs of persons with a wide range of physical and mental handicaps.

(4) A Community System of Protective Services to the Aged and an Information Center for the Aging. The first of these projects includes a proposal to develop and demonstrate a method to pinpoint older impaired persons and plan for their needs. The second includes the development and maintenance of an information pool of available health care services for the aging.

The Welfare Council is engaged in two additional joint projects which will greatly influence the future of health planning in Chicago. The first of these includes the establishment of a unified health information, referral, and counseling service intended to identify unmet health care needs and guide persons with such needs to the appropriate place.

---

[1]Interview with Mr. Robert Adams, Director of Planning and Research Division, Welfare Council of Metropolitan Chicago, December, 1969.

The second effort, which is closely tied to the first, is the participation with other key health planning agencies in the region in the formation of a comprehensive agency to carry out the goals of P. L. 89-749.

Northeastern Illinois Planning Commission

This official urban planning agency for the Chicago region has traditionally left many aspects of hospital planning in the hands of the Hospital Planning Council for Metropolitan Chicago, particularly the review of applications for hospitals. The Northeastern Illinois Planning Commission (NIPC) is concerned presently with health problems as they relate to the environment with particular reference to waste, water, air and noise.[1]

NIPC has engaged in studies related to the social and health aspects of substandard housing in suburban ghettos, but the health problems were viewed as a manifestation of larger environmental problems, e.g., inadequate sewage disposal. Also, NIPC had worked jointly with the Welfare Council for Metropolitan Chicago on a study pertaining to the establishment of multi-purpose health centers in southern Cook County.

Much attention recently has been given by NIPC to the establishment of an agency for the implementation of P. L. 89-749. NIPC is another of the several Chicago region agencies which have made contribution to the development of a comprehensive health planning agency. The latter agency is viewed by the former as a potential coordinating agency as well as a central data center for health care information.

Comprehensive Health Planning, Inc.

In keeping with the requirements of P. L. 89-749, an agency has been developed in the Chicago area through the combined efforts of many agencies. Known as Comprehensive Health Planning, Inc., this organization came into being late in 1969. The major purpose of the agency will be to review grant applications for the Public Health Service in the Chicago area and generally coordinate the activities of various other agencies.[2] The major emphasis of this organization will thus be administrative.

Some steps toward the actual development of health care planning have already been started. Comprehensive Health Planning has started to assist the Mid South Side Health Planning Organization (one of 16 such subregional groups in the metropolitan area)

---

[1] Interview with Dr. Robert Ducharme, Deputy Director, Northeastern Illinois Planning Commission.

[2] Interview with Mr. Thomas Mitchell, Research Department, Comprehensive Health Planning, Inc., December, 1969.

in the development of a plan. In keeping with P. L. 89-749, emphasis will be upon dealing with the consumer aspects of health care. Although hardly geographically comprehensive in nature, this first start represents a very different facet in health care planning.

Illinois Regional Medical Program (IRMP)

Established in July, 1967, as Chicago's response to P. L. 89-239, the Illinois Regional Medical Program is centered in Chicago. The efforts of this organization are complementary to the Partnership for Health organization in that they are developing other aspects of delivering patient care. As in many other Regional Medical Programs, the medical schools are the key to the operation. Establishment of the IRMP led to the formation of the Coordinating Committee of Medical Schools and Teaching Hospitals.[1] The educational aspects are clearly important in this program to offer the best possible care for heart disease, cancer and stroke.

The IRMP has, in addition, become engaged in at least two additional projects. One of these is a delivery improvement study in conjunction with the North Suburban Association for Health Resources (another of the 16 subregional groups) under the direction of Dr. Sheldon Waldstein. This program will also offer h spital morbidity data to the Hospital Planning Council for Metropolitan Chicago in the second of these projects. The latter agency is developing a series of delivery system alternatives for the IRMP, and this background study represents one in the series.

Now operational, the Illinois Regional Medical Program (IRMP) includes in its territory the entire State. However, many of its plans will be for parts of the State. Several broad objectives have been spelled out:

(1) Develop a continuing education program for health care practitioners.

(2) Enlarge diagnosis delivery projects.

(3) Improve screening techniques.

(4) Generate more public interest in problems of these diseases.

(5) Develop systems correlating health service patterns to demographic and socioeconomic data.

(6) Assist health care facilities to improve the provision of services.

(7) Expand electronic data processing in the area of research, patient care, and preventive services.

(8) Develop cooperative endeavors with voluntary societies related to RMP categorical diseases.

(9) Cooperate with public health programs.

---

[1]Illinois Regional Medical Program, Statement of Purpose (pamphlet).

In order to implement some of these objectives the central office of the IRMP has established a number of internal staff task forces. In addition, several voluntary and other Chicago area agencies will be developing alternative plans for many of the objectives. The Hospital Planning Council for Metropolitan Chicago has undertaken a morbidity-centered approached in developing several of these plans. The chapters which follow this background study are a result of some of the Hospital Planning Council's studies, and they are primarily concerned with items (5), (6), and (7) above.

CHAPTER II

THE SPATIAL APPROACH TO ANALYSIS OF HEART DISEASE, CANCER, AND STROKE

Proper planning of health care facilities inevitably must rely heavily upon the analysis of spatial and temporal aspects of disease incidence. Since the major biological breakthroughs in the latter nineteenth century many contributions related to health, civilization and cities have been made. A selective review of this literature indicates that three ostensibly contrasting, but fundamentally complementary, approaches to the study of disease and cities can be identified: medical environmentalism, epidemiology, and geosocial pathology (Fig. 5).[1]

The first of these approaches postulates that the physical environment is paramount in understanding the spatial variability of disease. Jacques M. May has clearly explained the intricate connections of disease and environment from the geographical point of view,[2] and a committee of the National Academy of Sciences is now beginning to explore the medical consequences of the geochemical environment.[3] Studies of this nature now appear to be most appropriate to developing nations, but differences between city and rural health patterns can be quite striking. For example, in parts of Africa and other tropical areas people are exposed to a wide variety of "temperate" diseases as well as ailments more common to their own climates. As technological advances contribute to

---

[1]Gerald F. Pyle, "Some Aspects of Urban Medical Geography" (unpublished Master's dissertation, Department of Geography, University of Chicago, 1968). There are several international efforts currently under way aimed at increasing our understanding of medical geography in general. Yu. V. Medvedkov, Chief of Ecology Unit, Division of Research in Epidemiology and Communicative Science, World Health Organization, is heading several studies of urban areas as well as other more traditional studies of medical geography. Prof. A. T. A. Learmonth is heading up the Commission of Medical Geography of the International Geographical Union. Also an international journal of medical geography is published in Hungary (Geographia Medica: Section on medical geography of the Hungarian Geographical Society and the Commission on Medical Geography of the International Geographical Union).

[2]Jacques M. May, The Ecology of Human Disease (New York: M.D. Publications, 1958), and idem, Studies in Disease Ecology (New York: Hafner Publishing Company, Inc., 1961).

[3]News Report (National Academy of Sciences), April, 1970.

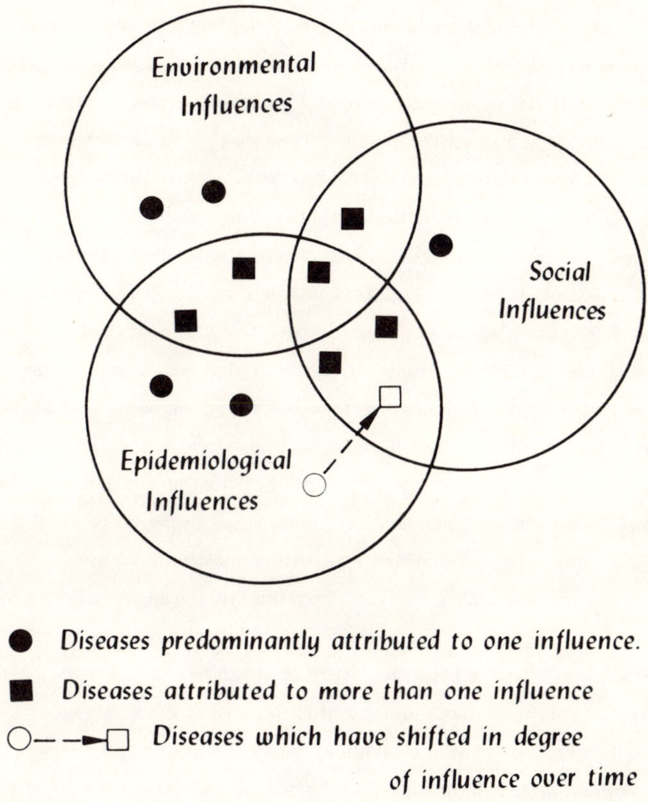

Fig. 5.--Approaches to urban medical geography

increased urbanization people emigrate from the rural countryside to cities. The destination of many is the raw slum which usually does not yet possess modern municipal facilities. Lack of immunity due to former isolation, the increased probabilities of infection because of crowding due to sheer densities and generally unhealthy habitations all contribute to a physical environment which generates tremendous urban health problems.

Evidence of environmental problems is also to be found in large cities. In addition to the rather obvious carcinogenic results of polluted air it is possible to identify direct or indirect effects of polluted water. In Chicago, for example, there is a distinct pattern of high incidence of infectious hepatitis in areas immediately adjacent to open bodies of water. The pattern is more than coincidental, for the hepatitis health measure demonstrated independence of 18 others in a 19-variable factor analysis.[1] Furthermore, evidence resulting from the research endeavors of James Mosley indicate that of all known waterborne viral diseases, infectious hepatitis is one of the most clearly identified as such, and that further transmission is possible through subsequent contact.[2]

Epidemiological variables demonstrate several kinds of patterning that call for a different approach to the study of disease incidence. First, epidemics of diseases with a distinct temporal cycle, such as rubella, can show spatial variations which parallel the distribution of more youthful populations or pockets of dense population clusters. As a result, until recently the greatest incidence of rubella was in the more youthful suburban and ghetto neighborhoods. But epidemiological patterns of this kind are shifting as more affluent people obtain new innoculations against particular diseases, and as a result concentrations of these diseases show up most strongly in poverty neighborhoods.

The third approach important to the study of urban health has been loosely termed geosocial pathology. This term has global implications, and when viewed at a metropolitan scale it is the geographic version of medical sociology.

As technological advances bring more environmental and epidemiological control, all areas of the urban settlement do not benefit equally. Neighborhoods representing social groups of differing status have tended to receive sanitary and medical innovations on the basis of ability to pay. Classical examples of how poverty and ill health are related in a growing urban system can be seen in the works of Snow, Rowntree, Banks, Stamp,

---

[1] Gerald F. Pyle and Joyce Lashof, "Geography of Disease and Death in the Two Chicagos," in Slum Medicine: Chicago's Apartheid Health System, by Pierre de Vise et al., (Chicago: University of Chicago Community and Family Study Center, 1969).

[2] James W. Mosley, "Transmission of Viral Diseases by Drinking Water," in Transmission of Viruses by the Water Route, ed. Gerald Berd (New York: Interscience Publishers, 1967), pp. 5-23.

and Rosenburg that explained nineteenth-century relationships in Britain and the United States.[1]

In Chicago health differences between poverty and non-poverty areas are extremely pronounced. In addition to the higher occurrence of once-common communicable diseases, many "social" diseases show up most clearly in poverty areas. Also, it is presumed that the general debilitating syndrome of inadequate diet, generally lower physical resistance, inability and/or unwillingness to seek medical aid until crucial periods, and inadequate access (not proximity) to health treatment all lead to higher probabilities of chronic illness.[2]

The Need to Link Spatial Analysis of Disease to Health Care Facilities Planning

Much urban medical geography has either merely described spatial patterns or at best suggested possible associations among diseases and/or other social and environmental causes. In consequence, and not unexpectedly, morbidity patterns of urban communities have not been included as major inputs in the health planning process. The traditional approach to hospital planning thus has relied primarily upon measures such as patient days, admissions per 1,000 population, average length of stay, or number of beds required on the basis of population projections. Only recently have attempts been made to consider socioeconomic and demographic variables in the planning process. In a 1964 study for the American Hospital Association, Gerald Rosenthal developed an analytical model geared to the utilization of key "sociodemographic" and economic variables.[3] The study utilized Hill-Burton State Areas as unit areas with the following linear regression model:

$$Y^i = a + b_1 X_1{}^i + \ldots + b_n X_n{}^i + e \qquad (1)$$

Where: Y^i = utilization of hospital facilities in State Area i,

X^i = independent socioeconomic and demographic variables characterizing State Area i.

---

[1]John Snow, B. W. Richardson, and Wade Hampton Frost, Snow on Cholera (New York: The Commonwealth Fund, 1936); B. Seebohm Rowntree, Poverty, A Study of Town Life (London: Macmillan and Co., Ltd, 1901); A. Leslie Banks, "The Study of the Geography of Disease," Geographical Journal, CXXV (June, 1959), 199-210; L. Dudley Stamp, Some Aspects of Medical Geography (London: Oxford University Press, 1964); and Rosenburg, Cholera Years.

[2]Pierre de Vise et al., Slum Medicine: Chicago's Apartheid Health System (Chicago: Community and Family Study Center, University of Chicago, 1969).

[3]Gerald D. Rosenthal, The Demand for General Hospital Facilities, Hospital Monograph Series No. 14 (Chicago: American Hospital Association, 1964).

The model served two purposes: to demonstrate to what extent the various independent variables influenced hospital use, and to predict future demand. The results of the analysis showed high positive regression coefficients for higher income persons (over $5,999 annual) utilizing hospitals and the reverse for per cent nonwhite and low income persons.

If the study of characteristics of communities is to be linked to the need for health care as well as demand, more systematic studies of intraurban health patterns and relationships are required. In an exploratory study of this nature in Chicago, health data were utilized as dependent variables and socioeconomic characteristics of persons grouped by Community Areas as independent variables.[1] The model was similar to the one used by Rosenthal:

$$Y_n = a + b_1X_1 + b_2X_2 + \ldots b_nX_n + e \qquad (2)$$

Where: Y_n = communicable disease rates and other health measures,

X_n = socioeconomic characteristics.

The study showed some strong relationships within poverty areas regarding infant deaths, venereal disease, and measles, but the model inputs needed refinement on several counts. As with the Rosenthal study, several distinct age groups should have been utilized. For more accurate results, the health measures should have been studied over time. And most important of all, measures requiring more hospital utilization needed to be tested. In Chapter III of this study the model mentioned above is refined for predicting heart disease, cancer, and stroke incidence; however, before the accomplishment of such a task, the ways in which these diseases are apt to vary spatially must be examined.

Authors dealing with the spatial variability of the diseases of the Regional Medical Program (hereafter abbreviated RMP) frequently imply that the results of such studies aid in planning future treatment as often as they help extricate etiological agents. In either case some familiarity with causative agents is necessary to accomplish a meaningful analysis of differences from place to place. The two crucial elements of studies reviewed are analysis of methods of reporting and the actual handling of reported statistics. Furthermore, some studies claim that reporting criteria from one area to another are too "artefactual" and hence meaningless. Another attitude projected is that reporting differences alone are not enough to nullify this approach. It would appear that in terms of geographical scale there are still sufficient differences in reporting methods from country to country in spite of W. H. O. efforts toward standardization to make international studies difficult; however, reporting in the United States has been sufficiently standardized to make possible studies at the interstate level and smaller. Methods of analyzing patterns range from explanations resulting from visual examination to sophisticated contiguity tests.

---

[1]Gerald F. Pyle and Philip H. Rees, "Problems of Modeling Disease Patterns in Urban Areas: The Chicago Example," in Economic Geography (forthcoming).

The Spatial Variability of Heart Disease and Stroke

In 1964, the President's Commission on Heart Disease, Cancer, and Stroke defined the term heart disease, as commonly used, to include a large number of conditions affecting the heart and circulatory system.[1] The cardiovascular-renal diseases, of which there are many, were divided into three categories:

(1) Strokes (blood vessel damage affecting the central nervous system).

(2) A whole series of diseases of the heart and blood vessels serving the body.

(3) Kidney diseases which are related to circulation.

Different groups of the population display distinct death rates from heart disease and stroke from one part of the country to another. In addition, in 1963, 72 per cent of all heart disease deaths occurred in persons 65 and older, and there were at least one-third more deaths that same year for males than for females from these maladies. The heart disease groups and stroke have been separated into subcategories due to medical differences; however, studies of the spatial distribution of these diseases reveal similar distributions.

Heart disease

Although there are many kinds of heart disease, studies of the spatial variability of these reveal that of the three major kinds, two can serve as indicators for the larger group.[2] The two diseases which are clearly identified as ailments showing variability over space are Arteriosclerotic Heart Disease (Coronary Heart Disease) and Hypertensive Heart Disease. The third, Rheumatic and Infectious Heart Disease shows far less clustering by unit of observation (state, county, etc.) than the other two; however, differences in the nature of the disease and in methods of reporting combined with a lower incidence relative to the other two to suggest it is not a likely indicator of general heart disease occurrence by place.

---

[1] President's Commission on Heart Disease, Cancer and Stroke, Report to the President.

[2] The following references were used in formulating this discussion: Brendan Phibbs, The Human Heart (St. Louis: C. U. Mosby Company, 1967); Public Health Service, Cerebrovascular Disease Epidemiology (1966); Jeremiah Stamler, The Epidemiology of Hypertension (New York, 1967); Public Health Service, Genetics and the Epidemiology of Chronic Disease, Publication No. 1163 (Washington, D.C., 1965). Several other studies have been summarized in an earlier report completed for the Illinois Regional Programs, Gerald F. Pyle and Susan M. Davies, "Morbidity and Mortality: Sources of Data and Methods of Analysis," Chicago Regional Hospital Study, Working Paper No. VI.2, October, 1969.

A little more than half of the cardiovascular-renal deaths in the United States are caused by arteriosclerosis. The disease is especially dangerous because of the narrowing and blockage of arteries carrying blood to the heart, brain, and kidneys. This damming can lead to clotting and possible complete blockage of blood flowing to those vital organs. Arteriosclerosis is caused by plaques comprised of fat and eventually calcium which accumulate on the inside walls of arteries to cause the blockage. Chances of developing this condition generally increase with age, but it is often difficult to determine if this condition is a leading cause after 65 years.

The age distinction alone would seem to help cause differences from one place to another by virtue of the common demographic occurrence of clustering of population of various age categories. Marked differences in death rates do appear among the various demographic groups as well as from geographic place to place, but these distributions require very careful analysis. For one thing, not all of the reasons are clearly understood.[1] There is no agreement, for example, that differences recorded and reported are all real in the sense that there is not some artificiality due to problems of diagnosis. Accuracy of medical certification of cause of death obviously depends upon the amount of information available to the physician. Furthermore, there has been a clarification of diagnostic criteria since the 1920's about this disease. It would appear that the shortcomings due to artificial differences within the United States should be recognized, but it is assumed here that they are insufficient to offset assessments of geographic patterns.

The most common distinctions made in studies of the distribution of arteriosclerotic heart disease in this country in addition to the increase during and beyond middle age are those for race, sex, and occupation. When health data are separated by race, i.e., using "white" and "non-white" categories, areas with concentrations of Negroes frequently show higher mortality rates. The most important question to address when analyzing such statistics is the actual degree of racial correlation. In many respects the higher rates may be associated with income and status. Epstein holds to the view that the higher rates in the South and metropolitan areas, where most American Negroes reside, are perhaps more environmental than racial.[2] High rates for white people also show up in these areas. In general, there are proportionately fewer deaths among Negroes from coronary heart disease than for hypertensive heart disease and stroke thus making such studies even more difficult.

---

[1]Iwao Moriyama, "Factors in Diagnosis and Classification of Deaths from CVR Diseases," Public Health Reports, LXXV (March, 1960), 189-95.

[2]Frederick H. Epstein, "The Epidemiology of Coronary Heart Disease," Journal of Chronic Diseases, XVIII (August, 1965), 735-74.

Differences by sex also exist, but they are not apparently uniform from one region to another. Furthermore, they appear to be different for urban areas also. In the United States white males have the highest rates while white women have the lowest. The difference in rates has, however, not held constant over time in different regions. Between 1950 and 1960 two states actually showed a decline in rates (California 12 per cent; Utah 4 per cent).[1] All others showed an increase, but this also was variable (New York 1 per cent; Kentucky 40 per cent). Studies of coronary heart disease in relation to urbanization indicate much higher rates in more metropolitan counties by as much as 37 per cent for males and 47 per cent for females than in less metropolitan counties.[2] Friedman[3] studied the relationship of coronary heart disease, on a state basis, to cigarette consumption (based on tax revenues), urbanization and water hardness and found a high correlation to all of these. This indicates that numerous factors are involved in the distribution of this disease.

The aspect of hardness of water is of particular interest to many health researchers. In a 1960 study, Schroeder[4] demonstrated that a negative correlation existed between hardness of water and deaths from cardiovascular diseases (International Classification:[5] 330-334 and 440-468), malignant neoplasms (140-205), and vascular lesions (330-334). The statistics were $r = -0.560$ for heart disease, $r = -0.309$ for cancer, and $r = 0.334$ for stroke. The states with the harder water and the lower death rates for these diseases were in the East North Central, the West North Central, and the Mountain States.

Stamler has also carried out studies of heart disease mortality in Chicago in relation to age, race, sex, and occupation.[6] In studies of utility companies and other employment groups in the early 1950's several conclusions about Chicago's population could be

---

[1] H. H. Hechter and N. O. Borhani, "Mortality and Geographic Distributions of Arteriosclerotic Heart Disease," Public Health Reports, LXXX (January, 1965), 11-24.

[2] P. E. Enterline, "Death Rates for Coronary Heart Disease in Metropolitan and Other Areas," Public Health Reports, LXXV (August, 1960), pp. 525-34.

[3] G. D. Friedman, "Cigarette Smoking and Geographic Variation in Coronary Heart Disease Mortality in the United States," Journal of Chronic Diseases, XX (October, 1967), 769-79.

[4] Henry A. Schroeder, "Relations Between Hardness of Water and Death Rates from Certain Diseases in the United States," Journal of Chronic Diseases, XII (November, 1960), 586-91.

[5] References to the "International Classification" are in most of these reports to the World Health Organization, International Classification of Diseases (7th rev. ed.; Geneva, 1957).

[6] See J. Stamler, M. Kjolsberg, and Y. Hall, 'Epidemiologic Studies on Cardiovascular-Renal Diseases: I. Analysis of Mortality by Age-Race-Sex-Occupation," Journal of Chronic Diseases, Vol. XII (November, 1960).

drawn. Coronary heart disease was the leader among all cardiovascular-renal diseases in the cause of death for middle-aged white men. White collar workers generally had a higher risk of one of the cardiovascular diseases being the cause of death than did blue collar workers. Hypertensive heart disease death rates were much higher for non-whites than for whites, and there was little difference between the sexes. White and non-white death rates for stroke were similar, and female rates were slightly higher than those for males.

Many references consider hypertension to be a leading factor in coronary heart disease as well as in hypertensive heart disease. Phibbs explains hypertension essentially as a condition which can produce heart failure due to abnormal blood pressure.[1] Normal blood pressure lies between 120-130 systolic (i.e., when heart contracts) and 70-80 diastolic (i.e., when heart relaxes). Strain is put on the heart and arteries when pressure increases (220/130), and this could cause a variety of problems including heart failure, rupture of artery walls, stroke, hemorrhage, and kidney failure. Hypertension is believed to increase with age in the United States. Stamler found higher rates of hypertension in cities.[2] The President's Commission on Heart Disease, Cancer, and Stroke findings indicated much higher hypertensive heart disease mortality (440-443) rates for non-whites than for whites, with sex making little difference. Although chances of hypertensive heart disease mortality increase with age, the overall incidence of this disease has gone down over the last 20 years.

Definite patterns emerge when "hypertension" is mapped, but Rose has pointed out that it is more judicious to combine rubrics 440 to 447 from the International List because of poor agreement among physicians about particular categories in instances of fatal hypertension.[3] In a study of the racial and regional distribution of average hypertension mortality in the United States for the period 1949-1951, Rose came to the following conclusions:

(1) There was not the large male excess of deaths as found with coronary heart disease.

(2) The correlation between a measure of urbanization (U.S. Census: by State) and hypertension mortality was 0.490, but "older" states were even higher, and states similar to California were lower.

(3) When the white and non-white statistics are separated and mapped the patterns are similar even though the actual non-white rates were higher.

---

[1]Phibbs, Human Heart, Chapter XIII.

[2]Stamler, Kjolsberg, and Hall, "Epidemiologic Studies on Cardiovascular-Renal Diseases I."

[3]Geoffrey Rose, "The Distribution of Mortality from Hypertension Within the United States," Journal of Chronic Diseases, XV (November, 1962), 1017-24.

In general the patterns showed high incidence of death from this malady in the South and in the East.

Stroke

Stroke (Cerebrovascular Disease: Vascular Lesions Affecting the Central Nervous System) is the No. 5 killer of people in their most productive years in the United States.[1] It also accounts for about 20 per cent of all cardiovascular-renal deaths, and it ranks third as a cause listed for all deaths in this country. Unlike the other cardiovascular-renal diseases, stroke claims more female victims than male. However, part of this is due to the fact that 80 per cent of the victims are probably over 65 years old.

Strokes, often fatal, result when circulation of the blood fails due to disease of the blood vessels. There are generally three types of stroke:[2]

(1) Those due to occlusion by thrombosis or clotting of the diseased vessel,

(2) Those due to occlusion by a fragment of a clot which becomes dislodged from the heart or vessels of the neck and blocks the cerebral vessels, and

(3) Rupture of a cerebral vessel due to hypertension or fault of the vessel wall with hemorrhage into the brain.

The first two account for most deaths.

A survey of patterns of mortality in several countries indicates that climate has an important role in stroke mortality.[3] This includes the United States. Blood pressures tend to be higher in winter, and even survival from an initial stroke could lead to the introduction of other infectious complications such as pneumonia. Conversely, many parts of the United States with mild winters (the South) have the highest annual incidence of stroke mortality. However, there is also high stroke mortality incidence in the Upper Midwest, the Northwest, and New England.[4] When spatial patterns for white and non-white are examined separately, there is little difference.

---

[1]President's Commission on Heart Disease, Cancer and Stroke, Report to the President, pp. 11-14.

[2]Gerald F. Pyle and Susan M. Davies, "Morbidity Analysis of Heart Disease, Cancer, and Stroke," Chicago Regional Hospital Study, Working Paper V.6, October, 1969.

[3]Reuel A. Stallones, "Epidemiology of Cerebrovascular Disease: A Review," Journal of Chronic Diseases, XVIII (August, 1965), 859-72.

[4]Michael B. Shimkin, Science and Cancer, Public Health Service Publication No. 1162 (Washington, D.C., 1964), and President's Commission on Heart Disease, Cancer and Stroke, Report to the President, pp. 1-20.

Spatial Aspects of Cancer

Cancers have been defined as uncontrolled new growths which invade and destroy living tissue.[1] These growth are made up of cancerous cells which differ from normal cells in size, shape, growth rates, and many other ways. Malignant tumors or cancers differ from benign types in growth beyond the original organ. In general, malignant tumors share the following characteristics:[2]

(1) A higher rate of cell growth and multiplication than normal tissues.

(2) Complete lack of tissue and organ boundary maintenance.

(3) A microscopic appearance which suggests immature rather than mature cells.

(4) The spread in late stages to parts of the body far from the place of origin.

Due to the histological implications cancers have traditionally been considered a collection of diseases rather than a single type. Studies of the spatial variability of cancers are thus complicated by a wide variety of differential occurrence rates recorded by histological <u>site</u>. In addition, different rates by site have been attributed to differences in sex, age, race, place of residence, individual behavior, specific environment, and many other "non-medical" items.

In recent years about 16 per cent of all deaths have been due to cancer. This makes cancer second to heart disease as a leading cause of death (heart disease, 40 per cent; stroke, third, with 11 per cent).[3] There were nearly one million persons in the United States under treatment in 1969 and during the same year there were probably 615,000 cases diagnosed for the first time. In 1969 about 325,000 persons died of cancer.[4] The national death rate for cancer has gone up since 1930, the first time when really accurate records on any national scale were recorded. However, since 1950 the actual rate of increase has lessened. For the last 20 years more men than women have died of cancer. Furthermore, half of all cancer deaths were in persons over 65.

---

[1]John C. Bailar, Haitung King, and Marie Joy Mason, <u>Cancer Rates and Risks</u>, Public Health Service Publication No. 547 (Washington, D. C.: U. S. Department of Health, Education, and Welfare, Public Health Service, National Institutes of Health, 1964), p. 4.

[2]American Cancer Society, "1969 Cancer Facts and Figures" (pamphlet; New York: American Cancer Society, Inc., 1968).

[3]<u>Ibid</u>., p. 4.

[4]John C. Bailar and Susan S. Devesa, "Special Cancer Survey Section, National Cancer Institute" (paper presented at the Sixth National Cancer Conference, Denver, Colorado, September 18-20, 1968).

Variability of data sources

Sources of data for cancer differ somewhat from those for heart disease and stroke in that registers for mobidity exist in some places. The Connecticut Health Department has maintained a register on the basis of hospital-reported morbidity and mortality examination since 1935. Similar coverage in New York State dates to 1942. Some parts of California also have registries. The United States Public Health Service has made use of these and other sources in studies of the incidence of cancer nationally. However, for complete coverage of the country it is necessary to turn to mortality tables published annually by the Division of Vital Statistics.

Studies of cancer in relation to urban areas have been made in the past, and some of these studies still serve as assets in understanding incidence. The National Cancer Institute made a canvass of all diagnosed cases of cancer in 10 metropolitan centers in 1937-1938 and again in the same cities in 1947-1948. A similar study was conducted for the State of Iowa in 1950. An up-to-date survey is currently being undertaken by the National Cancer Institute under the direction of John C. Bailar III.[1] The survey covers most of the areas of the earlier studies, but in addition it includes Colorado and Puerto Rico (see Table 2). This sample is presumed to be 10 per cent of the U.S. population. The time period includes the three years 1969 to 1971. Data are being gathered from three sources: (1) physicians records; (2) hospitals and clinics; and (3) death certificates. The final reports will include morbidity and mortality by age, sex, race, and site.

Differences by site and sex are probably two of the most important ingredients necessary to the understanding of any study of the spatial variability of cancer. The sex occurrence differences are due to the marked differences in the male and female reproductive systems, for in women the genital and breast sites combined cause nearly half of all deaths from cancer. When the reproductive systems are excluded, rates by sex are nearly the same. Cancer of the digestive system accounts for the greatest number of newly diagnosed cases in both sexes.[2] In men the next leading sites are in the respiratory system. Figure 6 shows relative shares by site for Connecticut from 1935 to 1959.[3]

As mentioned already, chances of acquiring cancer increase with age. The one outstanding exception to this, of course, is leukemia. In the age group 2 to 14 cancer is

---

[1] Bailar et al., Cancer Rates and Risks, pp. 10-16.

[2] Connecticut State Department of Health, Cancer in Connecticut: Incidence Characteristics, 1935-1962 (Hartford, 1967).

[3] R. W. Miller, 'Environmental Agents in Cancer," Yale Journal of Biology and Medicine, Vol. XXXVII (June, 1965).

TABLE 2

AREAS CURRENTLY BEING STUDIED BY
THE NATIONAL CANCER INSTITUTE

Area	Counties Included	Projected 1970 Population	Estimated New Cancer Cases During 1969-1971
Atlanta (SMSA)	DeKalb, Fulton, Clayton, Cobb, Gwinnett	1,415,000	14,000
Birmingham (SMSA)	Jefferson, Shelby, Walker	749,000	7,500
Dallas-Forth Worth (SMSA)	Dallas, Collin, Denton, Ellis, Tarrant, Johnson, Kaufman, Rockwall	2,209,000	22,000
Detroit (SMSA)	Wayne, Macomb, Oakland	4,211,000	42,000
Minneapolis-St. Paul (SMSA)	Hennepin, Ramsey, Anoka, Dakota, Washington	1,742,000	17,500
Philadelphia (city)	Philadelphia	2,102,000	21,000
Pittsburgh (SMSA)	Allegheny, Beaver, Washington, Westmoreland	2,339,000	23,500
San Francisco-Oakland (SMSA)	Alameda, San Francisco, Contra Costa, Marin, San Mateo	3,188,000	32,000
Colorado	All	2,146,000	21,500
Iowa	All	2,757,000	27,500
Puerto Rico	All	2,489,000	25,000
Total		25,347,000	253,500

Source: Bailar and Devesa, "Special Cancer Survey Section."

second only to accidents as a cause of death. Furthermore, the children of higher income white families have a much higher mortality rate than children of lower income black families.[1]

There are other site differences attributed to racial differences. Some of the differences appear to be racial while others should perhaps be associated either with social status or sub-cultural traits. Only skin cancer has any definite racial basis owing to skin

[1]American Cancer Society, "1969 Cancer Facts and Figures," pp. 5-11.

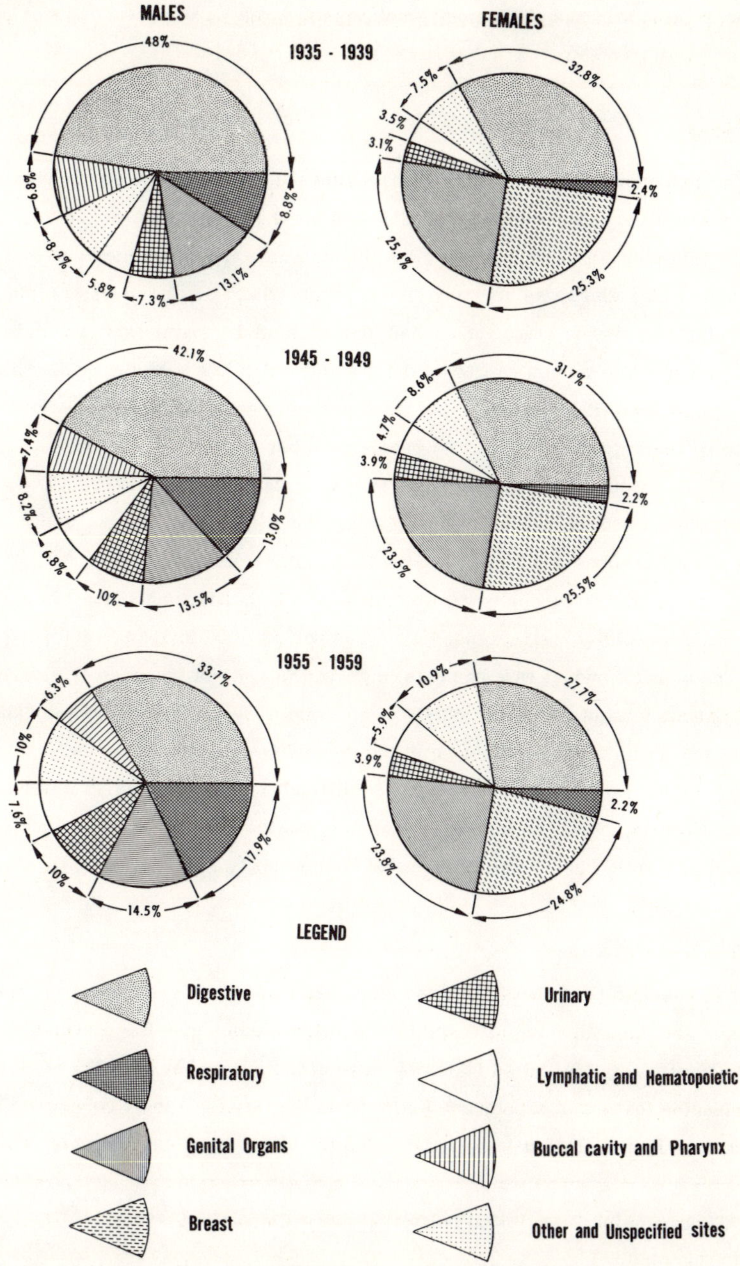

Fig. 6.--Distribution of various cancer sites in Connecticut, 1935 to 1959

pigmentation. Darker skin affords more protection from ultra-violet light. Higher cervical cancer rates are reported among black women while higher breast cancer rates are reported for white women.

Recent trends

The President's Commission on Heart Disease, Cancer, and Stroke published temporal trends by race and sex in the United States for the period 1930 to 1960. These trends are shown on Figure 7. In white men there was a sharp decline in stomach cancer while in non-whites there was not very much change. Both black and white male groups showed a startling rise in lung cancer, and blacks showed a significant growth in prostate cancer. Among white women cancer of the breast, which has been the leading site for many years, showed little change; rates were not quite so high among non-whites but seemed to be increasing slightly. The greater number of deaths from uterine cancers among non-white women (despite a decline in rates) stands out. This has always been the leading cause of death and contrasts sharply with rates for white women, and it suggests both cultural differences and lack of access to medical treatment.

In recent years, cancer mortality rates have been hovering above 100 per 100,000 persons while morbidity has increased from 200 per 100,000 in 1930 to 300 per 100,000 in 1967.[1] The actual survival rate has thus improved in spite of increased incidence and the National Cancer Institute expects this situation to improve. It has estimated that the mortality rate will remain fairly stable while the morbidity rate may be as high as 400 per 100,000 by 1985. However, these trends are difficult to specify by sites which have shown the greatest change, i.e., respiratory, stomach, uterus, and breast. Uterine cancer should decline, while lung cancer will probably continue to rise.[2]

Geographic variability

It is possible to study differences in cancer rates from one part of the country to another and get some meaningful results. Mortality studies give the best indication of regional variations in the United States because of the general availability of statistics. The outstanding feature of cancer deaths in the United States is their concentration in the Manufacturing Belt. This pattern is revealed to hold in many cancer sites, while others

---

[1]"Cancer on the Rise," Medical World News (December, 1967).

[2]U. S. Department of Health, Education, and Welfare, "Cancer Mortality Trends in the United States 1930 to 1955," Public Health Service Monograph No. 6 (Washington, D. C., 1961).

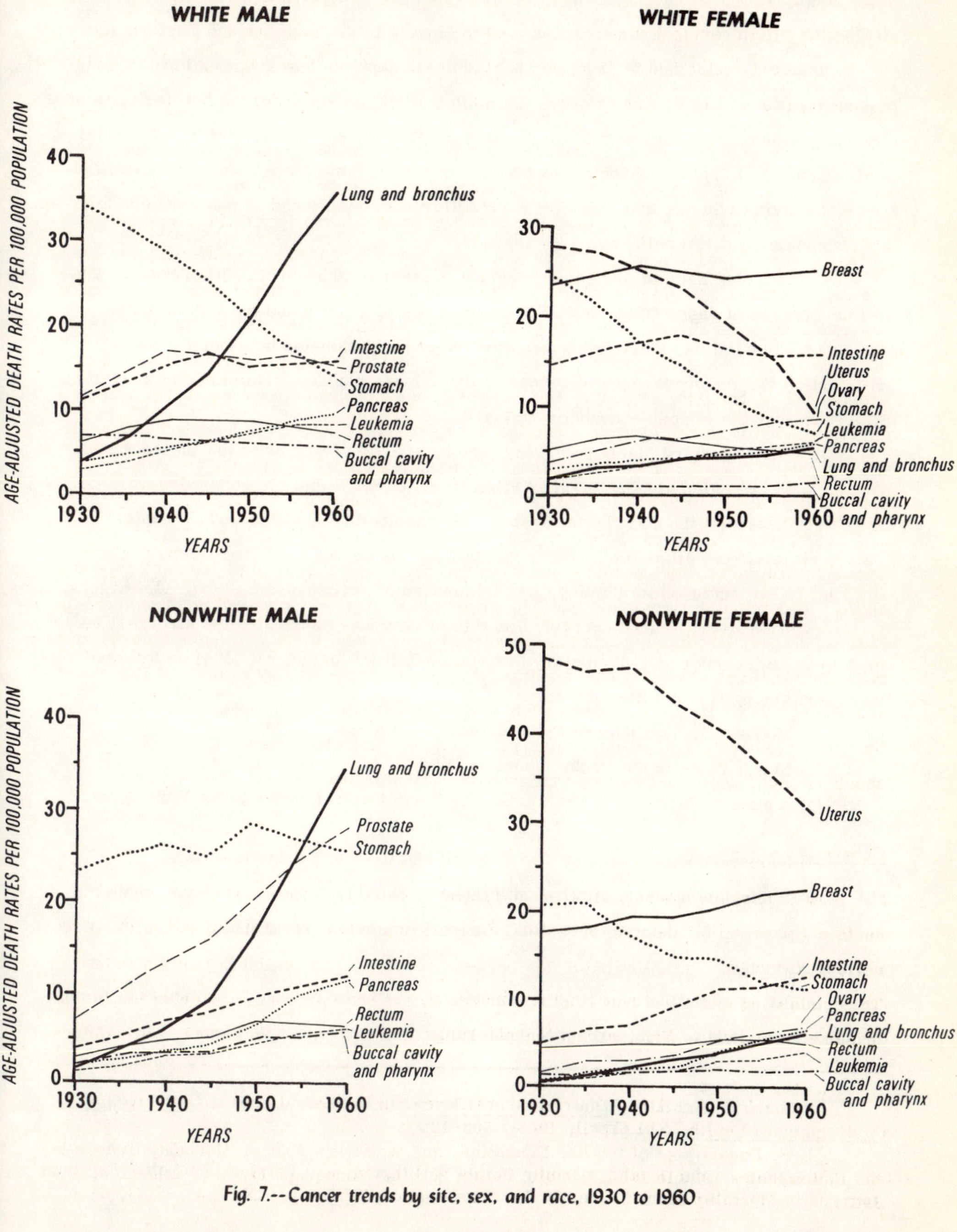

Fig. 7.--Cancer trends by site, sex, and race, 1930 to 1960

seem to cluster in other specific geographic patterns. The high incidence of skin cancer in the South, as a presumed response to climate, is the most obvious concentration in any single site. High cervical cancer rates tend to cluster in the Southern and Eastern states.

In a study published in 1968, Michael Shimkin explains how geographic variations in cancer patterns can be understood.[1] Shimkin explains to some degree how the current site categories of cancer appear to vary with sex, age, race, and nationality. A spatial implication is, of course, associated with each of the variable traits. In these spatial terms, Shimkin indicates that aside from the differences mentioned above there are few other consistent spatial patterns.

Conversely, Shimkin indicates evidence in favor of urban-rural differences. The high occurrence of respiratory cancer in urban areas of Britain and the United States stands out. In addition, there is some indication of a relationship between degree of urbanization and the occurrence of cancer of the urinary bladder. Shimkin also indicates differences related to socio-economic status.

In a 1967 study by MacDonald, Wellington, and Wolf, cancer in the United States was analyzed by region along with other ailments.[2] General disease subgroups were delineated as follows: (1) the circulatory system, (2) respiratory system, and (3) genito-urinary system, as well as total cancer mortality. This study indicated strong regional patterns. Also, included in the study was a measure of "urban density" (per cent of total state population living in urban areas), and this measure demonstrated the strongest relationship to total cancer and circulatory system mortality. In general all sites followed the pattern for total mortality:

(1) Moderately high Pacific Coast rates,

(2) Lower rates in the Rocky Mountain area,

(3) A general increase in rates from the North Central States to the East Coast, and

(4) Somewhat lower rates in New England and the South Atlantic area.

The above findings contrast somewhat with those of Shimkin, and this contrast further points out the need for detailed statistical analysis on several geographic scales or levels of areal coverage.

So far as variation over time is concerned, the basic pattern remained very much the same from 1930 to 1950, except that the range between higher and lower rates was

---

[1] Michael B. Shimkin, "Distribution of Cancer in the United States," Archives of Environmental Health, XVI (April, 1968), 503-12.

[2] Eleanor J. MacDonald, Dorothy Gaites Wellington, and Patricia F. Wolf, "Regional Patterns in Mortality from Cancer in the United States," Cancer, XX (May, 1967), 617-22.

reduced. Generally there was an increase in the rates of Southern states (probably owing to improved reporting and medical services as in 1930 a significant proportion of deaths were stated to be caused by "senility").

From work carried out in many surveys and studies of cancer it appears that urban residents have higher total cancer rates than rural residents. The highest urban-rural ratios appear to be cancers of the esophagus, intestine, rectum, bladder, and respiratory organs. This has been shown to be true in the 1950 Iowa study, the New York State and Connecticut registries, and by similar findings in Denmark, Finland, and Norway. A more detailed view of these differences shows that rural counties have lower rates than those which contain urban areas.

The study of cancer in 10 cities which took place in 1937 and again in 1947 on the basis of incidence showed great differences between cities for various cancer sites (the greatest differences are between the digestive system, skin, and female genital organs). It seems clear that the urban-rural ratio can only be one explanation for regional variations. Another contrast between the 1937 and 1947 surveys is the different growth rates or decline in various sites. In Denver, for example, the incidence in cancer of the ovary increased from 18.2 to 21.0 per 100,000 while in Atlanta there was a decrease from 4.1 to 3.4 per 100,000.

It is clear from work carried out thus far that much must still be accomplished regarding efforts to explain temporal and spatial variations in cancer on the basis of present knowledge. Few spatial patterns have been explained in such a way that prediction of future morbidity and hence hospital use can be made. However, it would appear that work relating cancer to urban ecological variables has at least begun.

Shimkin, for example, has done this in one study already mentioned.[1] A socio-economic ranking of five groups in accordance with education, income-occupation, residential location, and race was formulated, and cancer rates were compared for these groups. There appeared to be more cancers among lower classes, and the disease rates usually decreased with increased status. This relationship, of course, may relate a great deal to occupation, i.e., many lower status jobs expose workers more often to carcinogenic elements in the atmosphere. The same probably holds true for place of residence. Nor is the problem in any way restricted to respiratory problems. There appeared to be a social class differential of perhaps twice as much for gastric cancer in lower status men and three times for cervical carcinoma in lower status women.

Graham, Levin, and Lilienfield developed a socio-economic gradient in Buffalo for

---

[1]Shimkin, "Distribution of Cancer . . . ."

the period 1948-52.[1] Their definition of socio-economic status included ethnicity, religion, dietary habits, occupation, housing, and use of medical facilities. Their analysis postulated the following findings:

(1) For male patients, there was increasing incidence with decreasing socio-economic status for cancer of the esophagus, stomach, liver, lung, and larynx.

(2) For female patients, there was increasing incidence with decreasing socio-economic status for cancer of the stomach, liver, and cervix. An increasing incidence with increasing socio-economic status was noted for cancer of the female breast.

(3) Essentially no variations in incidence were observed for cancer of the buccal cavity, large intestine, rectum, pancreas, corpus uteri ovary, and prostate.

(4) These results were generally similar to those previously reported in Copenhagen, Denmark, New Haven, Connecticut, and Great Britain.

In addition, the only strong rate of cancer decrease with decreased status appeared to be female breast cancer.

A 1967 study by Greenburg of Staten Island shows noteworthy associations between environment, social status, and cancer.[2] A study relating cancer to air pollution had been completed for the period 1914-1920 by J. Meyers, and Greenburg developed a similar study in order to show temporal and spatial variations. In the earlier study Meyers showed that the highest cancer death rates were in the north and east of the island in locations adjacent to excessive industrial fumes or residential heating.

The Greenburg study showed for the Borough of Richmond during the period 1959-1961 some interesting similarities to the Meyers study and some differences partly due to changes in reporting, population composition, and increased emphasis in the more recent study upon socio-economic indices. Some areas termed "probably high air pollution" on the basis of the earlier study were areas of lower socio-economic status in 1960 and hence higher cancer rates were generally suspected. However, when consideration was given to sites other than respiratory, location became less important. The more recent study would indicate that social causes are now more important than environmental ones, but the latter should not be ignored.

Pittsburgh has also been studied at least twice. Two contributions, one in 1954 and one in 1967, show cancer patterns by small subareas for the city.[3] Both studies

---

[1]S. Graham, H. Levin, and A. H. Lilienfield, "The Socio-Economic Distribution of Cancer of Various Sites in Buffalo, 1948-1952," Cancer, XIII (1960), 80.

[2]Leonard Greenburg, Franklyn Field, Joseph I. Reed, and Marvin Glasser, "Air Pollution and Cancer Mortality," Archives of Environmental Health, XV (September, 1967).

[3]See Mary Ellen Patno, "Geographic Study of Cancer Prevalence Within an Urban Population," Public Health Reports, LXIX (August, 1954), 705-15, and Leonard Chiazze,

make use of census tracts to construct socio-economic scales; however, the methods of analysis of morbidity and mortality are sufficiently different to cause problems when comparing the two periods.

In the 1954 contribution, Patno utilized census tracts to build 16 similar areas on the basis of income, ethnicity (black/white ratio), and number of blue collar workers. The prevalence of cancer per 100,000 population was mapped by age, sex, and race, and areas of high and low prevalence were found and analyzed. The "downtown" and "hill" regions, areas of lower status, led all areas in cancer morbidity and mortality within the white population. Although Negro rates were high in those areas, they were high elsewhere also. High female breast cancer rates were also found in "Squirrel Hill," a white residential area of high status. Conversely, some low status white areas showed very low rates.

The 1967 study of Pittsburgh is partly negated because the decision was made to drop any consideration of the non-white population. Hence, a goodly portion of the lower social strata are not considered. The method of analysis is also different because incidence rather than prevalence rates are utilized. In spite of the problem of lack of compatibility some similar conclusions are reached.

On the basis of the 1960 population census, 15 homogeneous residential areas were developed. Variables utilized include income, education, per cent of housing sound, per cent of population white, per cent foreign born, and per cent blue collar workers. Contrasting areas of high and low rank were then selected. Although little correlation was established between the two periods, some patterns stand out for overall rates (all sites). The highest cancer rates continued to be in the poorer portions of the city, but possibly due to diffusion of the population other patterns related to sex started to become more pronounced.

Clearly, there is a case for studies of the spatial variability of heart disease, cancer, and stroke. As indicated above, demographic characteristics of populations help to explain some of this variability of the diseases, but age structure appears to be the strongest single element. A sample of the recent distribution of mortality from these diseases in relation to age groups demonstrates this association.

State-to-State Variations of RMP Diseases in 1967

Mortality data, the only information comparable for the entire United States for the RMP diseases are available annually with about a two-year time lag from the U. S.

Jr., and Antonio Ciacco, "Intracommunity Variation in Cancer Incidence for Pittsburgh," Public Health Reports, LXXXII (September, 1967), 759-70.

TABLE 3

CRUDE MORTALITY RATES FOR HEART DISEASE, CANCER, AND STROKE, 1967

Political Unit	Mortality/100,000, 1967			Population (1,000's)	Per Cent Distribution		
	Heart Disease[a]	Stroke	Cancer		Under 18	18 to 65	Over 65
Maine	666.2	130.2	192.4	973	36.0	52.6	11.4
New Hampshire	602.2	118.5	193.3	686	35.3	53.9	10.8
Vermont	613.4	117.5	173.9	417	36.2	53.0	10.8
Connecticut	602.1	106.5	192.2	5421	34.2	54.7	11.1
Rhode Island	615.9	93.8	188.9	900	33.3	55.9	10.8
Massachusetts	495.8	94.9	165.5	2925	34.5	56.2	9.3
New York	568.5	88.3	186.4	18336	33.0	56.6	10.4
New Jersey	537.4	85.1	175.3	7003	33.8	56.9	9.3
Pennsylvania	618.0	106.0	183.5	11629	33.5	56.1	10.4
Ohio	525.2	105.3	163.4	10458	36.3	54.4	9.3
Indiana	543.9	121.1	155.3	5000	36.7	53.8	9.5
Illinois	589.0	102.2	168.7	10893	35.2	54.7	10.1
Michigan	469.6	91.3	151.5	8584	37.6	53.7	8.7
Wisconsin	543.1	109.2	164.2	4189	37.1	52.2	10.7
Minnesota	517.8	122.9	163.2	3582	37.6	51.4	11.0
Iowa	617.3	136.0	172.3	2753	35.5	51.9	12.6
Missouri	617.2	133.5	178.3	4603	34.2	53.9	11.9
North Dakota	460.7	100.5	140.8	639	38.3	51.8	9.9
South Dakota	527.9	113.4	162.2	674	38.3	50.1	11.6
Nebraska	569.3	126.8	173.3	1435	36.1	51.6	12.3
Kansas	543.6	117.5	149.8	2275	35.3	53.3	11.4
Delaware	473.2	66.9	146.3	523	38.1	54.3	7.6
Maryland	443.6	65.6	153.0	3682	36.8	55.9	7.3
Washington, D. C.	514.5	96.8	185.0	809	34.7	56.5	8.8
Virginia	438.9	87.7	128.1	4536	36.1	56.6	7.3
West Virginia	592.3	117.1	168.6	1798	34.6	55.2	10.2
North Carolina	447.5	105.2	115.4	5029	36.6	56.0	7.4
South Carolina	449.8	114.9	110.5	2599	38.9	54.3	6.8
Georgia	451.7	122.0	122.5	4509	37.8	54.8	7.4
Florida	556.4	121.9	186.9	5995	34.2	52.9	12.9
Kentucky	564.5	123.3	151.4	3189	36.1	54.0	9.9
Tennessee	507.6	128.8	140.5	3892	35.3	55.8	8.9
Alabama	462.6	119.1	130.5	3540	37.4	54.3	8.3
Mississippi	482.2	126.8	132.8	2348	39.8	51.4	8.8
Arkansas	555.9	134.0	152.0	1968	36.1	53.0	10.9
Louisiana	447.8	92.1	138.9	3662	39.9	52.5	7.6
Oklahoma	542.8	127.4	157.6	2495	33.8	55.2	11.0
Texas	404.1	92.2	130.2	10869	37.7	54.0	8.3
Montana	472.3	96.7	142.9	701	37.9	52.5	9.6
Idaho	443.8	95.1	131.3	699	38.1	52.6	9.3
Wyoming	448.9	91.4	130.2	315	37.8	52.7	9.5
Colorado	422.9	82.1	125.2	1975	36.9	54.3	8.8
New Mexico	279.2	54.1	100.0	1003	43.3	50.3	6.4
Arizona	350.6	66.7	125.3	1634	39.5	52.7	7.8

TABLE 3--Continued

Political Unit	Mortality/100,000, 1967			Population (1,000's)	Per Cent Distribution		
	Heart Disease[a]	Stroke	Cancer		Under 18	18 to 65	Over 65
Utah	312.5	56.4	89.7	1024	42.0	51.0	7.0
Nevada	337.6	68.9	122.7	444	38.1	56.3	5.6
Washington	524.3	110.7	159.5	3087	35.4	54.9	9.9
Oregon	524.1	117.3	158.4	1999	34.2	55.3	10.5
California	429.4	88.5	145.6	19153	35.3	56.1	8.6
Alaska	148.2	30.9	56.3	272	43.4	54.0	2.6
Hawaii	231.0	44.2	98.5	739	39.0	55.6	5.4

Sources: U. S. Department of Health, Education, and Welfare, Vital Statistics of the United States, 1967 (Washington, D. C.: U. S. National Vital Statistics Division, 1969), pp. 1-36 to 1-39, and U. S. Department of Commerce, Statistical Abstract of the United States, 1968 (Washington, D. C.: Bureau of the Census, 1968), p. 25.

[a]Includes vascular lesions.

TABLE 4

UNIVARIATE STATISTICS FOR MORTALITY RATES AND AGE GROUPS, 1967

Variable	Mean	Deviation	Minimum	Maximum
Heart disease	492.61	102.86	148.20	666.20
Stroke	101.29	24.31	30.90	136.00
Cancer	149.76	28.95	56.30	193.30
% under 18	36.758	2.39	32.90	43.40
% 18 to 65	54.127	1.99	50.10	56.90
% over 65	9.313	1.99	2.60	

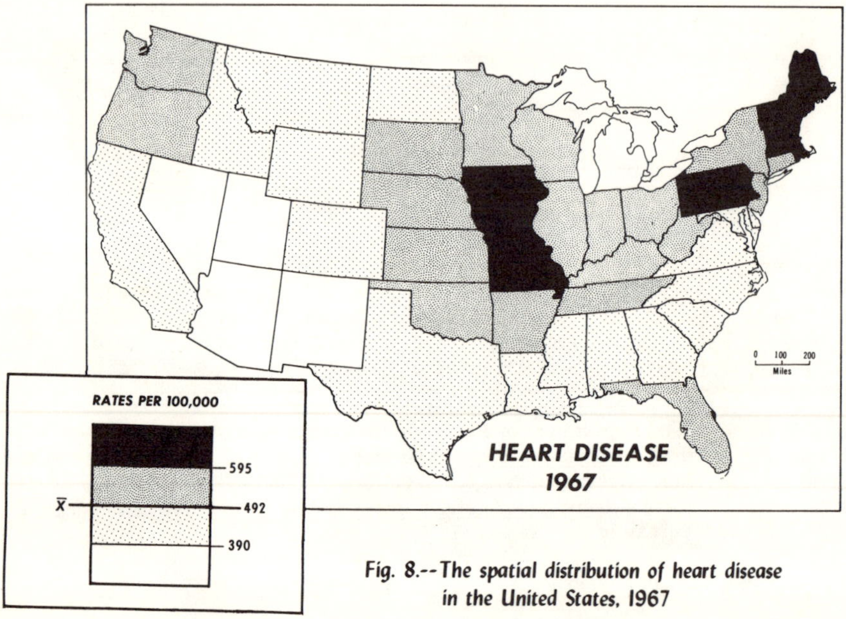

Fig. 8.--The spatial distribution of heart disease in the United States, 1967

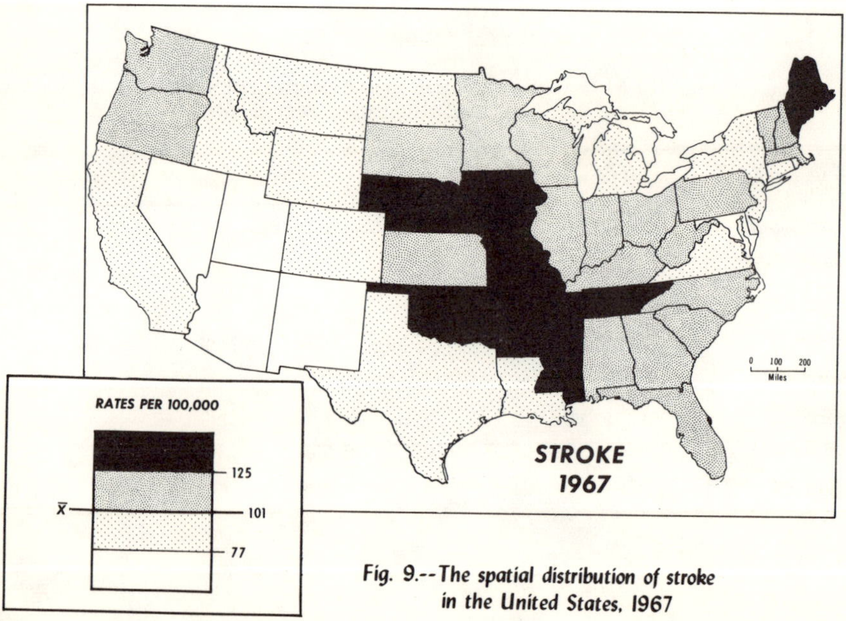

Fig. 9.--The spatial distribution of stroke in the United States, 1967

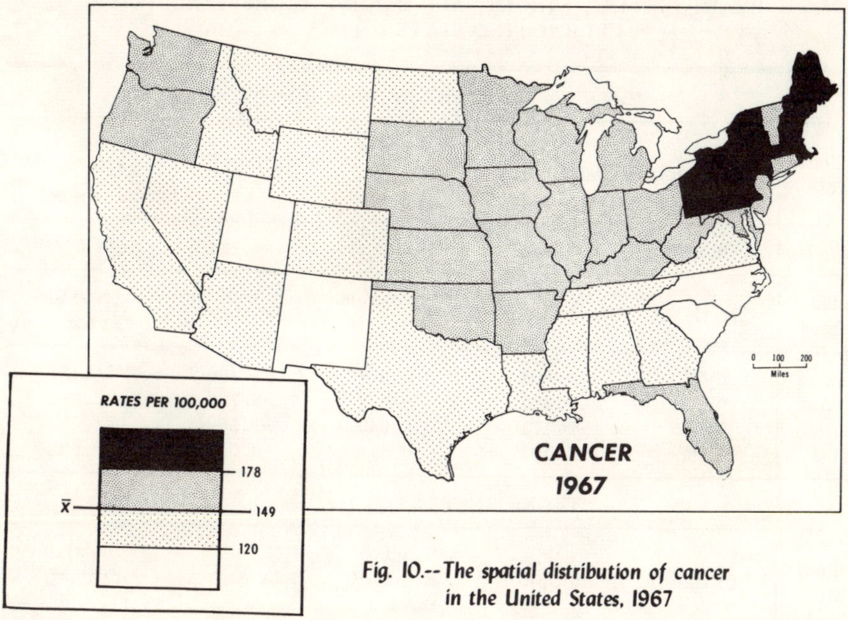

Fig. 10.--The spatial distribution of cancer in the United States, 1967

TABLE 5

ZERO-ORDER CORRELATION COEFFICIENTS FOR MORTALITY RATES AND AGE GROUPS, 1967

Variable	Heart Disease	Stroke	Cancer	Population	% under 18	% 18 to 65	% over 65
Heart disease	1.000						
Stroke	0.804	1.000					
Cancer	0.912	0.596	1.000				
Population	0.055	0.011	0.077	1.000			
% under 18	-0.775	-0.541	-0.804	0.115	1.000		
% 18 to 65	0.064	-0.120	0.150	0.530	-0.398	1.000	
% over 65	0.879	0.769	0.836	0.107	-0.652	-0.151	1.000

TABLE 6

HEART DISEASE, STROKE, AND CANCER REGRESSIONS
FOR UNITED STATES, 1967

HEART DISEASE REGRESSION (A)

Dependent Variable	Multiple R	Multiple R^2	Standard Error of Estimate	Intercept A	Standard Error of Intercept
Heart disease	0.919	0.844	42.271	-96.114	2444.739

Independent Variables	Partial R	Standardized B	Regression Error	Metric B	Regression Error
% over 65	0.240	0.804	0.474	41.439	24.457
% 18 to 65	0.051	0.171	0.492	8.796	25.289
% under 18	-0.045	-0.171	0.549	-7.352	23.580
Population	-0.039	-0.101	0.376	-0.001	0.002

STROKE REGRESSION (B)

Dependent Variable	Multiple R	Multiple R^2	Standard Error of Estimate	Intercept A	Standard Error of Intercept
Stroke	0.775	0.600	16.013	486.761	926.096

Independent Variables	Partial R	Standardized B	Regression Error	Metric B	Regression Error
% over 65	0.219	1.167	0.760	14.226	9.265
Population	-0.096	-0.400	0.605	-0.001	0.001
% 18 to 65	0.082	0.445	0.788	5.413	9.580
% under 18	0.073	0.443	0.879	4.499	8.932

CANCER REGRESSION (C)

Dependent Variable	Multiple R	Multiple R^2	Standard Error of Estimate	Intercept A	Standard Error of Intercept
Cancer	0.906	0.822	12.737	450.577	736.632

Independent Variables	Partial R	Standardized B	Regression Error	Metric B	Regression Error
% under 18	-0.148	-0.602	0.588	-7.272	7.105
% over 65	0.117	0.409	0.508	5.941	7.369
Population	0.059	0.164	0.404	0.001	0.001
% 18 to 65	-0.032	-0.115	0.526	-1.668	7.619

National Vital Statistics office.[1] Table 3 shows the distribution of total mortality from cardiovascular-renal (including stroke), stroke, and cancer for the year most recently available, 1967. The heart disease rates are somewhat inflated by the inclusion of vascular lesions, but it does present an accurate picture of the magnitude of the disease. The cancer figures include all sites, and in most instances the rates are somewhat higher than those forecasted for the United States in the early 1960's by the National Cancer Institute and the American Cancer Society.

Analysis of these data using a regression model identical with equation (2) may be used to demonstrate the spatial variability of these data on state-to-state variations. Univariate statistics for the health and age data[2] shown in Table 4 were developed from Table 3. When the disease data are mapped, the patterns shown on Figures 8 to 10 result. All diseases show clustering. Cardiovascular-renal types show the heaviest concentration in the Manufacturing Belt and the lowest in the Southwest. The pattern for stroke mortality shows the highest rates to be in the mid-central part of the country while the lowest are also in the Southwest. The distribution of cancer is similar to that of heart disease. All of these diseases are highly correlated (see Table 5), and the strongest associations are between heart disease and cancer (r = .912).

Table 5 also shows some rather significant associations between age groups and the diseases. For heart disease the per cent over 65 group displays high positive correlation (r = 0.879), and for the per cent under 18 group it shows the inverse with r = -0.775. The pattern also holds for stroke (r = 0.769; r = -0.541) and cancer (r = 0.836; r = -0.804) which does include leukemia mortality.

The regression model provides a more sophisticated test. Tables 6A to 6C show the multiple associations when all these groups are taken as causal variables. The results show fairly good fits and suggest that given a sufficient temporal sample, the regression model can be applied for predictive and planning purposes in metropolitan Chicago. This first step in building the IRMP model is taken in the chapter that follows.

---

[1] U. S. Department of Health, Education, and Welfare, Vital Statistics of the United States, 1967, pp. 1-36 to 1-39.

[2] U. S. Department of Commerce, Statistical Abstract of the United States, 1968, p. 25.

CHAPTER III

THE DISEASE INPUTS: NEED

A model for urban planning should, if it is to function in any sort of meaningful manner, consist of descriptive, predictive, and planning elements in that order.[1] This chapter handles the first two of the above phases, and Chapters IV, V, and VI each contribute elements for planning. The primary intent of the chapter is to build a calibrated sub-model which will function as the mechanism for providing morbidity and mortality inputs to the final allocation model for the treatment of heart disease, cancer, and stroke. The sub-model is built from disease data taken to be empirically derived input geared to produce empirically relevant output.

Recent Disease Patterns: Descriptions

The previous chapter examined studies of elements contributing to the spatial variability of the RMP diseases in general. From that base we can explore this variance in even greater detail by analyzing patterns of recent RMP disease occurrence in metropolitan Chicago.[2] The annual incidence of heart disease, stroke, and cancer for two years, 1960 and 1967, is taken to represent "recent" occurrence. The year 1960 is used because socio-economic and demographic data from the 1960 Census of Population are available. Data from 1967 represent the most up-to-date disease information available in complete form. The data are mapped and analyzed to be taken as the descriptive input to the sub-model. One of the most important aspects of the data turned out to be the source of the information, and a discussion of methods of collection and the shortcomings of the data at the source is of utmost importance in understanding the value of the disease input.

---

[1] Ira S. Lowry, "A Short Course in Model Building," in Spatial Analysis: A Reader in Statistical Geography, ed. Brian J. L. Berry and Duane F. Marble (Englewood Cliffs: Prentice-Hall, Inc., 1968), pp. 53-67.

[2] The study area consists of the Chicago SMSA as defined by the U. S. Bureau of the Census in 1960.

Sources of health data

There are at least a half-dozen important sources of health data which can contribute to major studies of this nature in Chicago. Health data are collected for specific purposes by several different agencies, and as a result the data vary in terms of geographical coverage and categories of health problems. The information provided by many of these agencies has rarely been utilized for urban health studies, and it is for that very important reason that Appendix A has been included with this study. Appendix A explains in detail the kinds of data available from these several agencies as well as some of the problems associated with the data actually used for analysis in this study.

The final sources of data selected for this study are the Illinois Department of Public Health and the Chicago Board of Health. The discussion in Appendix A explains why data from these two sources are not totally reliable; however, it was necessary to utilize these agencies for the following reasons:

(1) The methodology of this study requires reasonably comprehensive geographical coverage of the population of the Chicago SMSA, and the public health agencies are the only ones which cover the entire area when data are combined.

(2) Data were required for fairly small subareas, and, once again, the public health agencies were able to provide such coverage.

(3) It was necessary to have a common set of subareas within a fairly high degree of compatibility with collection units for demographic and socioeconomic information, and the public agencies could also accomplish this.

The sources of error in the data have been recognized, but they are hardly sufficient to nullify this study. Until such time that carefully controlled studies with predetermined and standardized methods of diagnosis are used in the Chicago SMSA, the public health departments are the best sources of data when it is necessary to consider the entire area and the entire population.

The Illinois Department of Public Health has charge of data for the entire Chicago SMSA, including the City of Chicago; however, only totals for the entire city are published by that agency. Figure 11 shows general trends since 1920 for the RMP diseases in the entire state.[1] The rates from 1960 to 1967 have been much the same for all of these maladies. Total deaths for 1967 in Illinois and Chicago by age groups are shown on Tables 7A and 8A. Also, included are the 1967 crude mortality rates (Tables 7B and 8B). Many of the age-group and racial differences discussed in Chapter II also appear within these tabulations. The very high stroke rates for older populations stand out particularly.

The state agency also publishes more detailed breakdowns by type of disease for cities over 10,000 population, but age-specific rates have not been published. Also,

---

[1]Illinois Department of Public Health, "Vital Statistics, Illinois," Springfield, February, 1969.

TABLE 7A

NUMBER OF DEATHS ATTRIBUTED TO HEART DISEASE, CANCER, AND STROKE FOR ILLINOIS, 1967
(INCLUDES DEATHS OF ILLINOIS RESIDENTS OCCURRING OUTSIDE THE STATE)

Cause and Race	All Ages	0-4 Years	5-14 Years	15-24 Years	25-44 Years	45-64 Years	65-84 Years	85 and Over
Illinois, all causes	110,030	5,344	894	1,957	6,474	27,769	54,716	12,876
White	97,065	3,731	712	1,532	4,546	23,652	50,605	12,287
Nonwhite	12,965	1,613	182	425	1,928	4,117	4,111	589
1. Heart disease	48,023	28	11	63	1,456	11,866	27,430	7,169
White	43,453	21	9	44	927	10,110	25,511	6,831
Nonwhite	4,570	7	2	19	529	1,756	1,919	338
A. Arteriosclerotic	40,090	1	1	13	1,051	9,959	23,251	5,814
White	36,822	1	1	7	708	8,743	21,812	5,550
Nonwhite	3,268	--	--	6	343	1,216	1,439	264
B. Other	7,933	27	10	50	405	1,907	4,179	1,355
White	6,631	20	8	37	219	1,367	3,699	1,281
Nonwhite	1,302	7	2	13	186	540	480	74
2. Malignant neoplasms	18,439	83	159	163	1,098	6,850	9,144	942
White	16,562	77	139	133	900	5,992	8,433	888
Nonwhite	1,877	6	20	30	198	858	711	54
3. Vascular lesions affecting central nervous system	11,208	14	19	30	298	1,795	6,942	2,110
White	10,036	13	17	23	188	1,407	6,362	2,026
Nonwhite	1,172	1	2	7	110	388	580	84

Source: Ibid.

TABLE 7B

CRUDE MORTALITY RATES PER 100,000 FOR HEART DISEASE, CANCER, AND STROKE IN ILLINOIS, 1967
(ESTIMATED POPULATION IN EACH GROUP AS OF JULY 1, 1967)

Cause and Race	All Ages	0-4 Years	5-14 Years	15-24 Years	25-44 Years	45-64 Years	65-84 Years	85 and Over
Illinois, all causes	1,014.1	513.8	40.6	115.9	256.1	1,198.5	5,477.1	17,638.4
White	1,014.3	433.8	37.9	102.3	205.8	1,116.7	5,400.7	17,807.2
Nonwhite	1,012.9	896.1	56.2	221.4	604.4	2,068.8	6,630.6	14,725.0
1. Heart disease	442.6	2.7	0.5	3.7	57.6	512.1	2,745.7	9,820.5
White	454.1	2.4	0.5	2.9	42.0	477.3	2,722.6	9,900.0
Nonwhite	357.0	3.9	0.6	9.9	165.8	882.4	3,095.2	8,450.0
A. Arteriosclerotic	369.5	0.1	0.0	0.8	41.6	429.8	2,327.4	7,964.4
White	384.8	0.1	0.1	0.5	32.1	412.8	2,327.9	8,043.5
Nonwhite	255.3	-0-	-0-	3.1	107.5	611.1	2,321.0	6,600.0
B. Other	73.1	2.6	0.5	3.0	16.0	82.3	418.3	1,856.2
White	69.3	2.3	0.4	2.5	9.9	64.5	394.8	1,856.5
Nonwhite	101.7	3.9	0.6	6.8	58.3	271.4	774.2	1,850.0
2. Malignant neoplasms	169.9	8.0	7.2	9.7	43.4	295.6	915.3	1,290.4
White	173.1	9.0	7.4	8.9	40.7	282.9	900.0	1,287.0
Nonwhite	146.6	3.3	6.2	15.6	62.1	431.2	1,146.8	1,350.0
3. Vascular lesions affecting central nervous system	103.3	1.3	0.9	1.8	11.8	77.5	694.9	2,890.4
White	104.9	1.5	0.9	1.5	8.5	66.4	679.0	2,936.2
Nonwhite	91.6	0.6	0.6	3.6	34.5	195.0	935.5	2,100.0

Source: Ibid.

TABLE 8A

NUMBER OF DEATHS ATTRIBUTED TO HEART DISEASE, CANCER, AND STROKE FOR CHICAGO, 1967
(INCLUDES DEATHS OF ILLINOIS RESIDENTS OCCURRING OUTSIDE THE STATE)

Cause and Race	All Ages	0-4 Years	5-14 Years	15-24 Years	25-44 Years	45-64 Years	65-84 Years	85 and Over
Chicago, all causes	42,137	2,260	296	675	3,094	12,110	20,353	3,349
White	31,986	1,003	148	348	1,465	8,821	17,270	2,931
Nonwhite	10,151	1,257	148	327	1,629	3,289	3,083	418
1. Heart disease	19,137	15	5	42	864	5,396	10,794	2,021
White	15,499	9	3	29	389	3,959	9,334	1,776
Nonwhite	3,638	6	2	13	475	1,437	1,460	245
A. Arteriosclerotic	15,938	1	1	9	605	4,365	9,209	1,748
White	13,336	1	1	4	288	3,379	8,109	1,554
Nonwhite	2,602	--	--	5	317	986	1,100	194
B. Other	3,199	14	4	33	259	1,031	1,585	273
White	2,163	8	2	25	101	580	1,225	222
Nonwhite	1,036	6	2	8	158	451	360	51
2. Malignant neoplasms	7,021	19	42	63	395	2,793	3,469	240
White	5,514	14	25	37	226	2,090	2,922	200
Nonwhite	1,507	5	17	26	169	703	547	40
3. Vascular lesions affecting central nervous system	3,616	5	4	14	159	785	2,185	464
White	2,727	4	2	8	62	498	1,756	397
Nonwhite	889	1	2	6	97	287	429	67

Source: Ibid.

TABLE 8B

CRUDE MORTALITY RATES PER 100,000 FOR HEART DISEASE, CANCER, AND STROKE IN CHICAGO, 1967 (ESTIMATED POPULATION IN EACH GROUP AS OF JULY 1, 1967)

Cause and Race	All Ages	0-4 Years	5-14 Years	15-24 Years	25-44 Years	45-64 Years	65-84 Years	85 and Over
Chicago, all causes	1,187.0	610.8	43.0	141.8	360.6	1,531.0	5,865.4	17,626.3
White	1,260.3	436.1	34.8	106.4	242.5	1,389.1	5,756.7	17,241.2
Nonwhite	1,003.1	897.9	56.1	219.5	641.3	2,108.3	6,559.6	20,900.0
1. Heart disease	539.1	4.1	0.7	8.8	100.7	682.2	3,110.7	10,636.8
White	610.7	3.9	0.7	8.9	64.4	623.5	3,111.3	10,447.1
Nonwhite	359.5	4.3	0.8	8.7	187.0	921.2	3,106.4	12,250.0
A. Arteriosclerotic	449.0	0.3	0.1	1.9	70.5	551.8	2,653.9	9,200.0
White	525.5	0.4	0.2	1.2	47.7	532.1	2,703.0	9,141.2
Nonwhite	257.1	-0-	-0-	3.4	124.8	632.1	2,340.4	9,700.0
B. Other	90.1	3.8	0.6	6.9	30.2	130.3	456.8	1,436.8
White	85.2	3.5	0.5	7.6	16.7	91.3	408.3	1,305.9
Nonwhite	102.4	4.3	0.8	5.4	62.2	289.1	766.0	2,550.0
2. Malignant neoplasms	197.8	5.1	6.1	13.2	46.0	353.1	999.7	1,263.2
White	217.3	6.1	5.9	11.3	37.4	329.1	974.0	1,176.5
Nonwhite	148.9	3.6	6.4	17.4	66.5	450.6	1,163.8	2,000.0
3. Vascular lesions affecting central nervous system	101.9	1.4	0.6	2.9	18.5	99.2	629.7	2,442.1
White	107.4	1.7	0.5	2.4	10.3	78.4	585.3	2,335.3
Nonwhite	87.8	0.7	0.8	4.0	38.2	184.0	912.8	3,350.0

Source: Ibid.

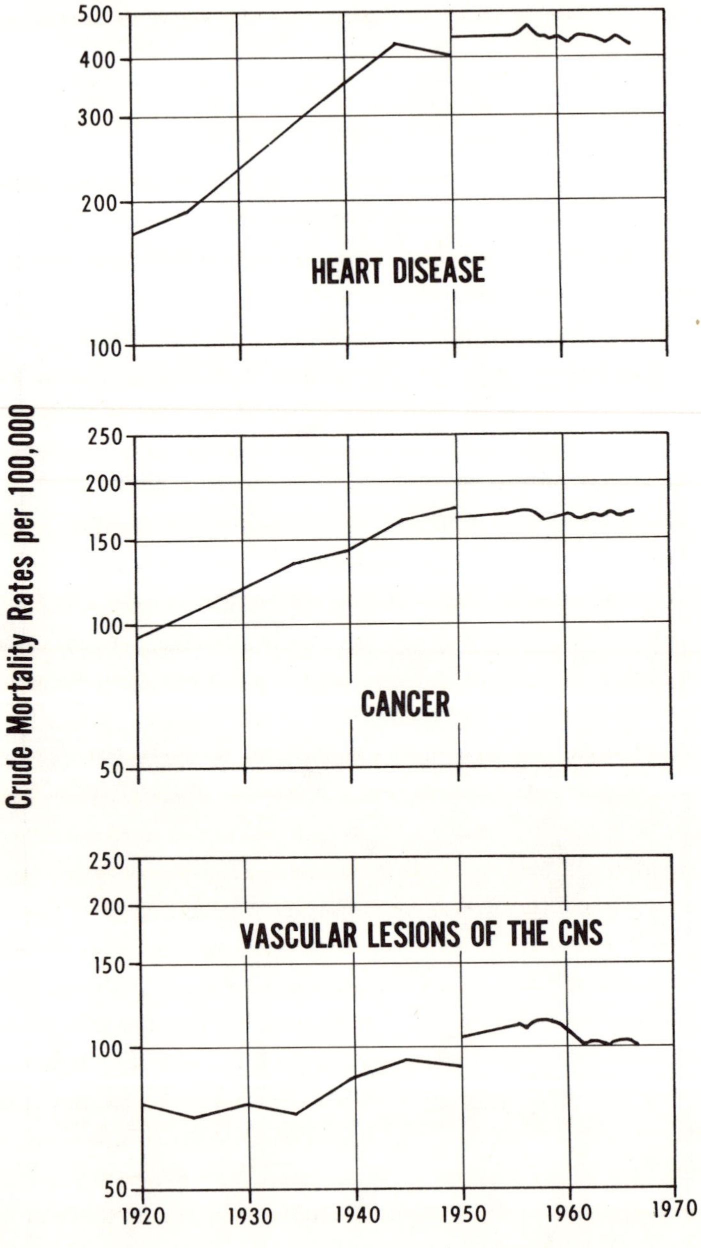

Fig. II.--Crude mortality rates for heart disease, cancer, and stroke in Illinois, 1920 to 1967

although detailed subdivisions of cardiovascular disease are determined, there are no breakdowns for specific cancer sites. As indicated by the discussion of spatial variability, there is much more variation among the cancer sites than among the various cardio-vascular-renal types.

Determination of disease types and units of data collection

In order to describe the spatial patterns of the RMP diseases, two important decisions had to be made. The first was to determine how to treat the diseases in order to demonstrate variability, and the second was the selection of modifiable areal units which would maximize the amount of variability to be shown.

It was decided that due to problems in diagnosis, particularly for hypertension and hypertensive heart disease, that all cardiovascular ailments except vascular lesions would be considered one category. Stroke deaths were considered as another disease. Cancer totals were considered as a group, but eight additional site groups were selected on the basis of possible patterns of spatial variability, the availability of actual site data from the Departments of Public Health, and on the basis of some previous investigations by the American Cancer Society in the Chicago area.[1] The diseases are shown on Table 9.

The method of analysis requires that the entire SMSA be subdivided into small areal units. It was possible to obtain from the Illinois Department of Public Health data for most towns of over 2,500 and either separate township totals where the population was over 2,500 in 1960 or groups of less populous townships. Similarly, it was possible to obtain data for the eleven disease groups shown on Table 9 from the Chicago Board of Health for 1960 and 1967 by Community Area. In addition, it was necessary that the data collection units be identical to areas for which 1960 Census data were available.

The resultant subareas are shown on Figure 12 and listed on Table 10 by name. They represent the units of discussion for the remainder of this chapter. Most incorporated municipalities in the Chicago SMSA are represented; however, those incorporated after 1960 are not shown. Also, health data for both periods were not available for some towns, two examples being Zion and East Chicago Heights. Only township totals were available, and it was necessary to subtract municipal totals to obtain differences. This condition resulted in some peculiar areas where one or more municipalities straddle township boundaries (e.g., units 201 and 250). A problem developed in determining boundaries in congested areas, and some rather large units such as 177 and 176 resulted. Also, some of the rural fringe areas are somewhat large; however, deaths are fewer by actual count.

---

[1] American Cancer Society, "1969 Cancer Facts and Figures."

TABLE 9

DISEASES SELECTED FOR AREAL INVESTIGATION

Name	International Classification
Total cardiovascular disease	400-468
Vascular lesions of C. N. S.	330-334
Total cancer	
Cancer site groups	
Digestive system*	150-154
Respiratory system	162, 163
Genitals, male and female	171, 172-174, 177
Breast	170
Leukemia and aleukemia	204
Buccal cavity and pharynx	140-148
Skin	190, 191
All other and unspecified	196-197, 155-160, 164-165, 175-176, 178-181, 192, 195, 198-199

*Data for the 75 Chicago Community Areas include only rectum and large intestine.

The data

The 1960 and 1967 mortality data are numerically listed on Tables 37 and 38 in Appendix B. Due to the fact that much more information related to mortality-morbidity comparisons for cancer types has been published, and because these diseases are presumed to demonstrate more spatial variability than the individual cardiovascular types, morbidity estimates have been made for mapping the former at this point in the study. The method used for making estimates for various sites is explained in Appendix B. For purposes of cartographic analysis, the maps can also be construed to reflect mortality, for they are simply crude mortality rates expanded by constant scalars for each site. Heart disease and stroke differentials are discussed in Chapter VI as they relate to the allocation model. The crude rates thus shown on Tables 41 and 42 are for heart disease and stroke mortality per 1,000 persons and estimated cancer morbidity per 1,000 persons for total cancer and those sites indicated by Table 9.

Univariate statistics were generated for the data shown on Tables 41 and 42, and these statistics are shown on Table 11. As indicated by Figure 11, the average rates for all of these diseases should have remained fairly constant from 1960 to 1967, and this is

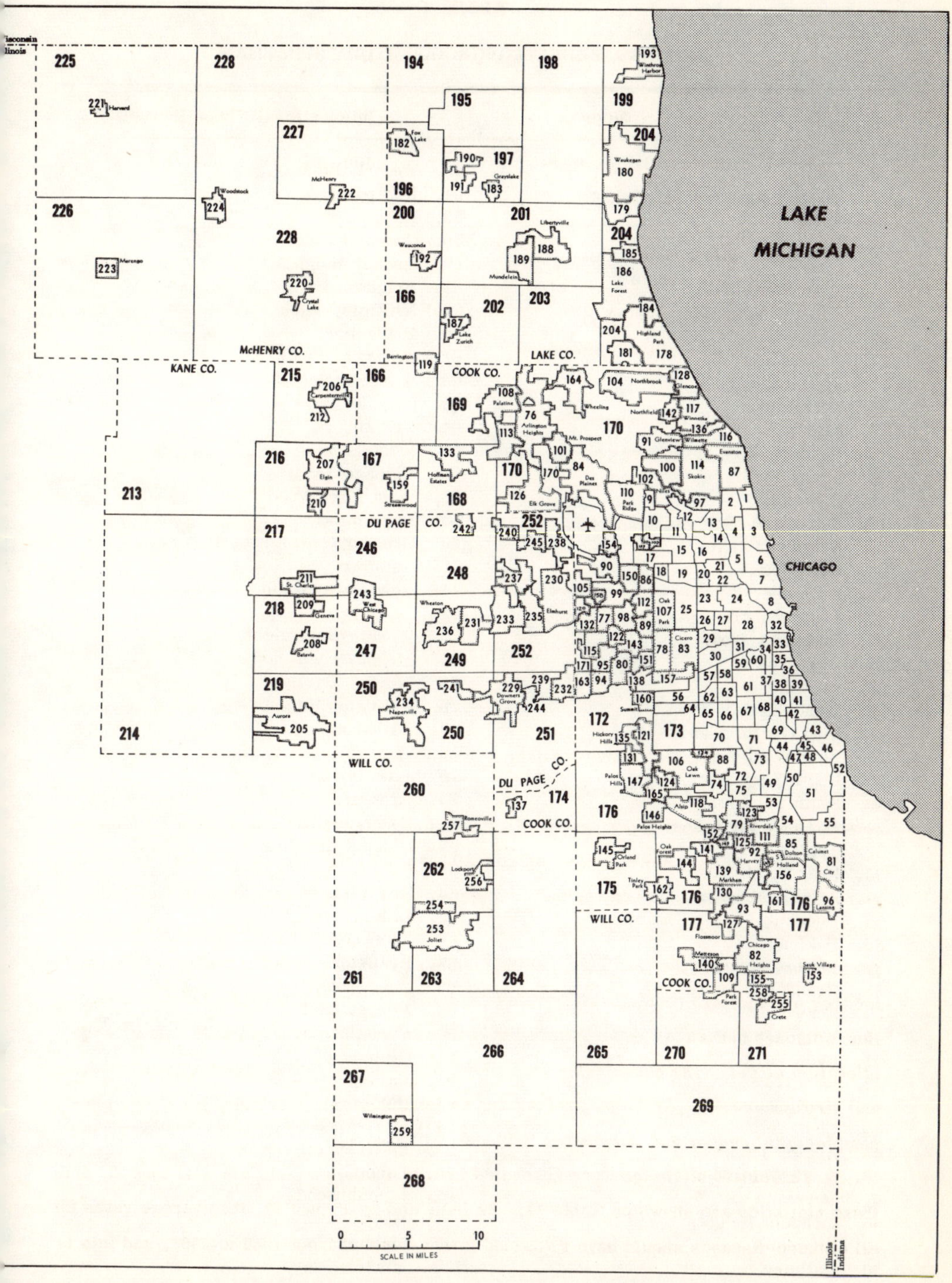

Fig. 12.--Regional medical program subareas for the Chicago SMSA

TABLE 10

REGIONAL MEDICAL PROGRAM STUDY SUBAREAS

1. Rogers Park
2. West Ridge
3. Uptown
4. Lincoln Square
5. North Center
6. Lake View
7. Lincoln Park
8. Near North Side
9. Edison Park
10. Norwood Park
11. Jefferson Park
12. Forest Glen
13. North Park
14. Albany Park
15. Portage Park
16. Irving Park
17. Dunning
18. Montclare
19. Belmont Cragin
20. Hermosa
21. Avondale
22. Logan Square
23. Humboldt Park
24. West Town
25. Austin
26. West Garfield Park
27. East Garfield Park
28. Near West Side
29. North Lawndale
30. South Lawndale
31. Lower West Side
32. The Loop
33. Near South Side
34. Armour Square
35. Douglas
36. Oakland
37. Fuller Park
38. Grand Boulevard
39. Kenwood
40. Washington Park
41. Hyde Park
42. Woodlawn
43. South Shore
44. Chatham
45. Avalon Park
46. South Chicago
47. Burnside
48. Calumet Heights
49. Roseland
50. Pullman
51. South Deering
52. East Side
53. West Pullman
54. Riverdale
55. Hegewisch
56. Garfield Ridge
57. Archer Heights
58. Brighton Park
59. McKinley Park
60. Bridgeport
61. New City
62. West Edison
63. Gage Park
64. Clearing
65. West Lawn
66. Chicago Lawn
67. West Englewood
68. Englewood
69. Greater Grand Crossing
70. Ashburn
71. Auburn Gresham
72. Beverly
73. Washington Heights
74. Mount Greenwood
75. Morgan Park
76. Arlington Heights
77. Bellwood
78. Berwyn
79. Blue Island
80. Brookfield
81. Calumet City
82. Chicago Heights
83. Cicero
84. Des Plaines
85. Dolton
86. Elmwood Park
87. Evanston
88. Evergreen Park
89. Forest Park
90. Franklin Park
91. Glenview
92. Harvey
93. Homewood
94. La Grange
95. La Grange Park
96. Lansing
97. Lincolnwood
98. Maywood
99. Melrose Park
100. Morton Grove

TABLE 10--Continued

101. Mount Prospect
102. Niles
103. Norridge
104. Northbrook
105. Northlake
106. Oak Lawn
107. Oak Park
108. Palatine
109. Park Forest
110. Park Ridge
111. Riverdale
112. River Forest
113. Rolling Meadows
114. Skokie
115. Westchester
116. Wilmette
117. Winnetka
118. Alsip
119. Barrington
120. Berkeley
121. Bridgeview
122. Broadview
123. Calumet Park
124. Chicago Ridge
125. Dixmoor
126. Elk Grove Village
127. Flossmoor
128. Glencoe
129. Harwood Heights
130. Hazel Crest
131. Hickory Hills
132. Hillside
133. Hoffman Estates
134. Hometown
135. Justice
136. Kenilworth
137. Lemont
138. Lyons
139. Markham
140. Matteson
141. Midlothian
142. Northfield
143. North Riverside
144. Oak Forest
145. Orland Park
146. Palos Heights
147. Palos Hills
148. Phoenix Village
149. Posen
150. River Grove
151. Riverside
152. Robbins
153. Sauk Village
154. Schiller Park
155. South Chicago Heights
156. South Holland
157. Stickney
158. Stone Park
159. Streamwood
160. Summit
161. Thornton
162. Tinley Park
163. Western Springs
164. Wheeling
165. Worth

166. Barrington and Cuba Townships excluding Barrington
167. Hanover Twp. exc. Streamwood
168. Schaumburg Twp. exc. Hoffman Estates
169. Palatine Twp. exc. Palatine and Rolling Meadows
170. Parts of suburban Northwest Cook Co. exc. cities previously listed
171. Parts of West Cook Co. not previously listed
172. Parts of Lyons Twp. not previously listed
173. Stickney Twp. exc. Stickney
174. Lemont Twp. exc. Lemont
175. Orland Twp. exc. Orland Park and Tinley Park
176. Southwest Cook Co. exc. previously listed cities
177. South Cook Co. exc. previously listed cities
178. Highland Park
179. North Chicago
180. Waukegan
181. Deerfield

TABLE 10--Continued

182. Fox Lake
183. Grayslake
183. Highwood
185. Lake Bluff
186. Lake Forest
187. Lake Zurich
188. Libertyville
189. Mundelein
190. Round Lake Beach
191. Round Lake Park
192. Wauconda
193. Winthrop Harbor
194. Antioch Twp.
195. Lake Villa Twp.
196. Grant Twp. exc. Fox Lake
197. Avon Twp. exc. previously listed cities
198. Newport and Warren Twps.
199. Benton Twp. exc. Winthrop Harbor
200. Wauconda Twp. exc. Wauconda
201. Fremont and Libertyville Twps. exc. Mundelein and Libertyville
202. Ela Twp. exc. Lake Zurich
203. Vernon Twp.
204. East Lake Co. exc. previously listed cities
205. Aurora
206. Carpentersville
207. Elgin
208. Batavia
209. Geneva
210. South Elgin
211. St. Charles
212. West Dundee
213. Northwest Kane Co.
214. West and South Kane Co.
215. Dundee Twp. exc. Carpentersville and West Dundee
216. Elgin Twp. exc. South Elgin
217. St. Charles Twp. exc. St. Charles
218. Geneva and Batavia Twps. exc. Geneva and Batavia
219. Aurora Twp.
220. Crystal Lake
221. Harvard
222. McHenry
223. Marengo
224. Woodstock
225. Northwest McHenry Co. exc. Harvard
226. Southwest McHenry Co. exc. Marengo
227. McHenry Twp. exc. McHenry
228. Eastern McHenry Co. exc. unit areas previously listed
229. Downers Grove
230. Elmhurst
231. Glen Ellyn
232. Hinsdale
233. Lombard

TABLE 10--Continued

234. Naperville
235. Villa Park
236. Wheaton
237. Addison
238. Bensenville
239. Clarendon Hills
240. Itasca
241. Lisle
242. Roselle
243. West Chicago
244. Westmont
245. Wood Dale
246. Wayne Twp.
247. Winfield
248. Bloomingdale Twp. exc. Roselle
249. Milton Twp. exc. Wheaton and Glen Ellyn
250. Naperville and Lisle Twps. exc. Naperville and Lisle
251. Downers Grove Twp.
252. Addison and York Twps. exc. previously listed cities
253. Joliet
254. Crest Hill
255. Crete
256. Lockport
257. Romeoville
258. Steger
259. Wilmington
260. Wheatland and Du Page Twps. exc. Romeoville
261. Plainfield and Troy Twps.
262. Lockport Twp. exc. Lockport and Crest Hill
263. Joliet Twp. exc. Joliet
264. Homer and New Lenox Twps.
265. Frankfort and Green Garden Twps.
266. West Southern Will Co.
267. Wilmington Twp. exc. Wilmington
268. Reed, Custer, Wesley Twps.
269. Peotone, Will, Washington Twps.
270. Monee Twp.
271. Crete Twp. exc. Crete and Steger

essentially what happened. Rates per 1,000 were used rather than the more conventional rates per 100,000 measure in order better to account for the rates for individual cancer sites. The range from minimum to maximum rate varies greatly. Some of the extremely high rates apply to inhabitants of the Loop, and thus do not represent a very realistic measure. At any rate, detailed comparisons can be made by consulting Appendix B.

Cartographic comparisons

The mortality and morbidity rates shown in Appendix B for each of the 271 subareas were mapped in an attempt better to understand the spatial variability of the diseases

TABLE 11

UNIVARIATE STATISTICS FOR RMP DISEASES: 1960 AND 1967

Reported Mortality per 1,000	Mean	Standard Deviation	Minimum Rate	Maximum Rate
Heart disease, 1960	3.522	.126	0.00	25.36
Heart disease, 1967	3.450	.123	0.05	20.63
Stroke, 1960	.752	.511	0.00	3.95
Stroke, 1967	.832	.880	0.00	7.84
Estimated Morbidity per 1,000				
Total cancer, 1960	2.709	1.347	0.00	10.68
Total cancer, 1967	2.780	1.450	0.00	12.75
Digestive cancer, 1960	.497	.344	0.00	1.68
Digestive cancer, 1967	.457	.349	0.00	2.21
Respiratory cancer, 1960	.234	.206	0.00	1.77
Respiratory cancer, 1967	.299	.211	0.00	1.17
Genital cancer (M & F), 1960	.419	.409	0.00	3.15
Genital cancer (M & F), 1967	.375	.317	0.00	1.67
Breast cancer, 1960	.366	.360	0.00	2.62
Breast cancer, 1967	.363	.328	0.00	1.98
Leukemia and aleukemia, 1960	.051	.105	0.00	0.95
Leukemia and aleukemia, 1967	.045	.071	0.00	0.31
Buccal cavity and pharynx, 1960	.042	.108	0.00	0.76
Buccal cavity and pharynx, 1967	.050	.127	0.00	1.04
Skin cancer, 1960	.032	.093	0.00	0.78
Skin cancer, 1967	.033	.084	0.00	0.70
Other and unspecified cancer, 1960	.419	.409	0.00	5.40
Other and unspecified cancer, 1967	1.062	1.064	0.00	10.35

in metropolitan Chicago. Some of the diseases repeatedly displayed patterns easy to interpret within the context of urban analysis while others displayed patterns requiring methods of analysis either beyond the context of this study or simply impossible to explain.

It is important to note that the cartographic method employed, while not new to disease mapping, has rarely been used, and this effort may be the first attempt to apply it to urban area disease mapping.[1] The method, trend surface analysis, was originally developed by geologists, and the method has since been utilized for a wide variety of purposes.[2]

---

[1] Howard C. Hopps, "Computer-Produced Distribution Maps of Disease," Annals of the New York Academy of Sciences, Vol. CLXI (September 30, 1969).

[2] See John W. Harbaugh and Daniel F. Merriam, Computer Applications in Stratigraphic Analysis (New York: John Wiley & Sons, Inc., 1968), pp. 61-100; R. J. Chorley and P. Haggett, "Trend-Surface Mapping in Geographical Research," in Spatial Analysis:

It was selected for this endeavor because of its ability to extrapolate and smooth surfaces. In fact, when used for such purposes it may be one of the most sophisticated surface smoothing methods yet developed.

It was possible to calculate the trend surfaces shown on the following 22 maps rapidly by using the University of Chicago's IBM 7094 computer. Initial line printer output was transferred by hand to produce the maps. The most significant feature in terms of cartographic interpretation is that in every instance the "reference contour" of the maps approximates the means shown on Table 11. Also, when possible the set of contour intervals was set to mesh with values of the standard deviation. Means on all maps are represented by the heaviest contour line, this enabling immediate recognition of where the average incidence of each disease is expected to occur.

Heart disease and stroke mortality

The patterns for heart disease mortality are shown on Figures 13 and 14. Deaths attributed to this leading killer in the Chicago area show similar patterns for 1960 and 1967. For both periods most of the inner suburbs and all of the City of Chicago demonstrate an incidence above the average, and the incidence of heart disease mortality decreases with distance from the center of Chicago. The northwestern part of the SMSA, which includes most of McHenry County, shows a high incidence for both periods. In general, the more youthful outer suburban fringe shows a lower incidence, as would be expected. The data from Will County vary more than those from other areas. In 1960, that county had some of the lowest rates, and in 1967 it had some of the highest. For parts of the metropolis other than Will County, the incidence of heart disease mortality was similar for both periods.

The patterns for death rates due to vascular lesions of the Central Nervous System (CNS) in many respects follow those for heart disease, although there is a noteworthy exception (Figs. 15 and 16). In terms of similarities, lower rates are reflected in outer suburbs, and higher rates in both the rural fringe and central city. The exception is that from 1960 to 1967 the area of highest stroke death rates "shifted" from the center of Chicago City to a long band running up the North Shore, consistent with the new types of residential construction in that area. Furthermore, a large portion of Chicago's South Side reflects a decreased rate in stroke deaths from 1960 to 1967. The latter area had ghettoized increasingly over the period, and the decreased number of deaths reported could be attributed in part to the more youthful makeup of the newer black population.

A Reader in Statistical Geography, ed. Brian J. L. Berry and Duane F. Marble (Englewood Cliffs: Prentice-Hall, Inc., 1968); and Peter Haggett, Locational Analysis in Human Geography (New York: St. Martin's Press, 1966), pp. 270-76.

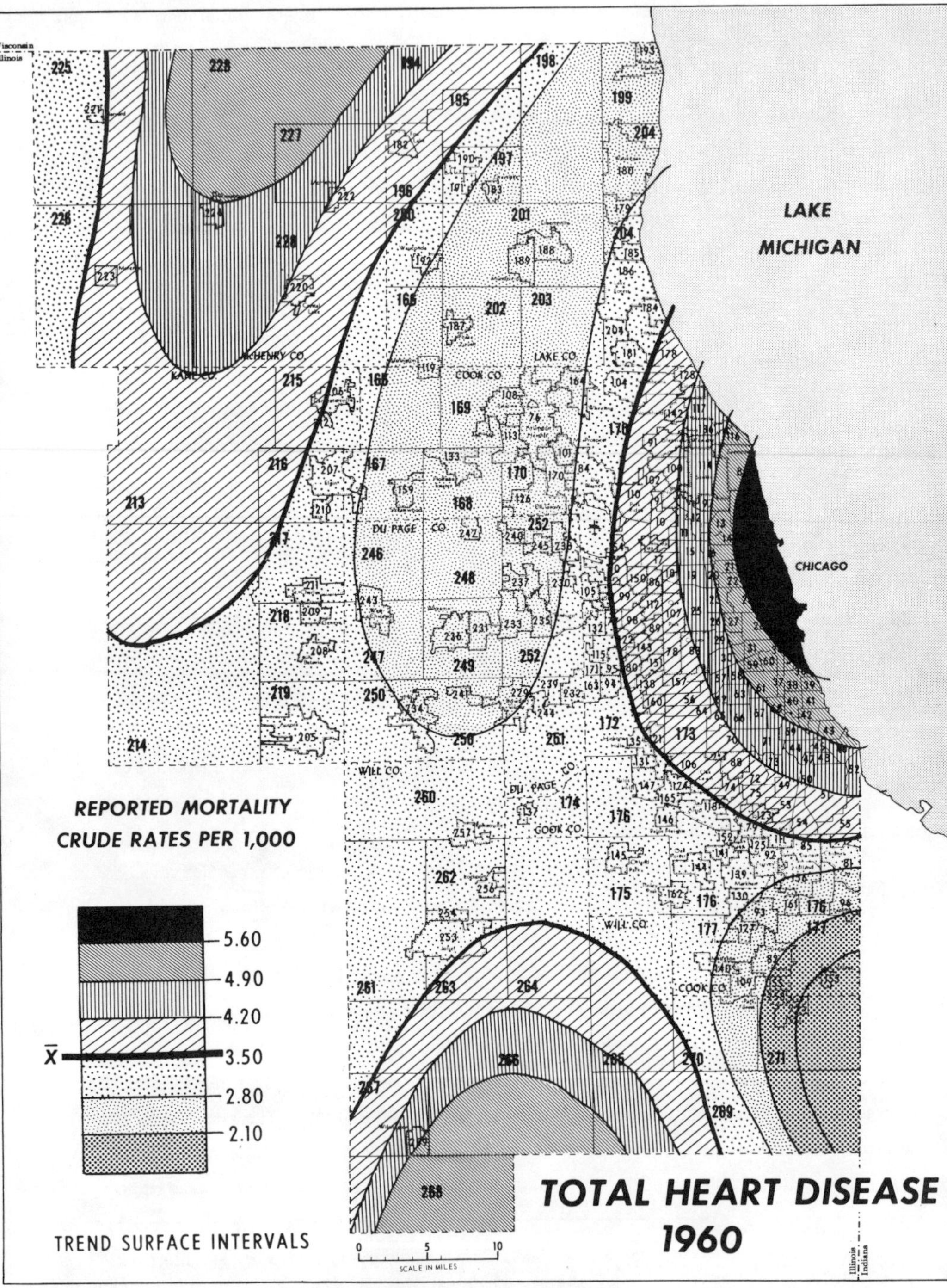

Fig. 13.--Total heart disease, 1960

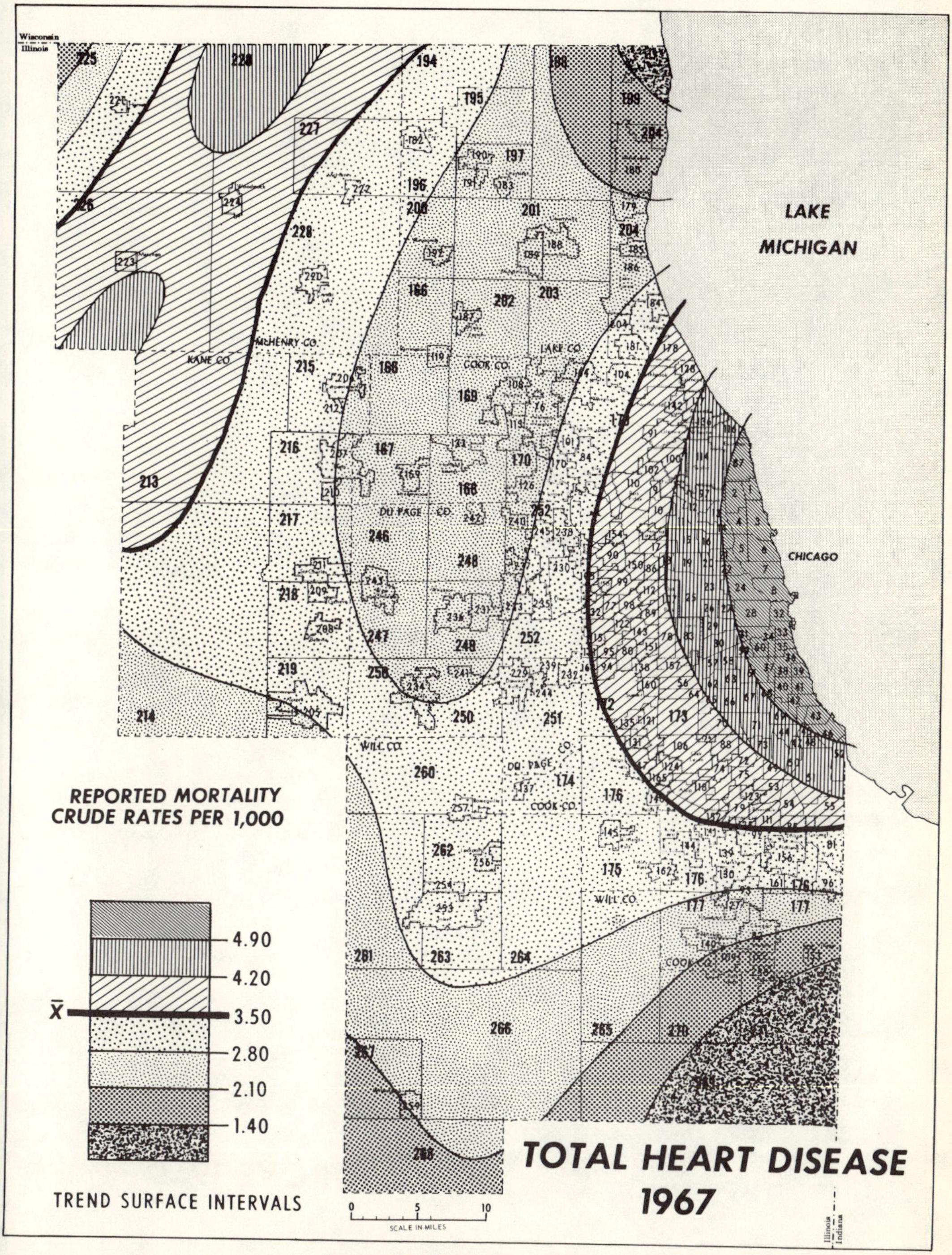

Fig. 14.--Total heart disease, 1967

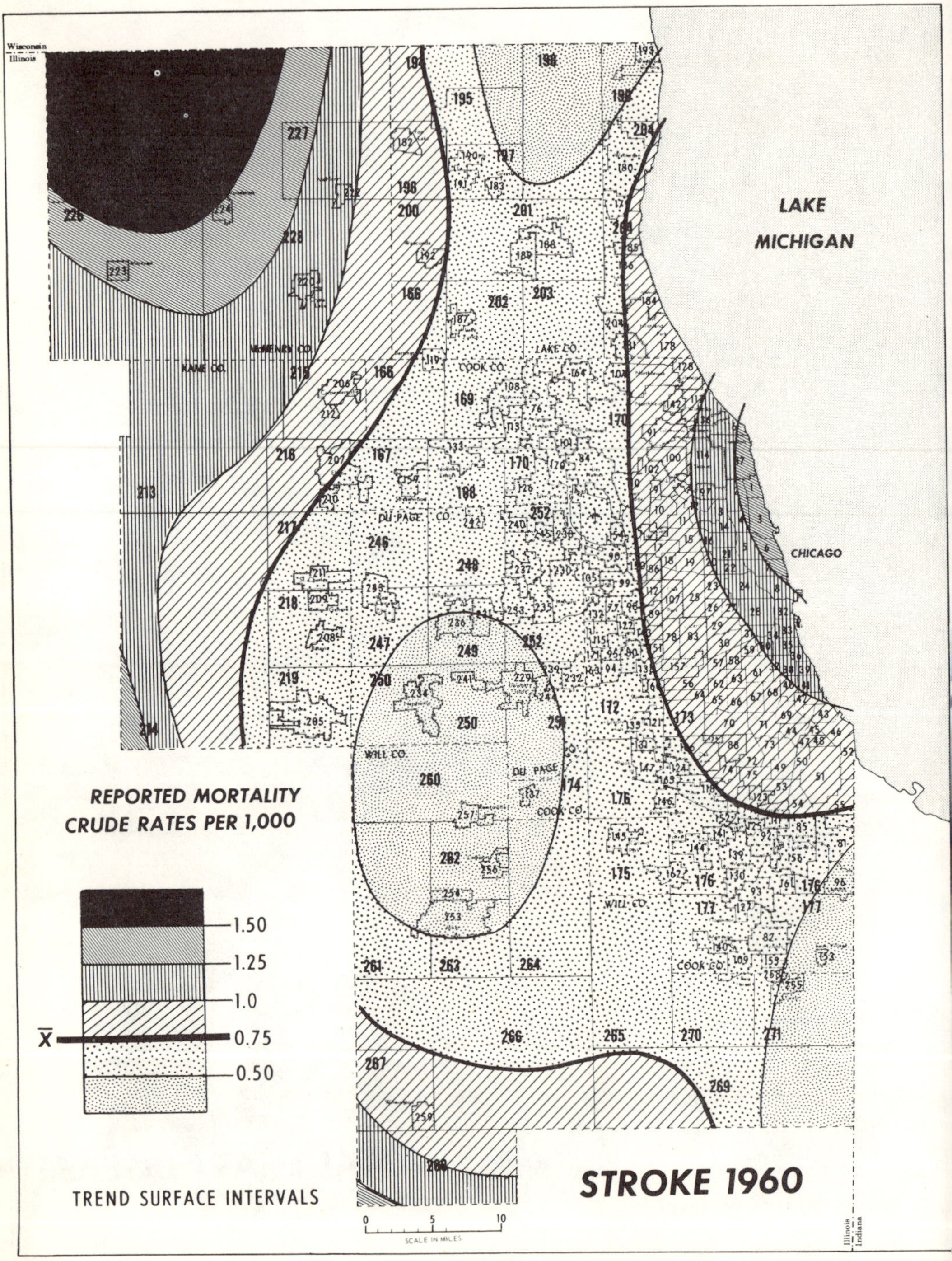

Fig. 15.--Stroke, 1960

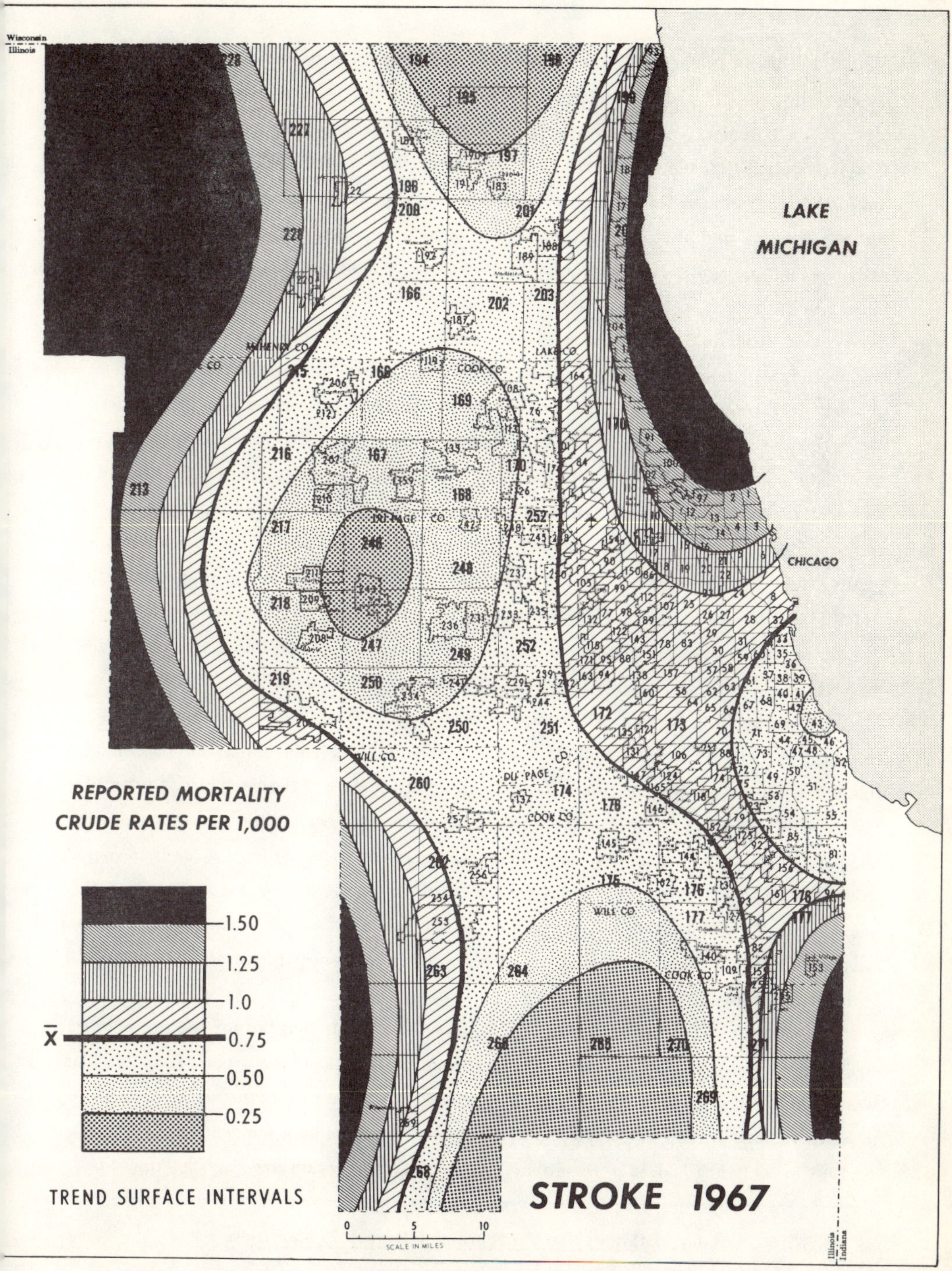

Fig. 16.--Stroke, 1967

Cancer sites

The trend surfaces for estimated total cancer morbidity in 1960 and 1967 are shown on Figures 17 and 18, and they are quite similar to the heart disease and stroke patterns. For both periods there are concentrations of higher cancer incidence in McHenry County, central Chicago, and parts of Will County. The youthful suburban fringe stands out for both periods as the band of lower rates. The most significant difference between the two patterns is that those for 1960 appear to be much more concentrated while the 1967 areas of high incidence are more broadly distributed. Also "pockets" of lower incidence appear in the suburban fringe in 1967.

Operating on the assumption already stated that the cancer sites when compared to one another vary more spatially than do the various heart disease types, eight "site groups" have been compared. The pie charts of Figure 19 give some idea of the relative share of each mortality group for 1960 and 1967. These charts were made with data obtained from Springfield. Digestive cancer, actually ten separate sites,[1] leads as a cause of death in all instances and in all general parts of the SMSA. Respiratory cancer is second in all areas and it persistently increased from 1960 to 1967. Male and female genital cancers were next, and the proportions were about the same for all areas and both times. Breast cancer percentages followed a course similar to genital cancers. The remaining sites also showed similar distributions; when these and the other site groups were mapped, however, a wide range of different patterns showed up.

Figures 20 to 35 show all the site group distributions for the two periods. The maps of "digestive" cancer should be viewed with caution (Figs. 20 and 21). The data for the maps, unlike the Figure 19 charts, includes only cancer of the rectum and intestines for the City of Chicago. Still, the maps can be compared because the same problem occurs on both maps. The 1960 and 1967 patterns in the southern part of the SMSA appear to be comparable. In the northern part, the patterns for the two periods are quite different. Table 12, which contains zero-order correlation coefficients for the 271 areas, has been added for further comparison and shows a correlation coefficient of only .407 for this leading site: only a fair relationship.

When the second leading site, respiratory cancer, is mapped for the two periods, the patterns are basically different (Figs. 22 and 23). In 1960, the areas of high incidence were restricted largely to the City of Chicago. By 1967 the former high incidence area appears to have spread westward and to the south. Another high incidence area developed by 1967 in McHenry and Lake Counties. The implication of outward "spread" must be

---

[1]E. V. Cowdry, Etiology and Prevention of Cancer in Man (New York: Appleton-Century-Crofts, 1968), pp. 39-118.

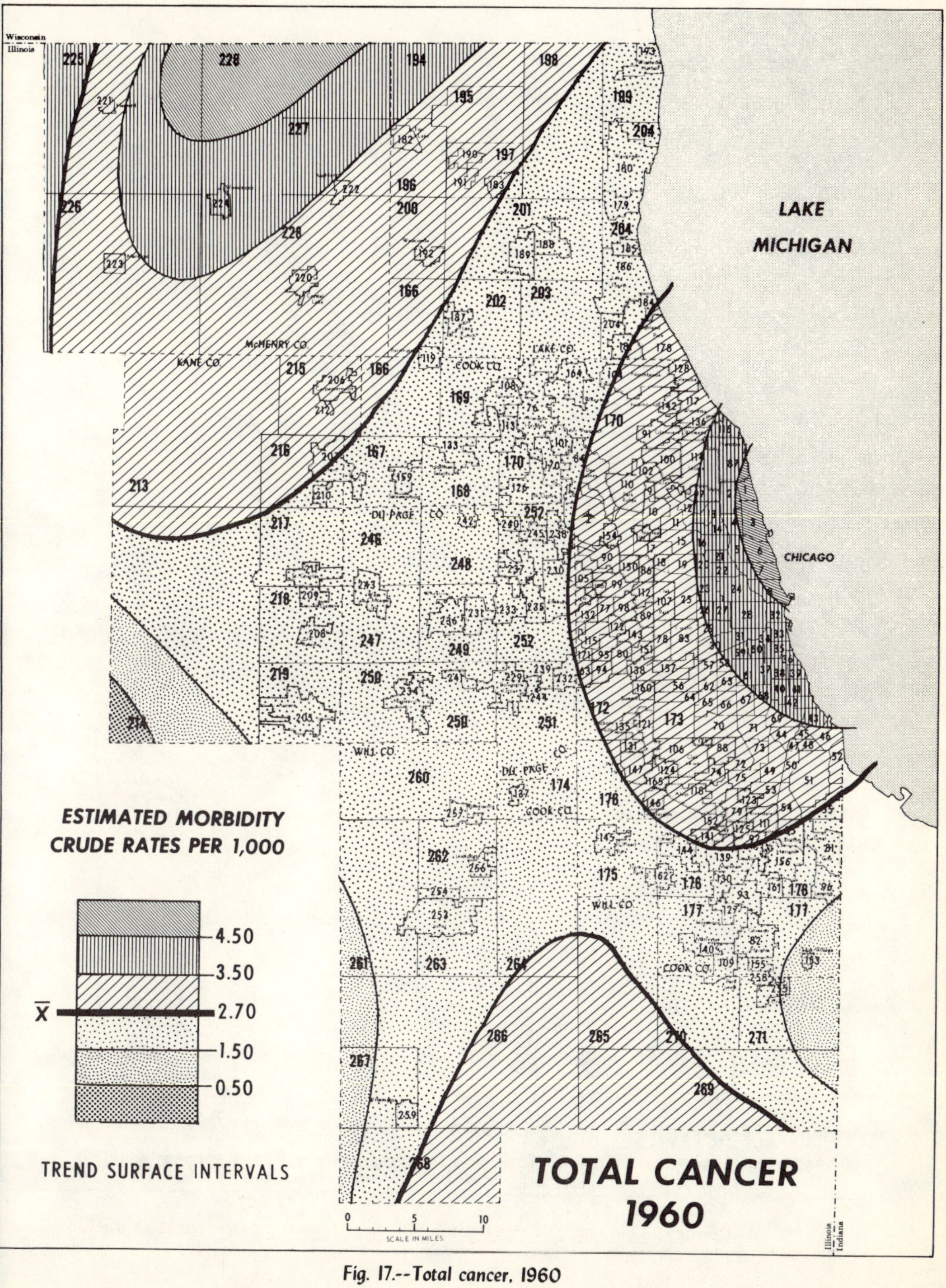

Fig. 17.--Total cancer, 1960

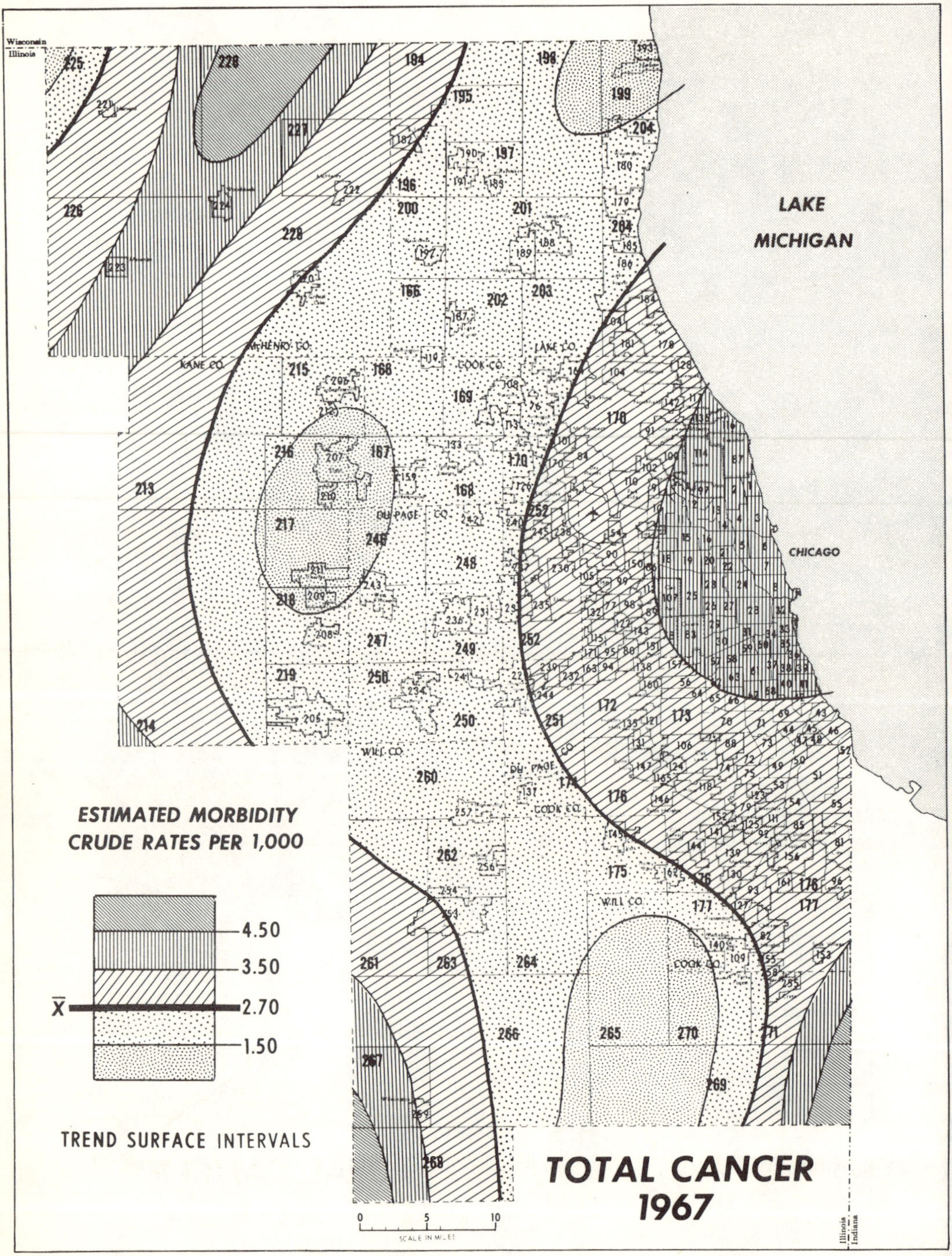

Fig. 18.--Total cancer, 1967

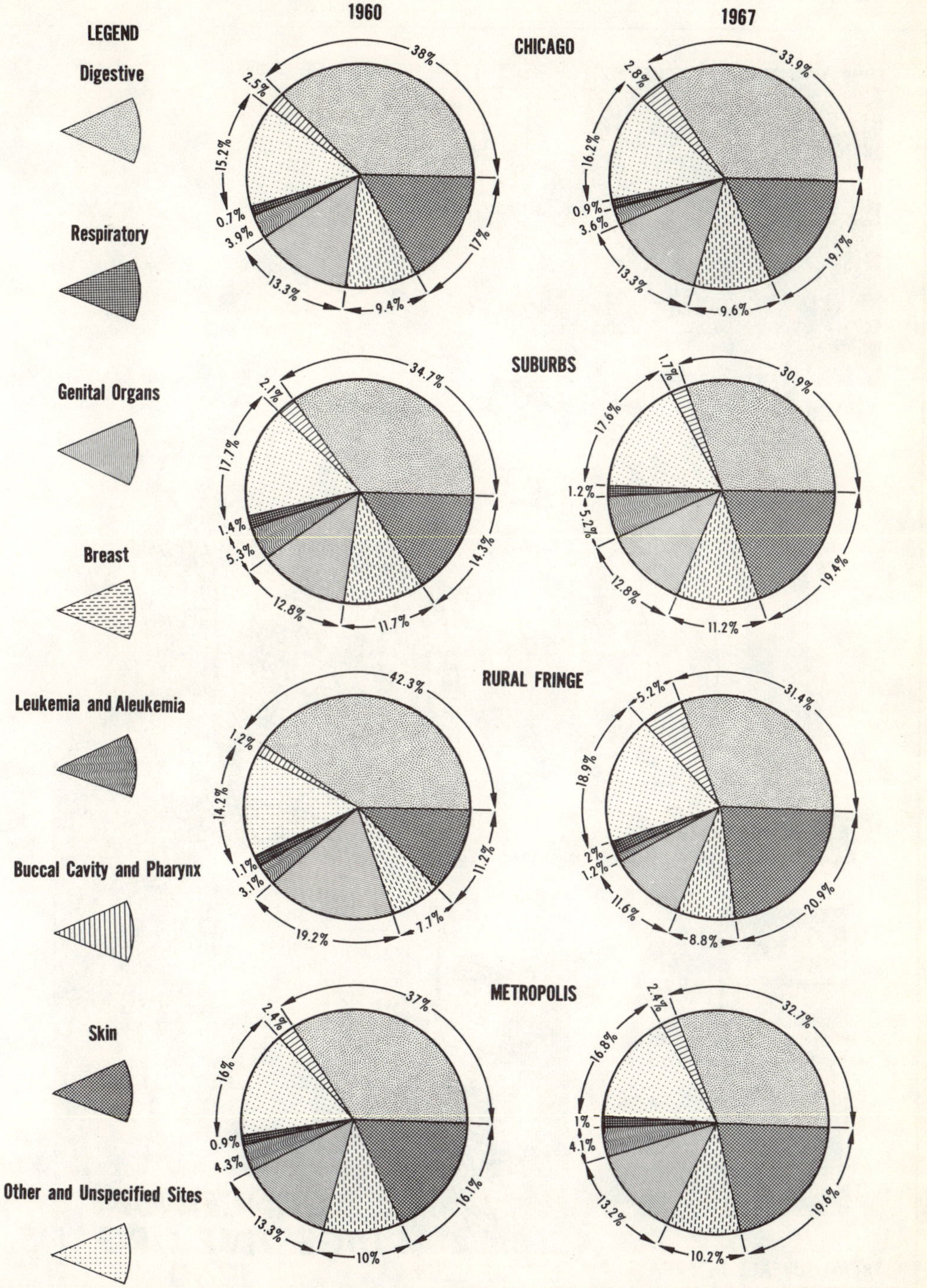

Fig. 19.--Relative shares for various cancer sites in the Chicago SMSA, 1960 and 1967

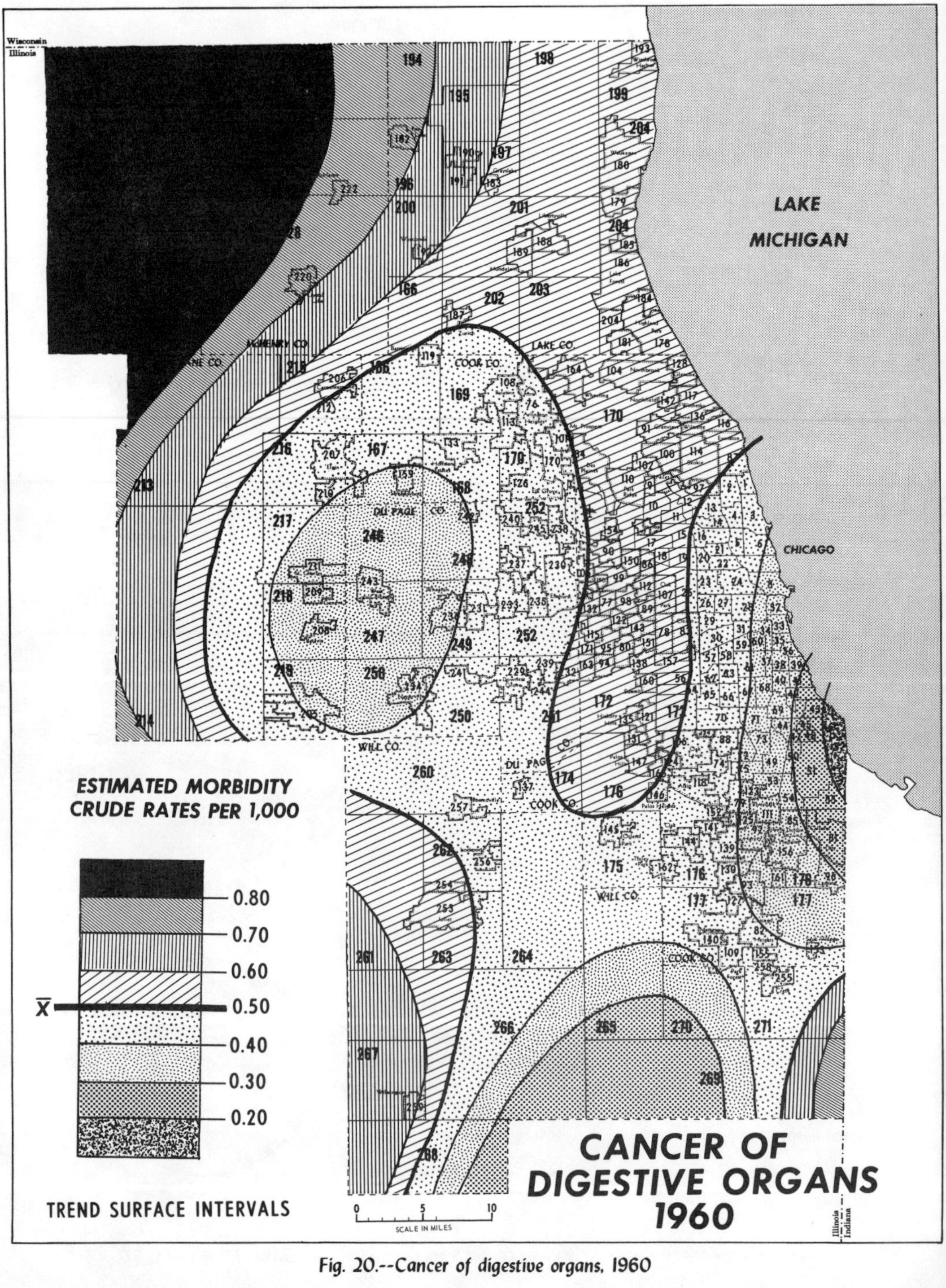

Fig. 20.--Cancer of digestive organs, 1960

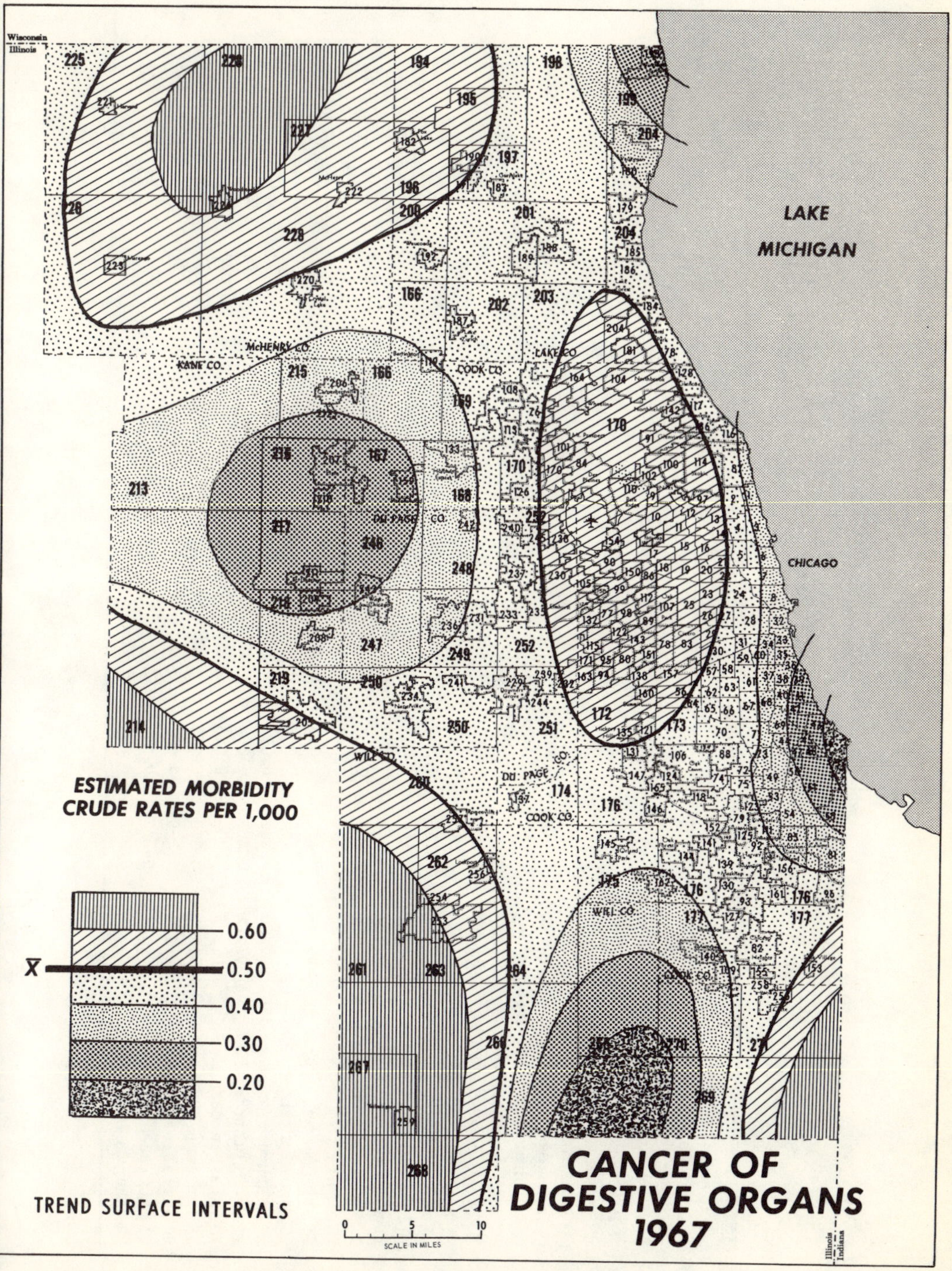

Fig. 21.--Cancer of digestive organs, 1967

TABLE 12

ZERO-ORDER CORRELATION COEFFICIENTS BETWEEN PAIRS OF DISEASES FOR THE 271 DATA COLLECTION SUBAREAS IN THE SMSA

Diseases	Diseases (Columnar Headings Correspond to Rows)										
	1	2	3	4	5	6	7	8	9	10	11
1 Heart disease, 1960	1.000										
2 Stroke, 1960	0.661	1.000									
3 Total cancer, 1960	0.718	0.593	1.000								
4 Digestive cancer, 1960	0.363	0.358	0.517	1.000							
5 Respiratory cancer, 1960	0.497	0.341	0.649	0.146	1.000						
6 Genital cancer, 1960	0.339	0.301	0.506	0.191	0.226	1.000					
7 Breast cancer, 1960	0.280	0.286	0.512	0.184	0.166	0.248	1.000				
8 Leukemia, 1960	-0.000	-0.048	0.190	0.150	0.004	0.096	0.032	1.000			
9 Buccal cavity, etc., 1960	0.137	0.180	0.157	0.095	0.119	0.075	-0.005	0.111	1.000		
10 Skin cancer, 1960	0.154	0.147	0.230	0.047	0.095	0.138	0.046	-0.048	0.129	1.000	
11 Other cancer, 1960	0.569	0.413	0.669	-0.065	0.450	0.131	0.242	-0.122	-0.003	0.241	1.000
12 Heart disease, 1967	0.638	0.491	0.638	0.290	0.474	0.260	0.294	-0.002	0.080	-0.002	0.540
13 Stroke, 1967	0.355	0.451	0.363	0.389	0.207	0.092	0.202	0.021	0.258	0.024	0.158
14 Total cancer, 1967	0.569	0.470	0.585	0.313	0.382	0.146	0.249	-0.057	0.089	0.197	0.548
15 Digestive cancer, 1967	0.340	0.199	0.289	0.407	0.163	0.190	0.076	0.039	0.052	0.051	0.045
16 Respiratory cancer, 1967	0.350	0.261	0.311	0.126	0.242	0.055	0.115	-0.050	0.081	0.139	0.337
17 Genital cancer, 1967	0.272	0.265	0.362	0.272	0.243	0.139	0.222	0.078	0.103	-0.001	0.190
18 Breast cancer, 1967	0.285	0.299	0.326	0.196	0.175	0.142	0.270	0.069	0.124	-0.003	0.199
19 Leukemia, 1967	-0.122	-0.072	-0.016	0.139	-0.068	-0.021	0.061	0.206	0.157	-0.002	-0.184
20 Buccal cavity, etc., 1967	0.151	0.159	0.051	0.225	-0.077	-0.016	-0.040	0.020	0.224	0.158	-0.045
21 Skin cancer, 1967	0.147	0.263	0.147	0.087	0.009	0.062	0.001	-0.058	0.264	0.240	0.181
22 Other cancer, 1967	0.511	0.392	0.489	0.013	0.365	0.034	0.181	-0.198	-0.043	0.215	0.727

	12	13	14	15	16	17	18	19	20	21	22
1 Heart disease, 1960											
2 Stroke, 1960											
3 Total cancer, 1960											
4 Digestive cancer, 1960											
5 Respiratory cancer, 1960											
6 Genital cancer, 1960											
7 Breast cancer, 1960											
8 Leukemia, 1960											
9 Buccal cavity, etc., 1960											
10 Skin cancer, 1960											
11 Other cancer, 1960											
12 Heart disease, 1967	1.000										
13 Stroke, 1967	0.371	1.000									
14 Total cancer, 1967	0.644	0.489	1.000								
15 Digestive cancer, 1967	0.296	0.265	0.599	1.000							
16 Respiratory cancer, 1967	0.465	0.306	0.647	0.203	1.000						
17 Genital cancer, 1967	0.391	0.249	0.472	0.193	0.269	1.000					
18 Breast cancer, 1967	0.314	0.308	0.442	0.246	0.093	0.160	1.000				
19 Leukemia, 1967	0.039	0.058	0.155	0.151	0.226	0.140	0.007	1.000			
20 Buccal cavity, etc., 1967	0.063	0.205	0.136	0.105	0.047	0.076	0.058	0.065	1.000		
21 Skin cancer, 1967	0.113	0.177	0.216	0.032	0.177	0.055	0.094	-0.034	0.212	1.000	
22 Other cancer, 1967	0.515	0.339	0.764	0.136	0.418	0.191	0.219	0.140	-0.043	0.181	1.000

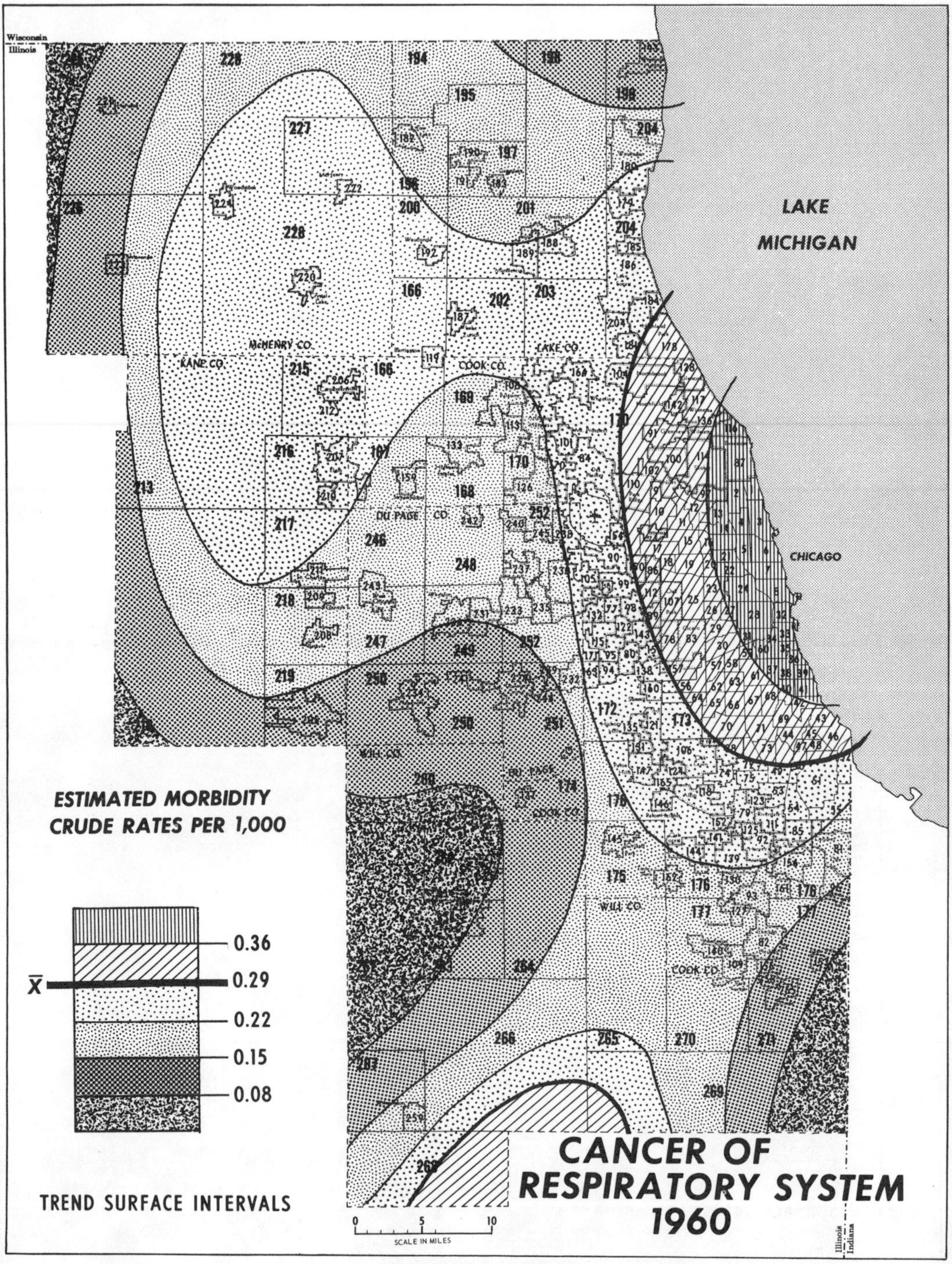

Fig. 22.--Cancer of respiratory system, 1960

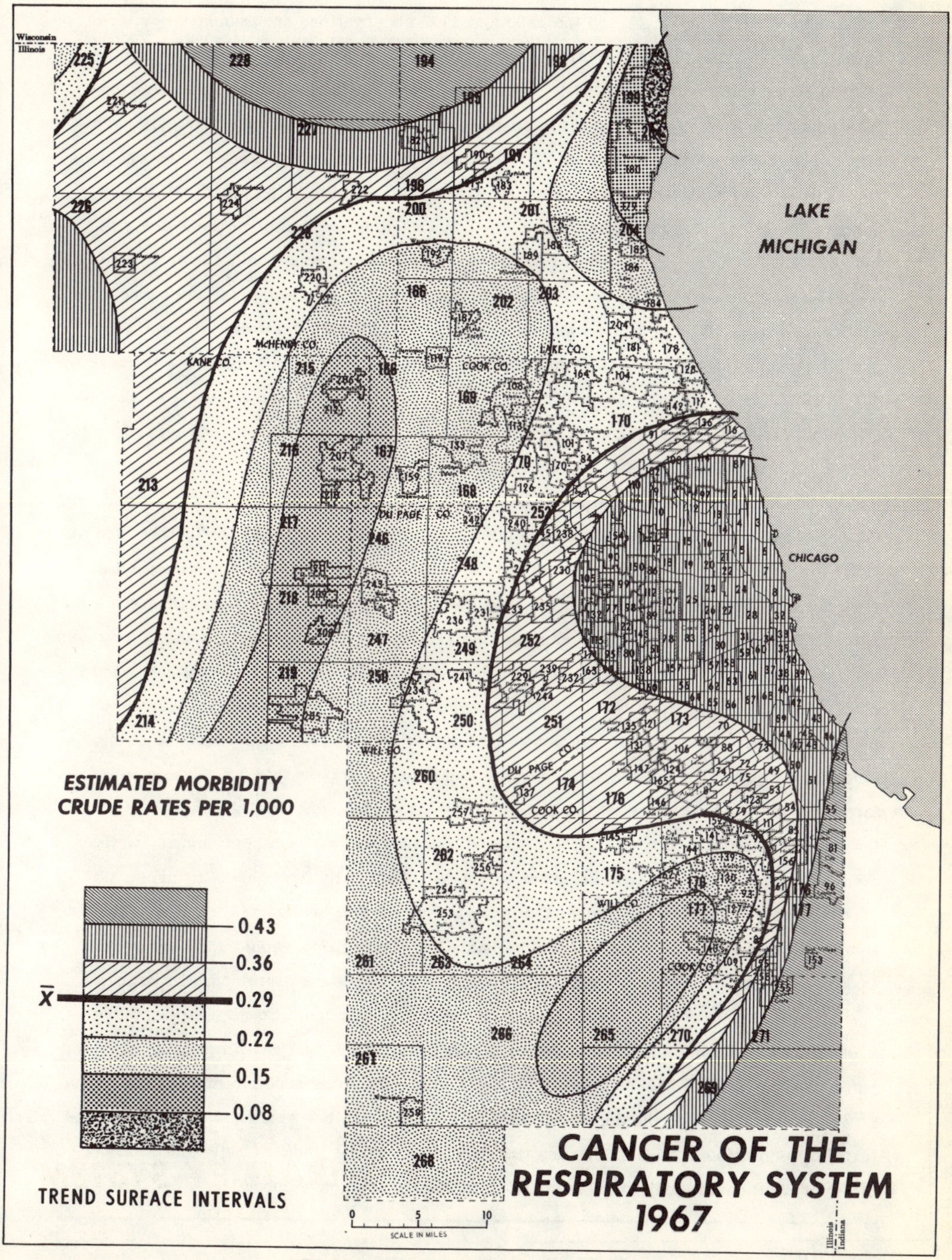

Fig 23.--Cancer of respiratory system, 1967

taken with caution, and this is best explained by examination of the correlation coefficients shown on Table 12. When the 1960 and 1967 observations are compared, r = .242; however, when each site distribution is compared to total cancer within each period, r = .649 in 1960, and r = .647 in 1967. In other words, the sites tend to be spatially correlated much more with total cancer for respective temporal distributions than with each other over the seven-year time gap. Spatial patterns are changing, and in different ways.

A similar statistical-cartographic situation occurs with both genital and breast cancers (male and female distinctions are not made within the data, but the latter site is insignificant for males). The visual patterns for these site groups do not even begin to match each other over the temporal spread (Figs. 24-27). Furthermore, the correlation coefficients are only significant when sites are compared to the total distribution. For genital cancers the temporal coefficient is .139, and the same relationship for breast cancer is .270. However, the same-period correlation coefficients are as follows: Breast Cancers to total, 1960 = .512, and the same site for 1967 = .442; Genital Cancers to total, 1967 = .472, and the same site for 1960 = .506.

The situation for leukemia is somewhat the converse to the previous relationships, but none of the numerical measures are strong. When 1960 and 1967 distributions are statistically compared, r = .206. In addition, the within-time coefficients are even lower: r = .190 when the 1960 distribution is compared to the total, and the same comparison for 1967 gives .155. In fact, visual examination of the maps reveals that the general patterns for both years are the reverse of the patterns for Total Cancer (Figs. 28 and 29). Past studies have concluded that there is a lower distribution of this basically childhood malady in ghetto areas, and that it is common to find higher rates of leukemia among higher income families. The geographical distribution appears to bear this out. The most similar patterns over the time spread show up in the higher incidence in Du Page County and the lower rates in the City of Chicago. Were it not for the cartographic "static" in the remainder of the SMSA, the correlation might be statistically more meaningful.

Comparisons for the Buccal Cavity and Pharynx site group show a statistical situation similar to Leukemia, but there is no basis for visual cartographic analysis in this instance (Figs. 30 and 31). When maps for the two periods are examined, the patterns appear to be wildly chaotic and unlike any of the previous maps. Cowdry explains this group as actually nine sites exposed to both external and internal carcinogens.[1] Common patterns from 1960 to 1967 are not to be found, and part of the problem may be due to the above aspect; however, the digestive sites with a large number also have a stronger pattern for comparison. A map showing the distribution of the Buccal Cavity and Pharynx sites for 1980 could easily be dissimilar to the two years now mapped.

---

[1] *Ibid.*, pp. 1-38.

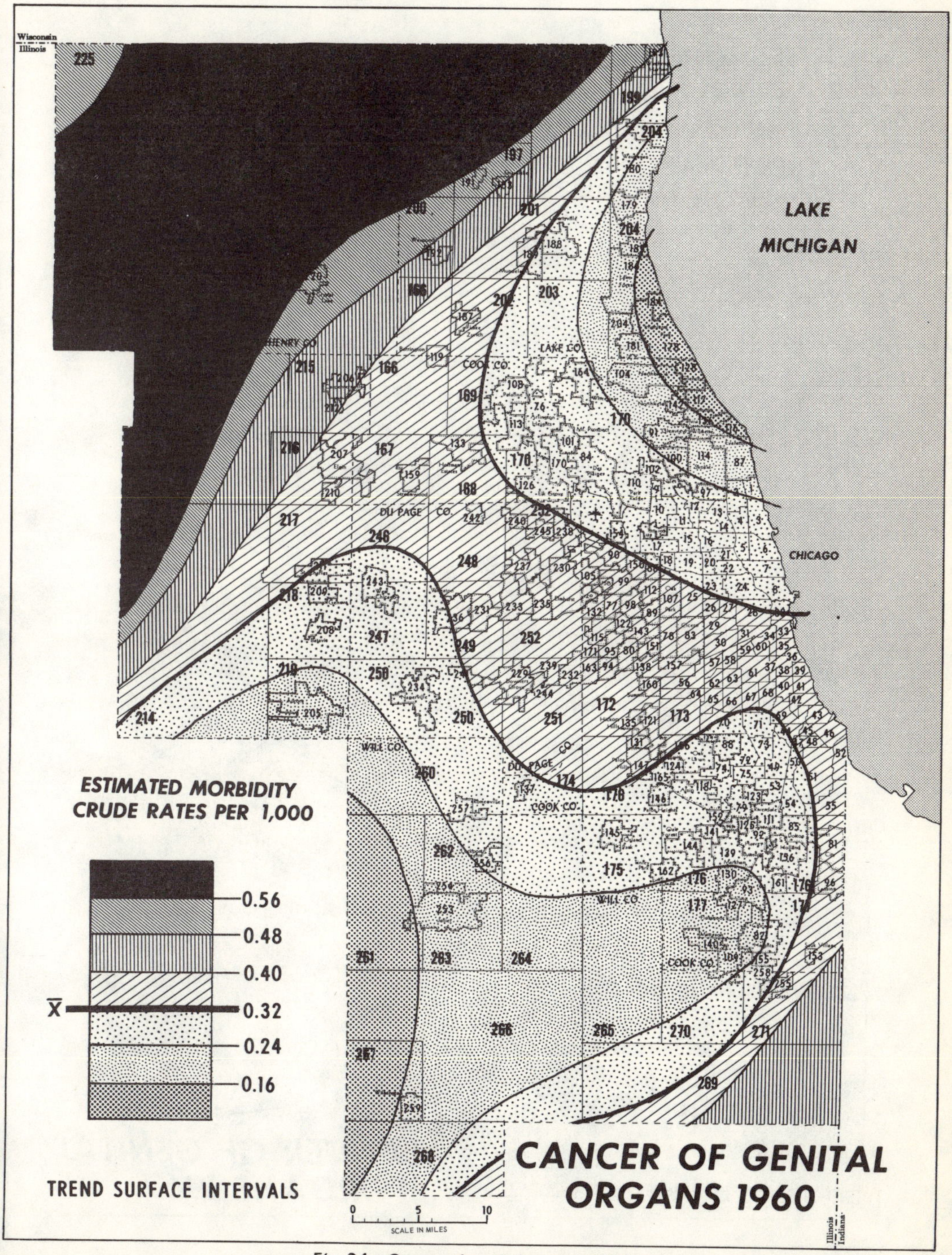

Fig. 24.--Cancer of genital organs, 1960

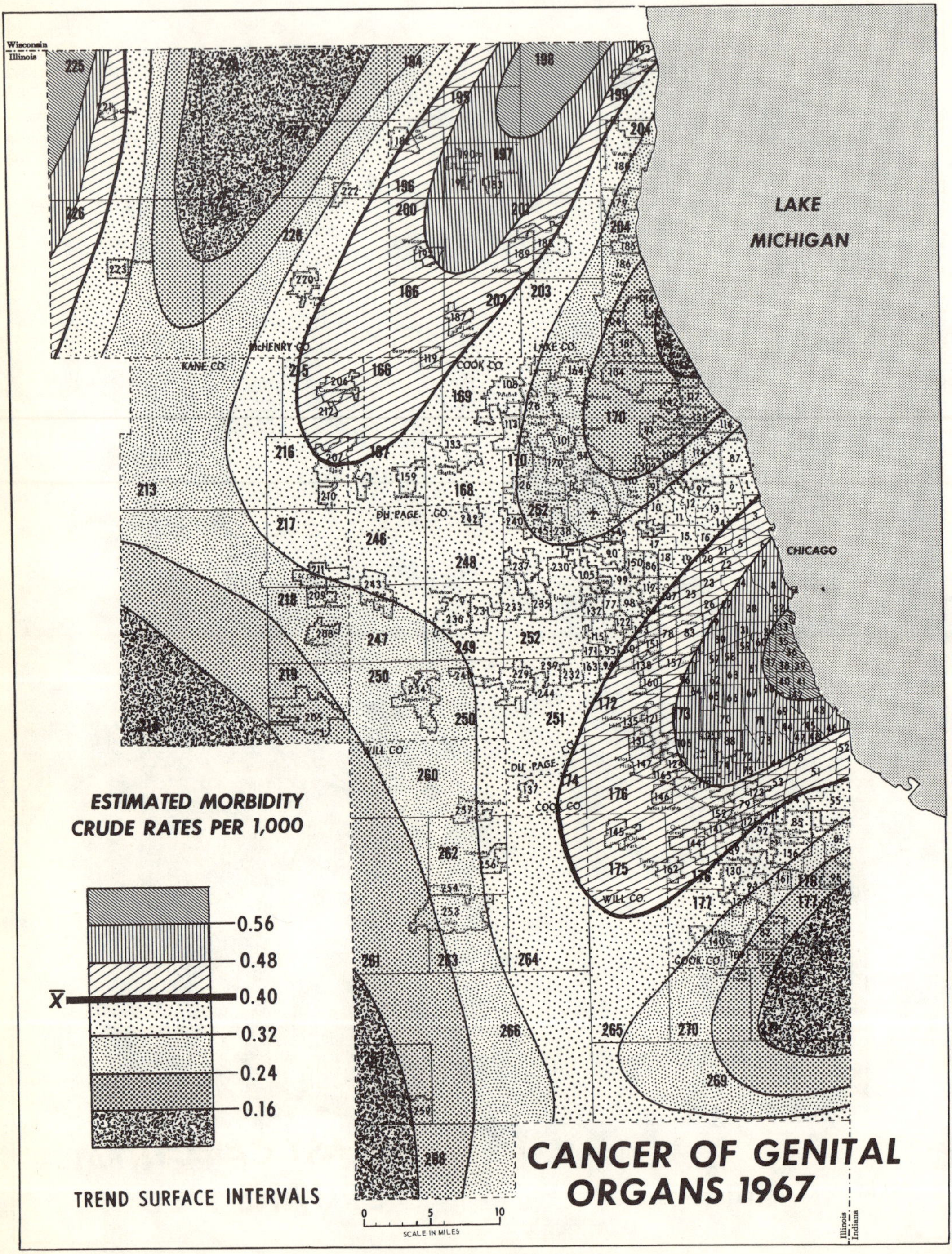

Fig. 25.--Cancer of genital organs, 1967

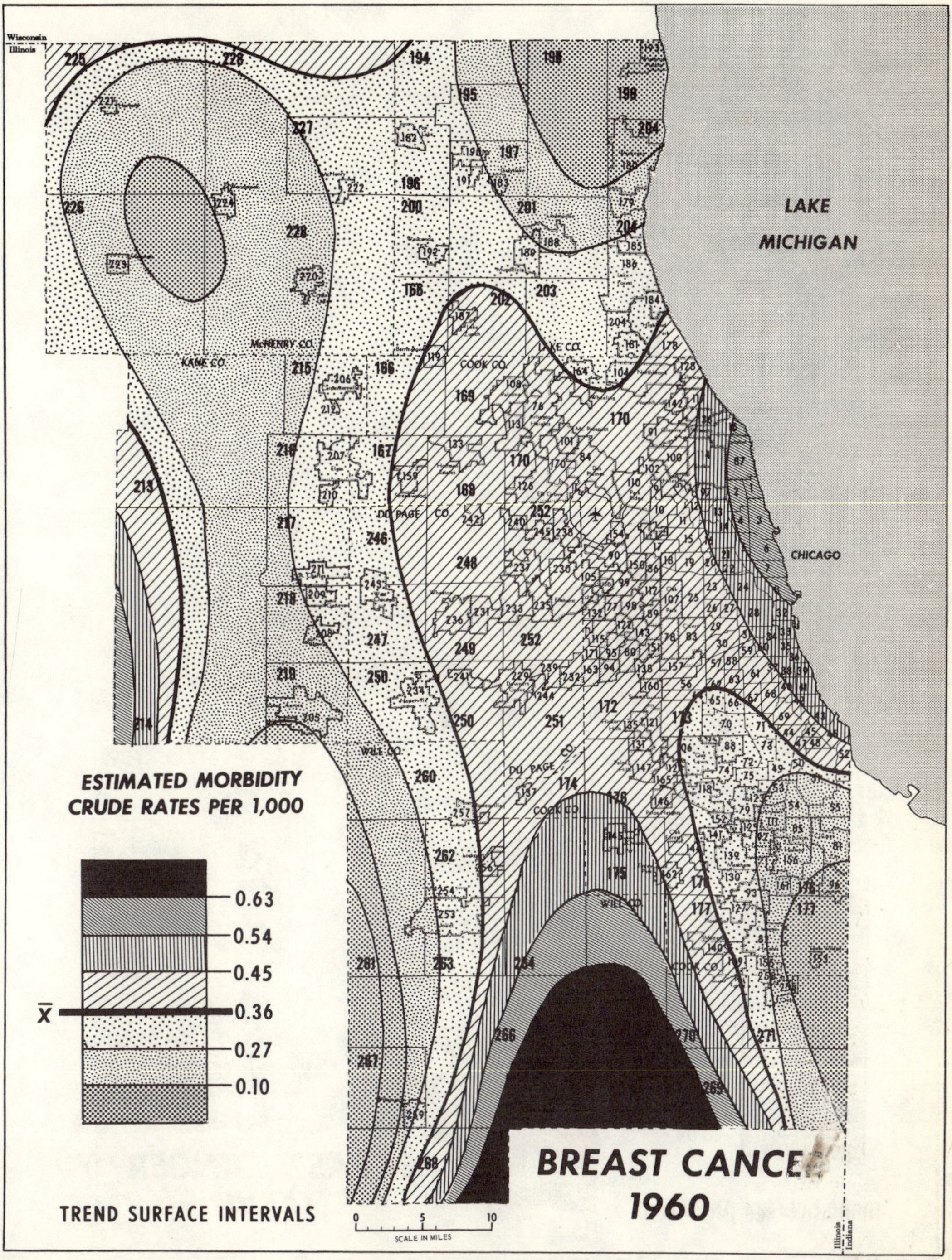

Fig. 26.--Breast cancer, 1960

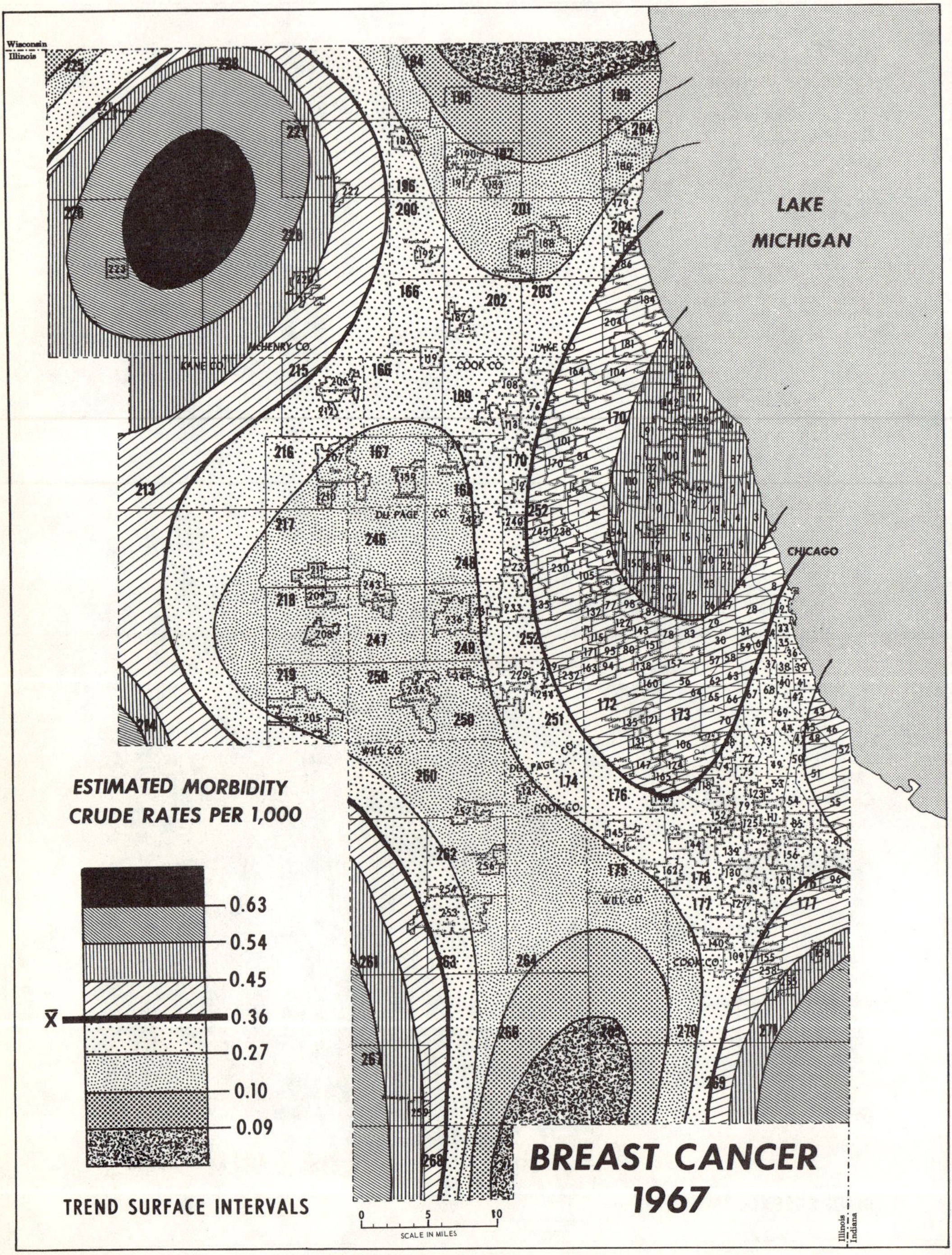

Fig. 27.--Breast cancer, 1967

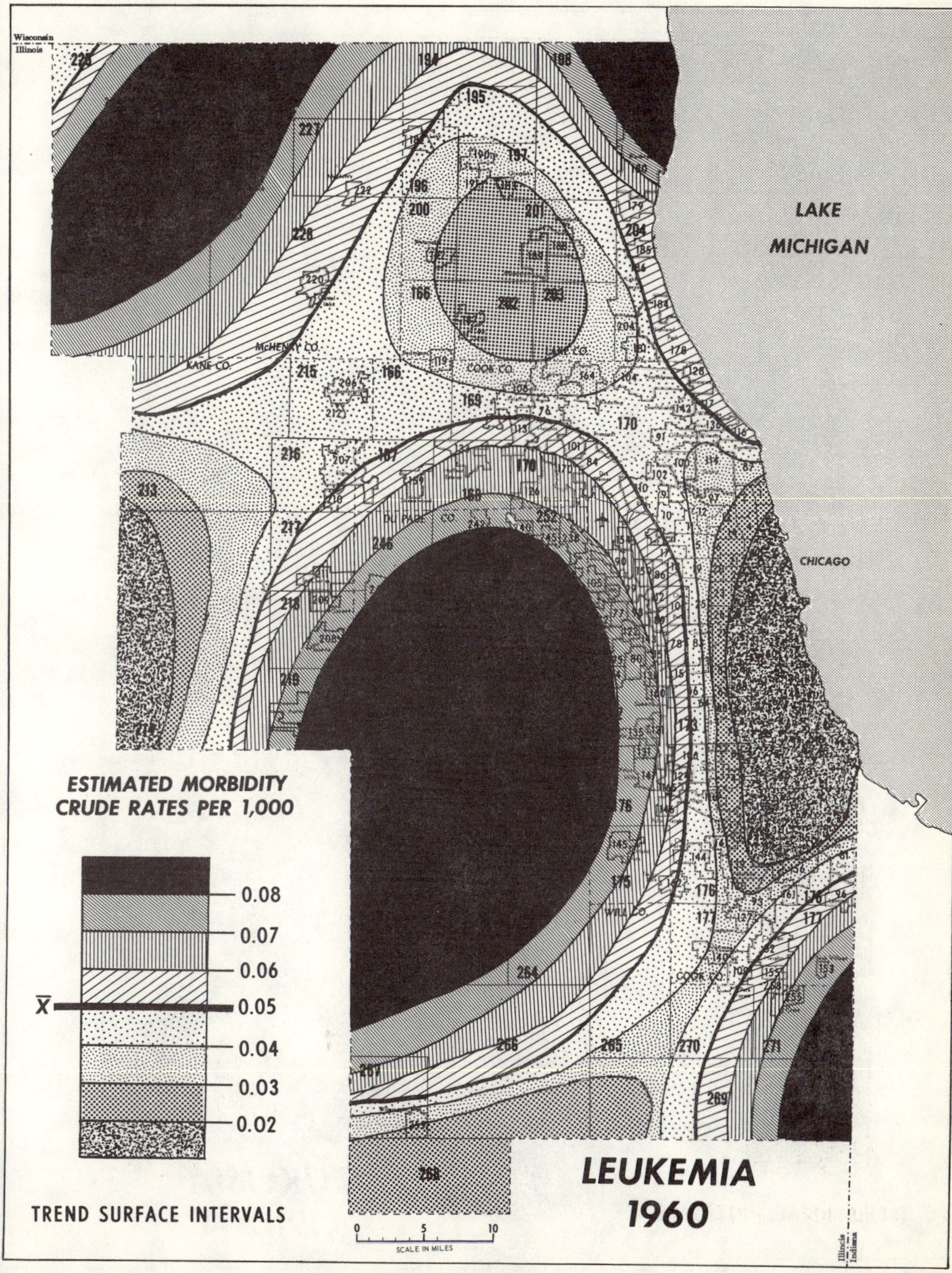

Fig. 28.--Leukemia, 1960

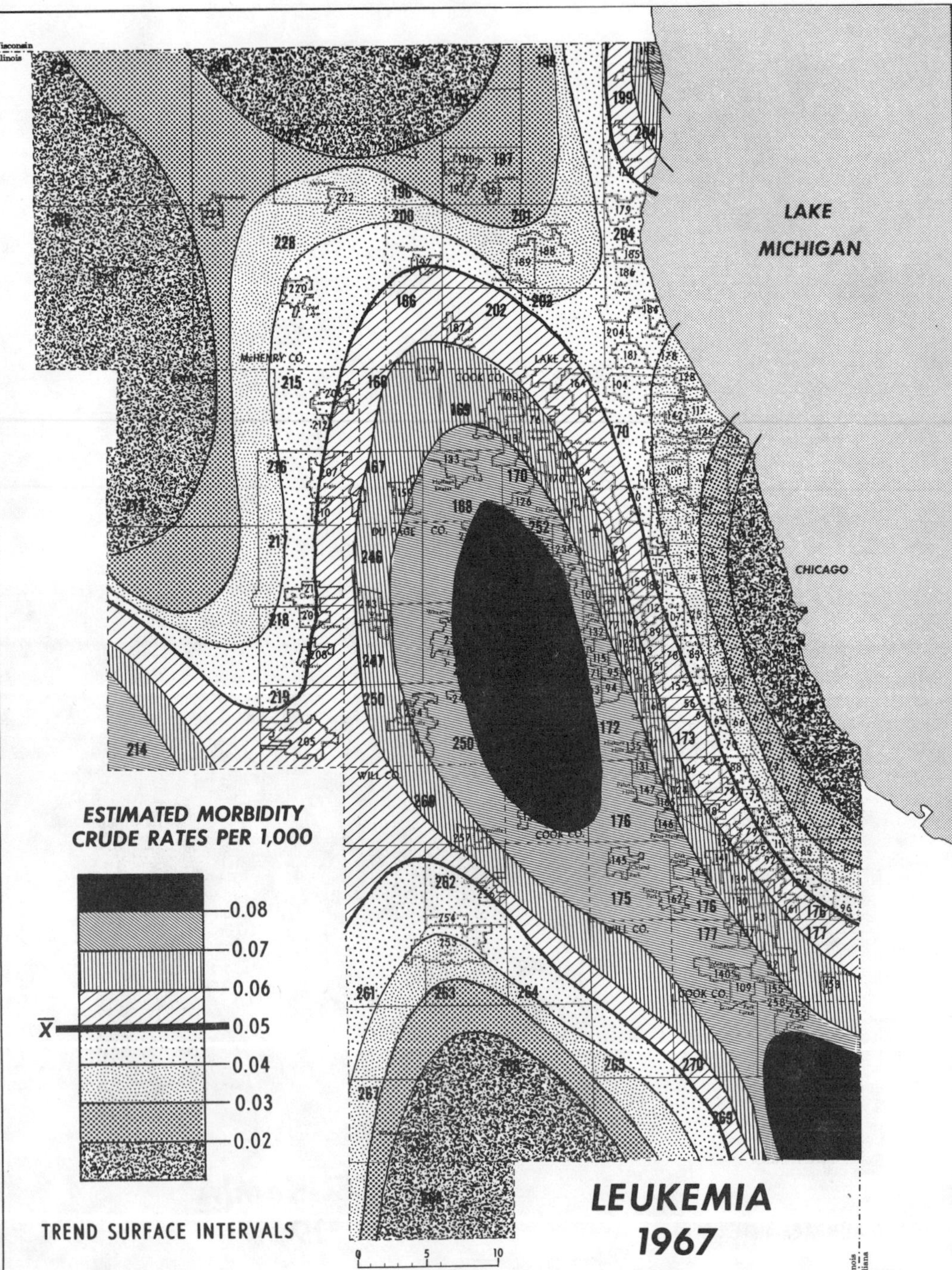

Fig. 29.--Leukemia, 1967

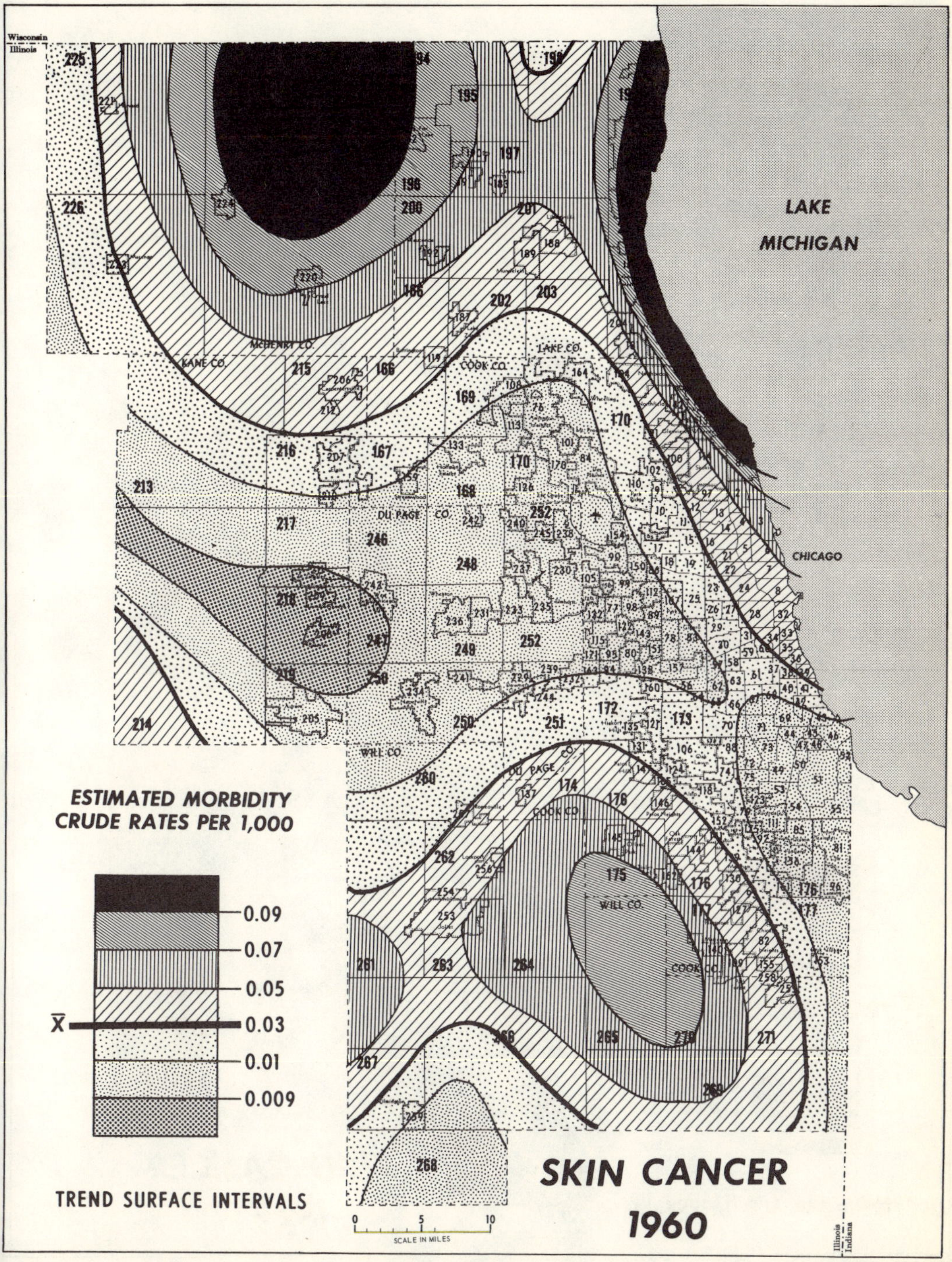

Fig. 30.--Skin cancer, 1960

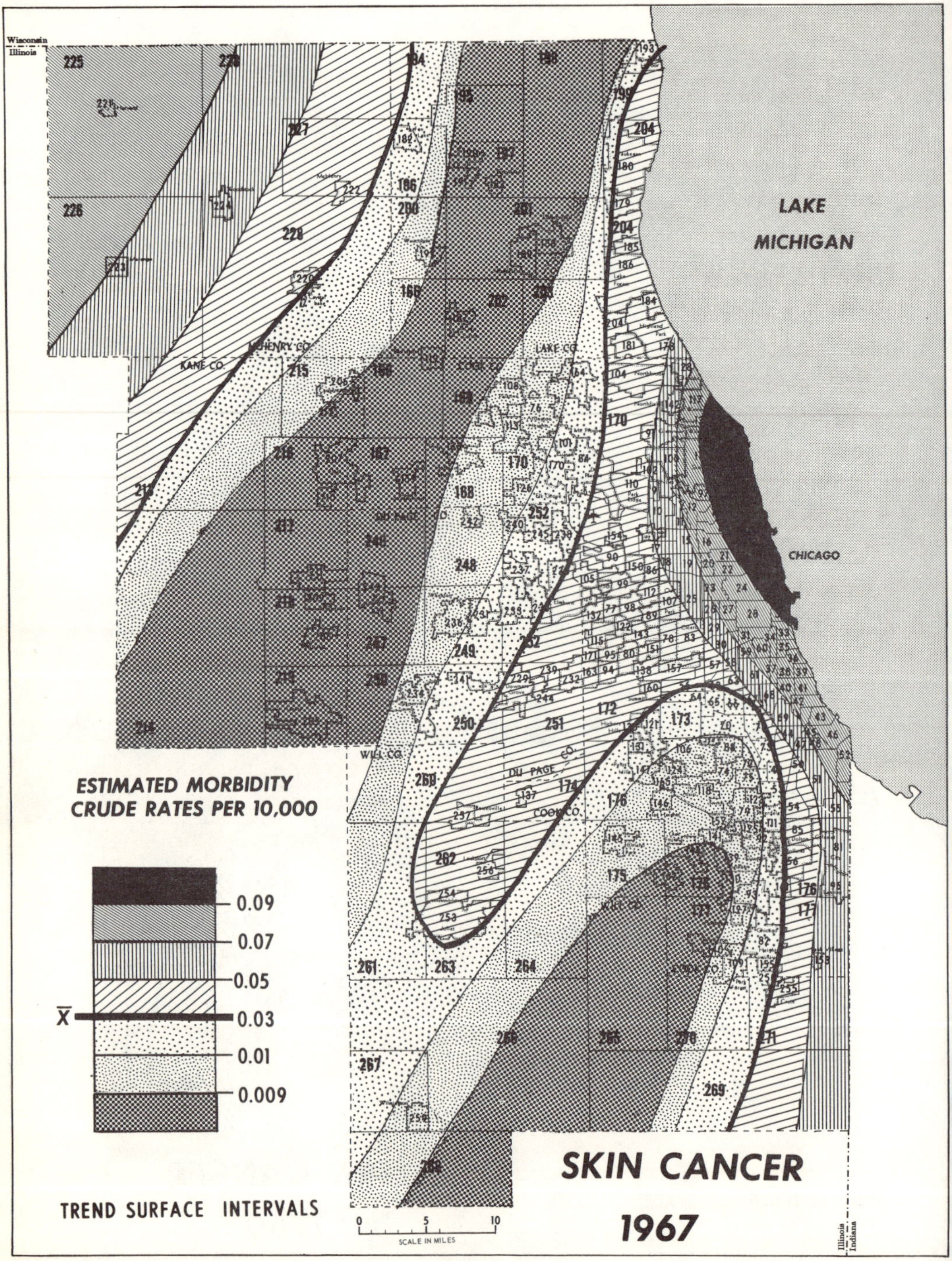

Fig. 31.--Skin cancer, 1967

The statistical comparisons for Skin Cancer are basically weak for both site-to-site and site-to-total tests (Figs. 32 and 33). Visual examination of the patterns for both years reveals that only the North Shore and part of McHenry County have high rates for both periods. Taking Shimkin's premise that this site is most prevalent in white persons frequently exposed to the sun's rays or other sources of ultraviolet radiation, it is possible to speculate an environmental association.[1] The rural population in McHenry County could easily be exposed to the sun, as could the farmers of Will County, but in the latter area, reporting is not consistent from period to period. There could be two reasons for the North Shore patterns. First, the area is inhabited by persons who frequent Florida beaches during colder months. Second, in parts of the Near North Side there has been an influx of Appalachian whites, and Shimkin has pointed out the high risk of this cancer in Southern males. Examination of the data also shows that rates of Skin Cancer incidence went up in both the Near North Side and Rogers Park from 1960 to 1967. Part of this increase could easily be attributed to further internal migration of former Southern whites within Chicago. This presents an interesting intraurban health problem for further investigation.

Some of the stronger statistical and cartographic associations show up when the site group "Other or Unspecified" is mapped (Figs. 34 and 35). The visual patterns are strikingly similar when compared to some of the previous maps, and the correlation coefficients follow suit. Comparison of 1967 to 1960 data yields an r of .727. When the sites are related to totals within each year, the results are r = .669 for 1960, and r = .764 for 1967. In general, the distributions are shown to follow the pattern set by Total Cancer for both years. It is unfortunate in many respects that the strongest site-to-site and temporal associations are for cancers not specified, but these diseases do account for about 16 per cent of all deaths reported for cancer in the metropolitan area. We can at least by process of elimination assume that the 1980 distribution will show up to be much the same.

Conclusions about mapping cancer sites

The following important conclusions regarding the mapping of cancer from data currently available should be noted:

(1) Such mapping should be approached with a great deal of caution. Some of the maps shown should be viewed with a degree of skepticism. It may be that it is easy enough to identify cancer *per se*, but site identification in advanced cases is difficult.

(2) There appear to be reporting inconsistencies which go beyond actual changes in distribution of difficult diagnoses. The data from Will County and southern Cook County appear to fluctuate more than the data from other parts of the SMSA.

---

[1] Shimkin, "Distribution of Cancer in the United States."

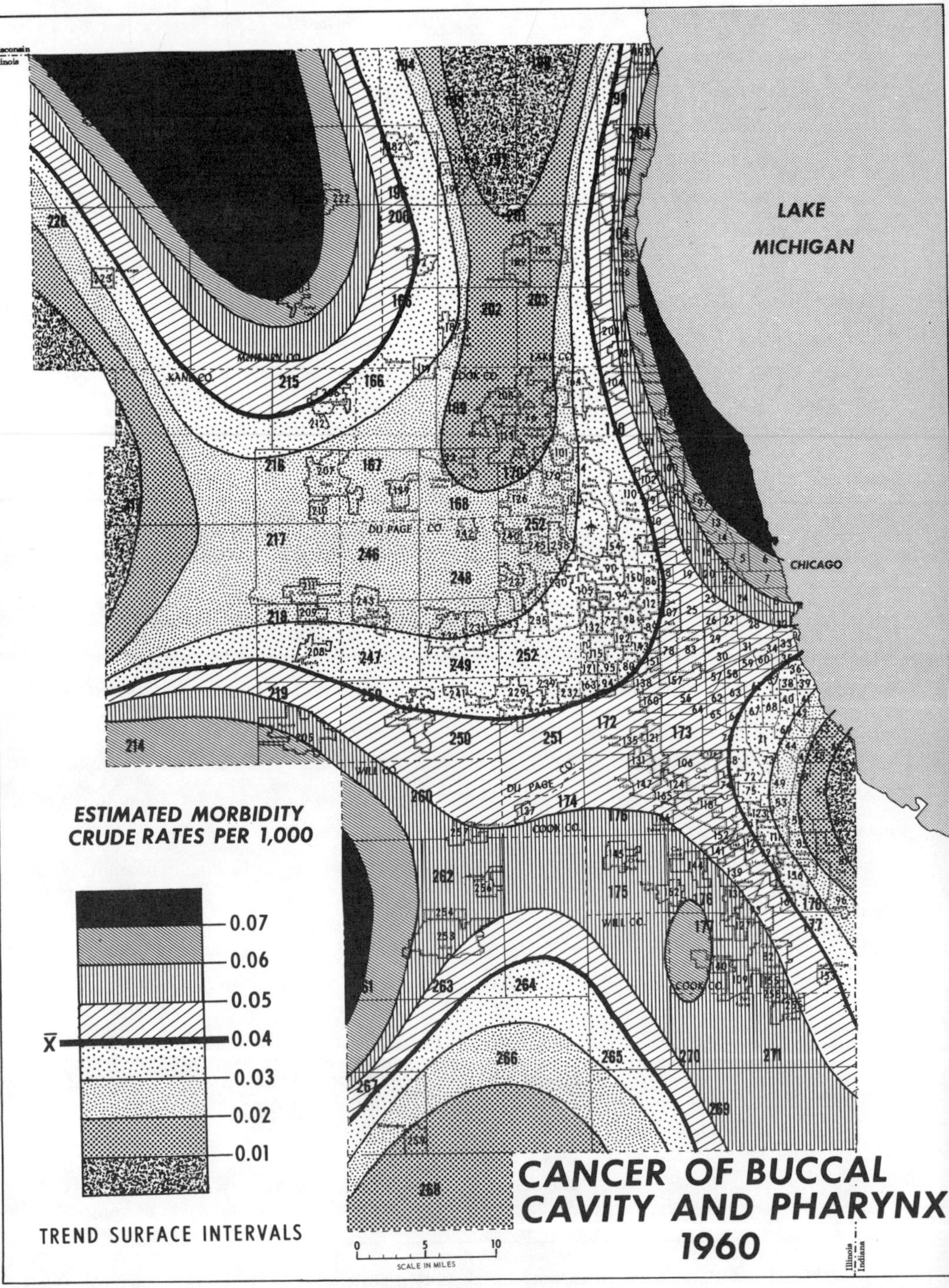

Fig. 32.--Cancer of buccal cavity and pharynx, 1960

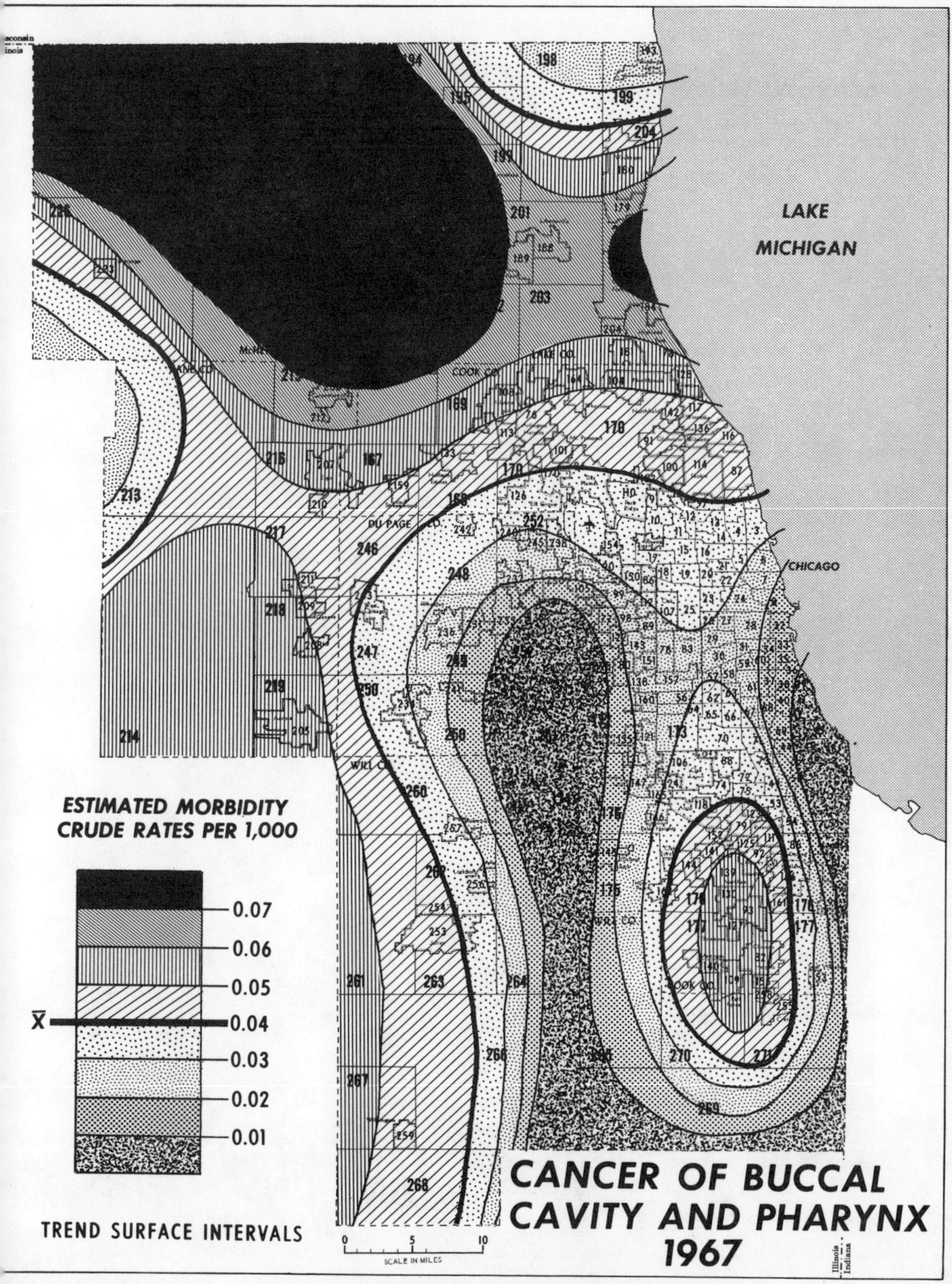

Fig. 33.--Cancer of buccal cavity and pharynx, 1967

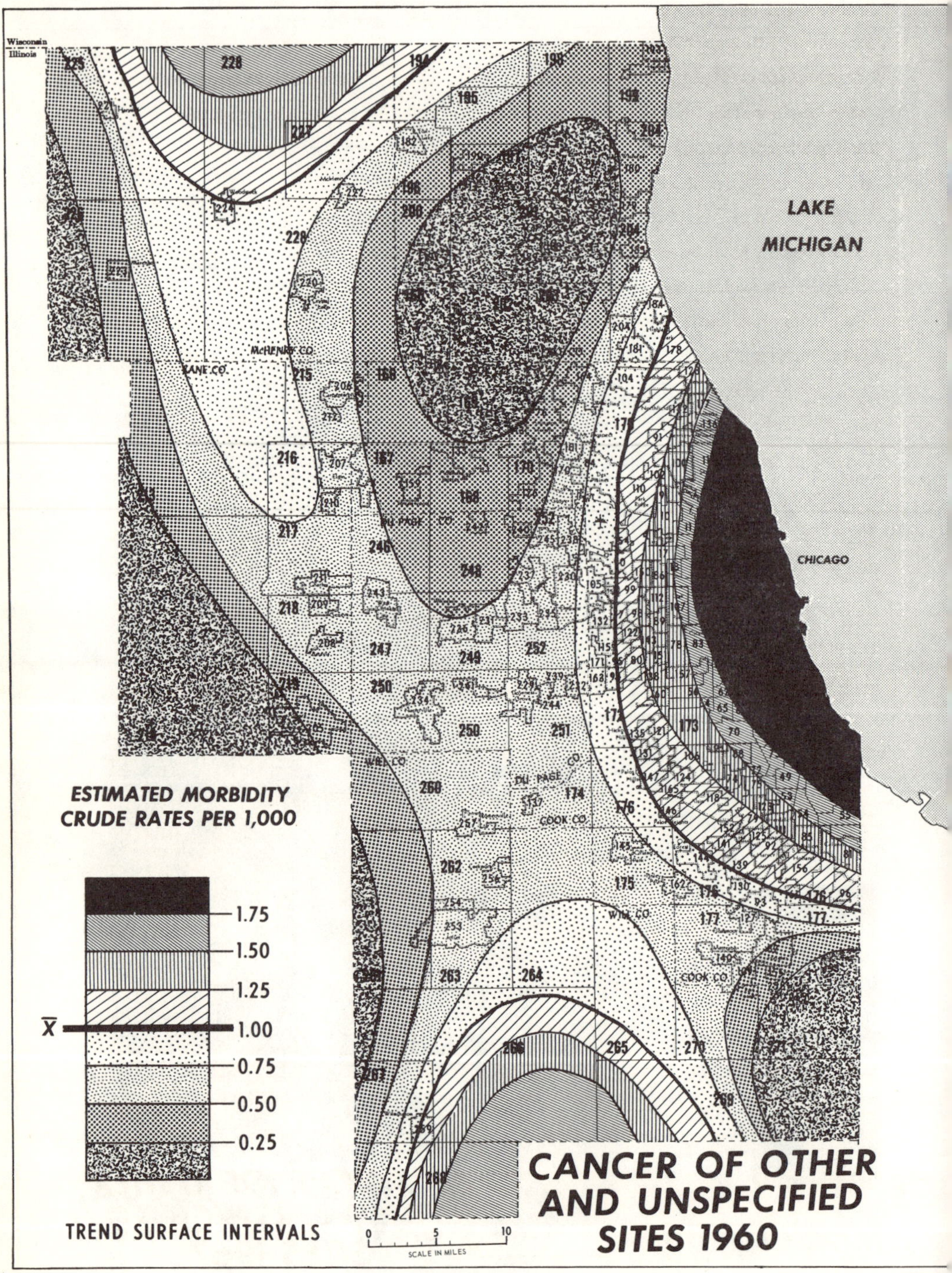

Fig. 34.--Cancer of other and unspecified sites, 1960

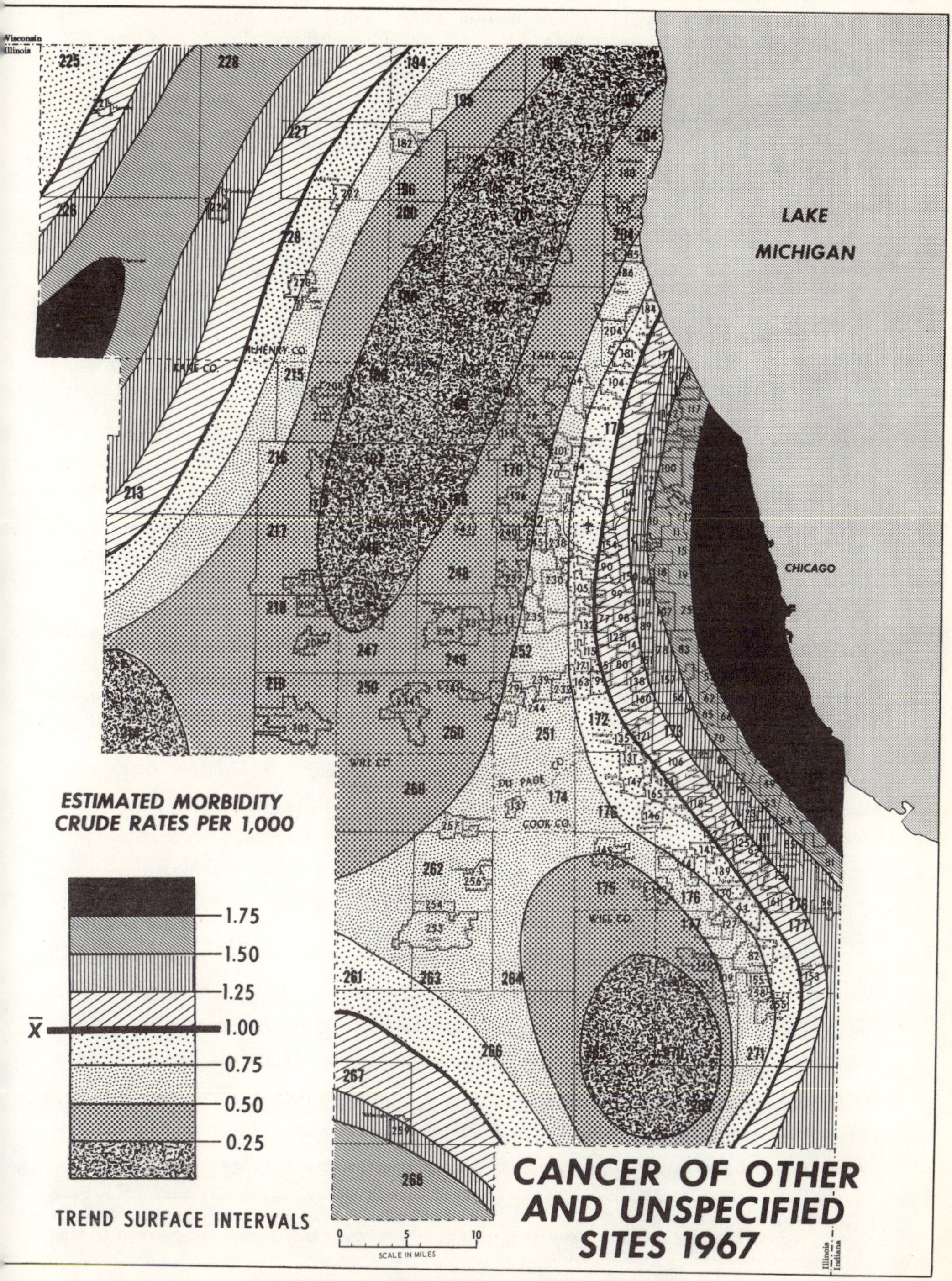

Fig. 35.--Cancer of other and unspecified sites, 1967

(3) The distribution of all cancers definitely changed from 1960 to 1967, and the individual sites, in spite of the two reasons listed above, follow patterns more closely related to the change in the distribution of the total incidence than to previous individual site patterns.

(4) For purposes of developing a forecasting model, it is sufficient to forecast the total distribution of cancer and speculate from that distribution about special sites. In fact, forecasting the total incidence of cancer over space may be the only method of determining specific sites.

The implication should not be that the future incidence of cancer cannot be determined from past patterns established, either. The correlation coefficient between 1960 and 1967 for Total Cancer is .585. However, in the following discussion it becomes apparent that cancer, as well as heart disease and stroke, are more highly inter-correlated with socio-economic and demographic characteristics of community populations than the diseases are with each other.

Disease Patterns in 1980: Forecasts

It is possible to use the results of the above descriptions in several ways during the construction of the actual forecasting model. Although some diseases were correlated better across the time span, the strongest correlations were within each time period, and this was especially true with the cancers. At least two relationships are suggested, and these serve as points of departure for the model development: first, knowledge of a number of socioeconomic and demographic characteristics of the inhabitants of the 271 data collection subareas might help explain the disease patterns better than mere comparisons with other disease patterns; and second, changes in these variables over the time span might aid in explaining changes in disease patterns to varying degrees. With these hypotheses in mind, a number of population-related variables have been statistically compared to disease patterns.

Selection of independent variables

The most convenient test for the above hypotheses is the regression equation (2). The assumption is that the diseases are dependent variables acted upon by a variety of independent socioeconomic and demographic variables, that, in turn, can be selected so that they describe the urban structure. Fortunately, we have in the literature a recently assembled compendium of many studies of the "Factorial Ecology" of communities.[1] These studies help us to understand the most significant variables which combine to form measures of social status, life style, and minority residential segregation--the most

---

[1] A forthcoming special issue of Economic Geography is exclusively devoted to such studies.

important aspects of urban social structure. The variables which form these measures were therefore collected along with additional information about age groups for the 271 subareas of this study, to be used as independent variables in the analysis. The combined group of variables includes:

Population
Population Density
Per Cent Substandard Housing
Per Cent White Collar Workers
Average Annual Income
Per Cent Unemployed
Median Education
Population per Household
Per Cent Black
Per Cent Foreign Born
Age Groups (Per Cent of Community)
    Less than 15 Years
    15 to 45 Years
    46 to 65 Years
    Over 65 Years

In order to obtain the disease forecasts essential as inputs to the allocation model (1960 to 1967 and 1967 to 1980), it was necessary to project each of the above variables. Initially, correlations between paris of variables were developed, and these are shown on Table 13. On the basis of these correlations and knowledge of which variables could be forecasted with any degree of confidence, a series of models showing associations among independent variables was developed.

These models were based upon the linear multiple regression equation, and methods of path analysis were used to help explain the results. For the past 50 years path analysis has built up around the work of Sewall Wright, a geneticist.[1] Early applications are summarized in his 1934 work and his 1960 contribution brings the method to date with newer regression techniques. The method is widespread now in both the biological and social sciences. Application of the former in population genetics are exemplified by Li and those in sociology by Duncan.[2]

The method essentially offers a diagrammatic interpretation of regression results, with particular emphasis upon the differences between simple correlations and standardized regression coefficients. However, definite causal flows are postulated.

---

[1] Sewall Wright, "The Method of Path Coefficients," Annals of Mathematical Statistics, V (September, 1934), 161-215, and idem, "Path Coefficients and Path Regressions: Alternative or Complementary Concepts," Biometrics, XVI (June, 1960), 189-202.

[2] C. C. Li, Population Genetics (Chicago: University of Chicago Press, 1955), Chapter XII, and Otis Dudley Duncan, "Path Analysis: Sociological Examples," The American Journal of Sociology, LXXII (July, 1966), 1-16.

TABLE 13

CORRELATIONS BETWEEN PAIRS OF SOCIOECONOMIC AND DEMOGRAPHIC VARIABLES, 1960 DATA

Variables[a]	1	2	3	4	5	6	7	8	9	10	11	12	13	14
* 1 Population	1.000													
* 2 Density	0.753	1.000												
** 3 % Substandard Housing	-0.024	-0.086	1.000											
** 4 % White Collar	0.062	-0.126	-0.494	1.000										
*** 5 Income	-0.029	-0.107	-0.606	0.579	1.000									
* 6 % Unemployed	0.192	0.294	0.607	-0.691	-0.699	1.000								
7 Education	-0.203	-0.343	-0.474	0.777	0.604	-0.691	1.000							
*** 8 Population per Household	-0.407	-0.446	-0.245	-0.078	0.276	-0.244	0.236	1.000						
* 9 % Black	0.328	0.414	0.311	-0.316	-0.384	0.526	-0.316	-0.173	1.000					
*10 % Foreign Born	0.341	0.432	-0.177	0.011	0.096	-0.019	-0.272	-0.489	-0.147	1.000				
11 % <15 Years	-0.272	-0.234	-0.060	-0.092	0.061	-0.043	0.215	0.698	-0.020	-0.452	1.000			
***12 % 15-45 Years	-0.100	-0.026	0.045	-0.270	-0.180	0.095	-0.157	0.300	0.069	-0.065	0.324	1.000		
13 % 46-65 Years	0.285	0.229	-0.057	0.230	0.103	-0.062	-0.056	-0.643	-0.003	0.378	-0.887	-0.471	1.000	
14 % >65 Years	0.169	0.160	0.182	0.082	-0.127	0.112	-0.211	-0.689	0.030	0.411	-0.772	-0.487	0.657	1.000

[a] Transformations have been made to approximate normal distributions: * = log; ** = log log; *** = $\sqrt{\ }$.

In the regression model, standardizer and therefore comparable regression coefficients for different variables are actually calculated by holding all other variables in the equation constant. It is thus necessary to express the variables in the form:

$$X_o = \frac{V_o - \bar{V}_o}{\sigma_{V_o}},\quad X_1 = \frac{V_1 - \bar{V}_1}{\sigma_{V_1}},\ \text{etc.} \qquad (3)$$

where V_n = the initial value of variable n

$\bar{V}_n$ = the mean value of n

σ_{V_n} = standard deviation of n

Wright originally used diagrams with two different kinds of arrows to indicate either causal paths (⟶) or simple correlations (↜↝). Thus in the diagram below the straight lines are causal paths originally determined by some chosen point of view regarding possible functional relationships among the observed variables. The double-headed curved arrows represented simple correlations.

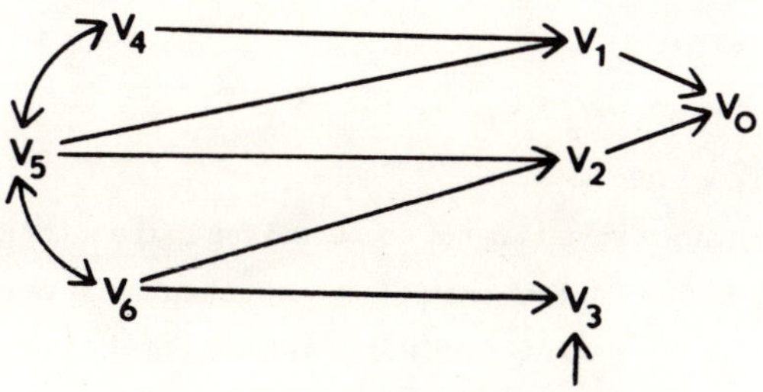

Fig. 36.--An early path diagram by Wright

Wright wrote the early path analysis equations:

$$\frac{(Vo - \bar{V}o)}{\sigma_{v_o}} = C_{o_1} \frac{(V_1 - \bar{V}_1)}{\sigma_{v_1}} + C_{o_2} \frac{(V_2 - \bar{V}_2)}{\sigma_{v_2}} + \ldots + C_{o_n} \frac{(V_n - \bar{V}_n)}{\sigma_{v_n}} \qquad (4)$$

where C_{o_1}, C_{o_2}, C_{o_n} represented the correlations, and the actual paths were explained in standard form as:

$$X_o = P_{o1} X_1 + P_{o2} X_2 + \ldots + P_{on} X_n \qquad (5)$$

where P_{o1} to P_{on} represented regression coefficients.

The basic premise of Wright has remained the same. Notations have changed with the streamlining of regression techniques. The equations and diagrams now most frequently used are indicated below.

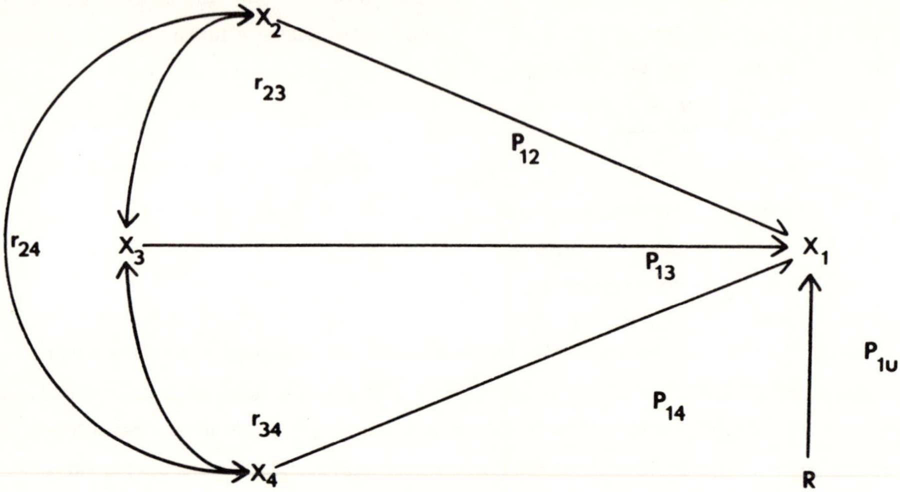

Fig. 37.--A simple path analysis model

The equation has developed as:

$$X_1 = P_{12} X_2 + P_{13} X_3 + P_{14} X_4 + P_{1u} R_u \quad (6)$$

where P_{1u} = path coefficients

R_u = explanatory variables not accounted for in the model.

The path coefficients are in fact the beta coefficients, which must be read back from X_1, so that $P_{12} = \beta_{12 \cdot 24}$, $P_{13} = \beta_{13 \cdot 24}$. Conversely, "spurious" relationships are indicated by the zero-order correlation coefficients, and are indicated as r_{24}, r_{23}, etc.

The idea of diagramming presumed causal flows to demonstrate relations between independent variables or possibly to search out dependent variables actually has many possibilities. For example, Blalock has recently summarized several general notions of causal flows, and Figure 38 shows many of the possibilities.[1] Item (A) is the regression approach in its simplest form where an inventory of supposed unrelated causes (X's) explain the dependent variables, Y. In (B), the next logical step, some "independent" variables are highly correlated, so that they are able to make predictors of others. A set (I's) of intermediate variables is hence used to explain Y. Conversely, it is possible to have one variable with multiple consequences (C) fan out and cause several dependent variables--the basis for the factor analysis discussed earlier. Developed further, as in (D),

---

[1]Hubert M. Blalock, Theory Construction (Englewood Cliffs, N.J.: Prentice-Hall, Inc., 1969), Chapter III.

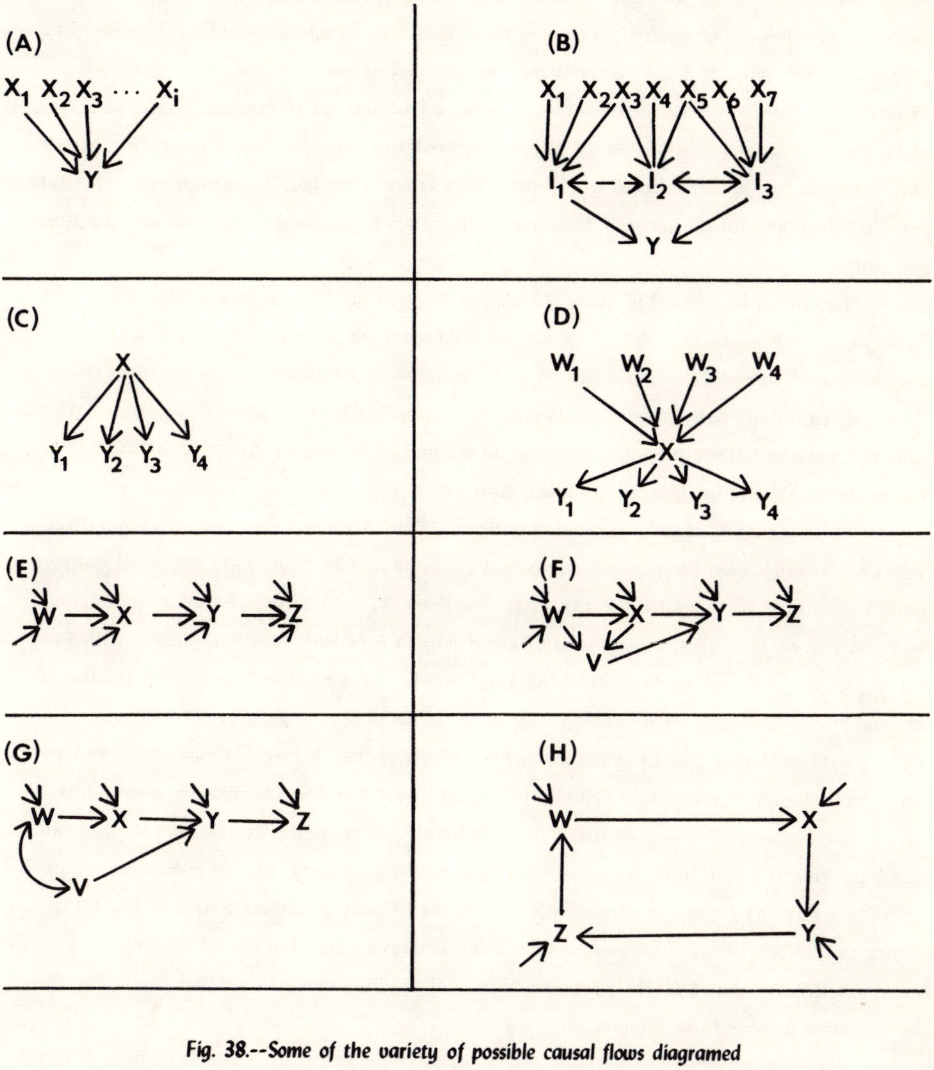

Fig. 38.--Some of the variety of possible causal flows diagramed

this reasoning can lead to a situation where there might be several independent variables (W's) contributing to one central variable (X) which in turn affects several dependent variables (Y's). This is perhaps a case for canonical analysis.

Related thinking includes causal chains and loops. In (E), each variable represents the building up of additional causes in a chain. A different variable, V, enters in (F), and either W or X could be the direct or indirect cause of V. Another possibility is shown in (G) where it may be that W and V are correlated but for possibly unknown reasons, and the curved line shows the "spurious" relationship. Finally, the entire relationship could be the causal loop shown in (H). Items (E), (F), (G), and (H) do not constitute a significant portion of the models developed below; however, they have been used by Hopps and Cuffey.[1]

The flows suggested by Item (B) appear to be best fitted to this study. On the basis of the correlations of Table 13 several regressions were attempted, and as a result the number of independent variables to be forecasted was trimmed from fourteen to eight. The final variables selected were: Population, Density, Income, Per Cent Black, and the four age groups. However, the other variables can be accounted for to some extent, and the models below indicate approximately how and how much.

The strongest of the regression models ($R^2 = .655$) was demonstrated by utilizing Per Cent Unemployed (W_1) as the dependent variable and Income (X_3), Per Cent Substandard Housing (V_1), Per Cent White Collar Workers (V_2), and Median Education (V_3) as independent variables. Unemployment is difficult to forecast, and it is, along with Population Density, one of the two variables most highly correlated with Per Cent Black. A second model was thus developed and added to the first (see Fig. 39). The new model ($R^2 = .351$) says that Per Cent Unemployed (and all of that variable's associated independent variables) and Population Density tell most about Per Cent Black--by community.

Conversely, Income by itself is most highly correlated with the four items used as independent variables in the regression diagrammed as Figure 40. These independent variables were Per Cent Unemployed, Substandard Housing, Education, and Per Cent White Collar Workers. The coefficient of determination for this model is .563, and this measure tells us that a fairly adequate degree of the variance of the other variables is known when income is accounted for.

Population per Household and Per Cent Foreign Born, also two variables difficult to forecast, are best accounted for by three of the age variables. These associations are shown on Figure 41. The regressions used in this model are not so strong as some of the

---

[1]Howard C. Hopps and Roger Cuffey, "Cause/Effect Relationships in Disease," International Pathology, X (January and April, 1969), 23-25.

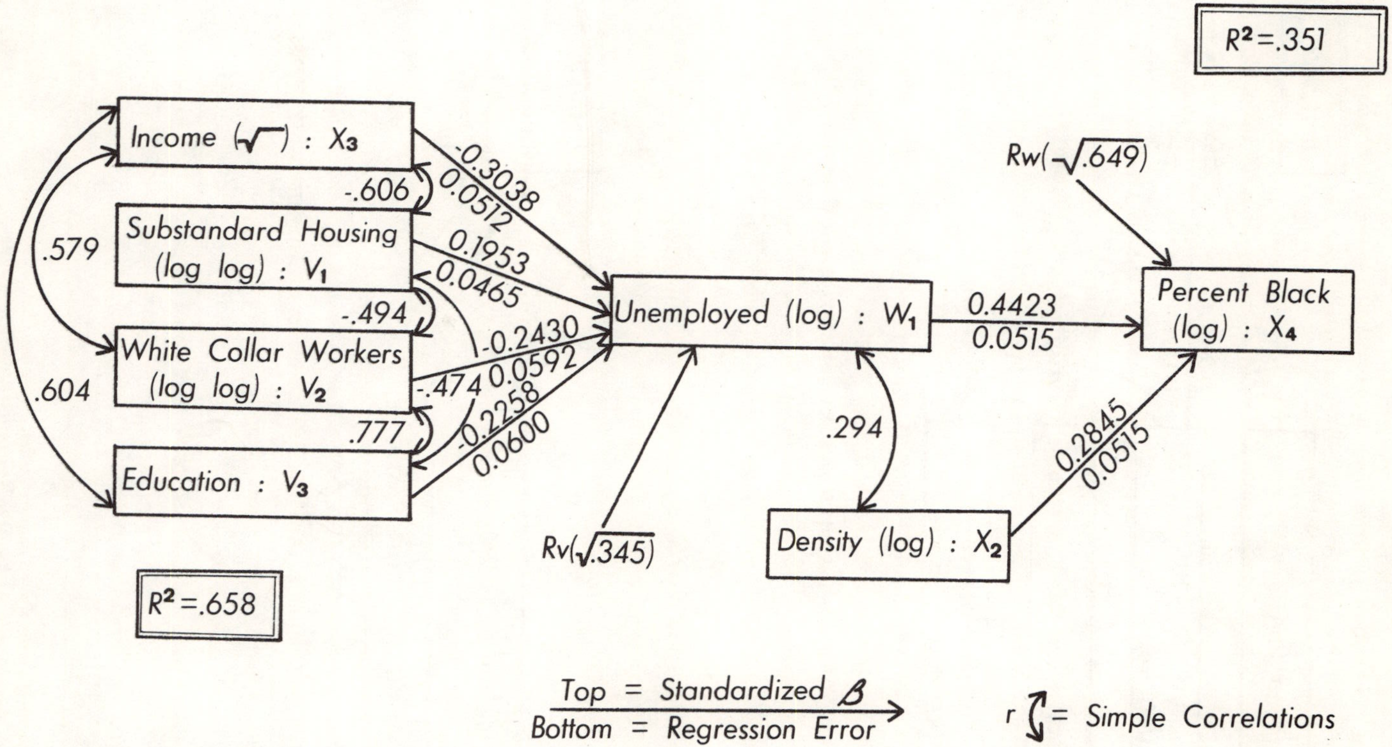

Fig. 39.--Path diagrams for the first alternative model for regression of 1960 socioeconomic variables

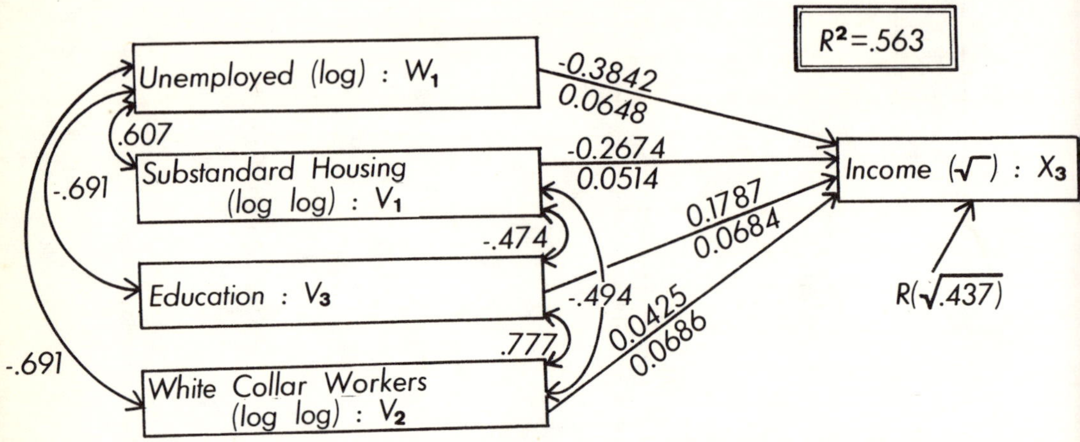

Fig. 40.--Independent variables explaining the most about income

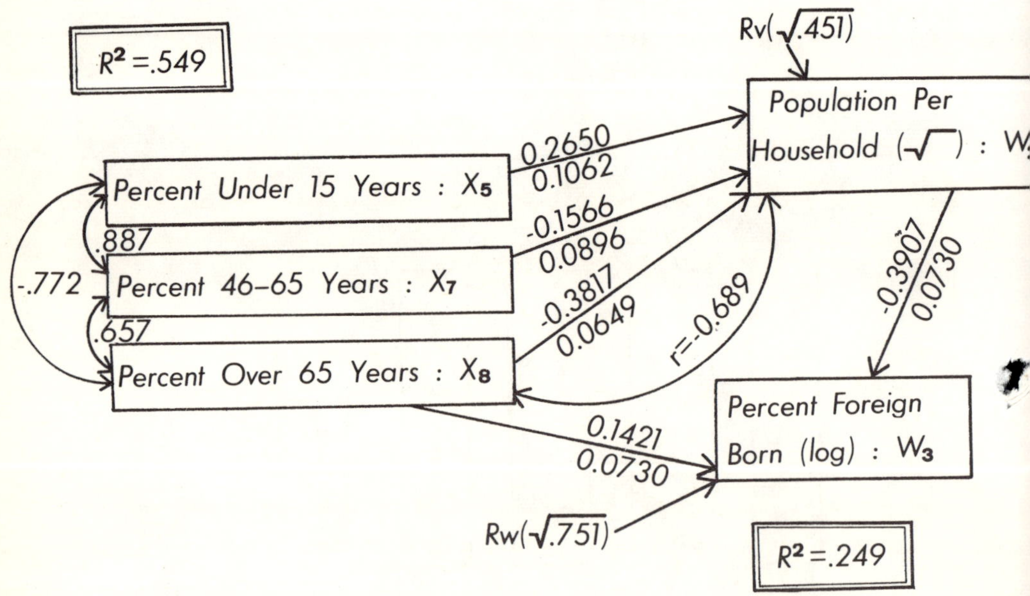

Fig. 41.--Best fitting model for age groups

previous tests, but knowledge of the simple correlations is at least helpful. In the first regression, an R^2 of .549 results when all age groups except Per Cent 15 to 45 are used as independent variables supposedly helping to determine Population per Household. The above is not a bad fit. However, for Per Cent Foreign Born, the strongest R^2 attained was .249 when Per Cent over 65 and Population per Household were used as independent variables.

As indicated by Figure 38, it would have been possible to construct many other, more elegant, models showing so-called causal flows. For the purposes of this study the important point is that methods of path analysis were used to show how a larger number of variables important to the urban ecology tie into the key variables to be used as independent elements in the construction of the morbidity-mortality models.

Regression results for 1960 diseases

When the 1960 disease rates were regressed against the eight key demographic variables some rather expected relationships resulted. The easiest way to approach these relationships is with the correlation coefficients shown on Table 14. Reading across the top of the table, we see that Heart Disease (variable 19) shows no strong single correlation with the first four variables, but does show a definite pattern with the four age groups. For Heart Disease and the more youthful group, r = -.527, and for Heart Disease and the more elderly group, r = .626. The other two age groups help form the negative to positive sequence. The relationship for Stroke is very close to that of Heart Disease.

The patterns for the various cancer groups, with the exception of Leukemia and Aleukemia, generally follow the Heart Disease and Stroke example. However, with the exception of the categories "Total Cancer" and "Other and Unspecified," the correlation coefficients are generally weak for cancer sites. The obvious implication is that many factors, probably mostly other than those factors related to the urban ecology, are influencing the distribution of various individual sites and site groups in Chicago. This observation in fact confirms the rather widely varying patterns seen on the maps earlier in this chapter (Figs. 20 to 35).

When all the disease variables were utilized as dependent variables in a linear multiple regression, only four of the eleven diseases showed a fairly significant coefficient of determination. Fortunately, three of these were Heart Disease, Stroke, and Total Cancer. Only one of the site groups, "Other and Unspecified," showed an adequate R^2. These relationships agree fairly well with previous cartographic and statistical information mentioned. The results of the three major regressions are shown on Tables 15 to 17.

TABLE 14

ZERO-ORDER CORRELATION COEFFICIENTS BETWEEN DEMOGRAPHIC VARIABLES AND RMP DISEASES, 1960

Variables[a]	1	2	3	4	5	6	7	8
* 1 Population	1.000							
* 2 Density	.753	1.000						
*** 3 Income	-.029	-.107	1.000					
* 4 Per Cent Black	.328	.414	-.384	1.000				
5 % >15 Years	-.272	-.234	.061	-.020	1.000			
*** 6 % 15-45 Years	-.100	-.026	-.180	.069	.324	1.000		
7 % 46-65 Years	.285	.229	.103	-.003	-.887	-.471	1.000	
8 % <65 Years	.169	.160	-.127	.030	-.772	-.487	.657	1.000
9 Total Cancer	.152	.317	-.146	.074	-.429	-.237	.434	.490
10 Digestive Cancer	.152	-.138	.061	-.101	-.143	-.189	.180	.290
*11 Respiratory Cancer	-.207	.312	-.171	.107	-.307	-.132	.311	.304
*12 Genital Cancers	-.026	.018	-.012	-.001	-.064	-.090	.093	.136
*13 Breast Cancer	.074	.181	.051	.020	-.214	-.169	.248	.206
*14 Leukemia	-.161	-.177	.120	-.153	.090	.066	-.064	-.114
*15 Skin Cancer	.067	-.037	-.131	-.018	-.098	-.028	.108	.100
*16 Buccal Cavity	.017	.023	.021	.030	-.038	-.031	.062	.050
17 Other Cancer	.438	.607	-.248	.218	-.477	-.173	.430	.455
*18 Stroke	.098	.218	-.194	.188	-.374	-.213	.355	.500
*19 Heart Disease	.182	.324	-.253	.194	-.527	-.243	.492	.626

[a] Transformations have been made to approximate normal distributions: * = log; *** = $\sqrt{\ }$.

TABLE 15

CANCER REGRESSION FOR CHICAGO SMSA, 1960

Dependent Variable	Multiple R	Multiple R^2	Intercept A	Standard Error of Intercept	
Total Cancer (Y_1)	.602	.363	2.1480	1.3830	
Independent Variables	**Partial R**	**Standardized B**	**Regression Error**	**Metric B**	**Regression Error**
Density (X_2)	0.325	0.4205	0.0753	0.8762	0.1569
% >65 Years (X_8)	0.294	0.3907	0.0781	0.1348	0.0269
Population (X_1)	-0.220	-0.2784	0.0760	-0.8236	0.2249
% 46-65 Years (X_7)	0.212	0.4026	0.1143	0.0781	0.0222
Income (X_3)	-0.134	-0.1168	0.0531	-0.0136	0.0062
% <15 Years (X_5)	0.121	0.2597	0.1308	0.0421	0.0212

TABLE 16

HEART DISEASE REGRESSION FOR CHICAGO SMSA, 1960

Dependent Variable	Multiple R	Multiple R^2	Intercept A	Standard Error of Intercept	
Heart Disease (Y_{11})	.717	.514	0.1801	0.2974	
Independent Variables	**Partial R**	**Standardized B**	**Regression Error**	**Metric B**	**Regression Error**
%>65 Years (X_8)	0.418	0.5867	0.0787	0.0261	0.0035
Density (X_2)	0.286	0.3296	0.0683	0.0885	0.0184
% 46-65 Years (X_7)	0.226	0.4225	0.1123	0.0106	0.0028
Income (X_3)	-0.212	-0.1779	0.0507	-0.0027	0.0008
Population (X_1)	-0.193	-0.2132	0.0670	-0.8129	0.0256
%<15 Years (X_5)	0.144	0.3001	0.1279	0.0063	0.0027
% 15-45 Years (X_6)	0.102	0.0969	0.0581	0.0435	0.0260
% Black (X_4)	0.051	0.0423	0.0516	0.0135	0.0165

TABLE 17

STROKE REGRESSION FOR CHICAGO SMSA, 1960

Dependent Variable	Multiple R	Multiple R^2	Intercept A	Standard Error of Intercept	
Stroke (Y_{10})	.570	.325	0.1518	0.1213	
Independent Variables	**Partial R**	**Standardized B**	**Regression Error**	**Metric B**	**Regression Error**
%>65 Years (X_8)	0.362	0.5072	0.0805	0.0418	0.0024
Density (X_2)	0.183	0.2412	0.0801	0.0427	0.0142
Population (X_1)	-0.165	-0.2130	0.0786	-0.0537	0.0198
% 46-65 Years (X_7)	0.150	0.2904	0.1181	0.0048	0.0019
%>15 Years (X_5)	0.128	0.2828	0.1355	0.0039	0.0018
Income (X_3)	-0.121	-0.1172	0.0593	-0.0012	0.0006
% Black (X_4)	0.106	0.1047	0.0607	0.0221	0.0127

The independent variables shown are those which either entered the model with a regression error less than half the metric B coefficient or close to that relationship. "Close to" means that if the independent variable entered no other model very significantly but was fairly close to a level of significant entry it was used. General measures and levels for the eight cancer sites are shown on Table 18.

TABLE 18

REGRESSIONS FOR VARIOUS CANCER SITE GROUPS, 1960

Dependent Variable	R^2	Independent Variables[a]
*Digestive Cancer (Y_{12})	.265	X_8, X_5, X_7, X_1, X_2
Respiratory Cancer (Y_3)	.199	X_2, X_3, X_7, X_8, X_5
*Genital Cancer (Y_4)	.267	X_8, X_5, X_7
*Breast Cancer (Y_5)	.095	X_7, X_2, X_1
*Leukemia (Y_6)	.054	X_2, X_6, X_3, X_4, X_5, X_7
*Buccal Cavity (Y_7)	.004	X_7
*Skin Cancer (Y_8)	.033	X_3, X_7, X_1, X_6
Other Cancer (Y_9)	.544	X_2, X_3, X_8, X_7, X_4

X_1 = Population (*) X_3 = Income (**) X_5 = % <15 Years X_7 = % 46-65 Years
X_2 = Density (*) X_4 = % Black (*) X_6 = % 15-45 Years (**) X_8 = % >65 Years

Transformations have been made to approximate normal distributions: * = log; ** = $\sqrt{\ }$.

[a]In order of importance in the model.

The three Heart Disease, Stroke, and Total Cancer models can then be said to replicate reality within the limitations imposed by the coefficients of determination, and the equations would be written:[1]

Given Y_1 = Total Cancer
Y_{10} = Total Stroke
Y_{11} = Total Heart Disease
X_1 = Population
X_2 = Density
X_3 = Income
X_4 = % Black
X_5 = % <15 Years
X_6 = % 15-45 Years
X_7 = % 46-65 Years
X_8 = % >65 Years

$$Y_{11} = 0.2974 + (0.0261 * X_8) + (0.0885 * X_2) + (0.01056 * X_7) - (0.0027 * X_3) - (0.8129 * X_1) + (0.0063 * X_5) + (0.0435 * X_6) + (0.0135 * X_4) \quad (7)$$

[1]Transformations indicated on the table are still held, so Y_{11}, for example, is actually $\log_{10} Y_{11}$, etc.

$$Y_{10} = 0.1213 + (0.0418 * X_8) + (0.0427 * X_2) - (0.0537 * X_1) + (0.0048 * X_7) + (0.0039 * X_5) - (0.0012 * X_3) + (0.0221 * X_4) \quad (8)$$

$$Y_1 = 2.1480 + (0.8762 * X_2) + (0.1348 * X_8) - (0.8236 * X_1) + (0.0781 * X_7) - (0.0136 * X_3) + (0.0421 * X_5) \quad (9)$$

Interestingly, Age over 65, Population Density, and Population have a leading part in all three models. To build the final forecasting model, however, it is necessary to examine the 1967 relationships and work from that point. Furthermore, in order to examine the 1967 relationships it is necessary through various means to gather in a number of forecasts and projections of the ecological variables to both 1967 and 1980, the latter, of course, being the target year for the mortality-morbidity inputs into the larger allocation model, because, of course, the data base for the ecological data is the 1960 Census.

Forecasting independent variables

A wide range of methods, both previously published as well as some presumably unique to this study, were used to develop a set of independent variables for the 1967 and 1980 regressions. The forecasts, projections, and estimates used should be viewed as capable of containing any of a number of errors which often accompany such attempts. Whenever possible, estimates and forecasts previously developed by specialized urban planning agencies and organizations were adapted to the subareas of this study. Population and Density could be adapted from two sources already dealing with those subjects. Income was also projected from two sources, and the ethnic and age variables were forecasted exclusively for this study.

Two of the urban planning agencies most actively engaged in forecasting population numbers are the Northeastern Illinois Planning Commission (NIPC) and the Real Estate Research Corporation (RERC). Some of the most recent forecasts produced by these agencies were synthesized to fit Hospital Planning Districts in 1969.[1] For the City of Chicago RERC forecasts were considered to be the most appropriate for this study, and for the suburban areas NIPC forecasts were utilized. In terms of the human ecology of the Chicago SMSA, these combined forecasts reflected the following characteristics pertaining to population growth:

(1) Most central city subareas (Chicago Community Areas) demonstrated a population growth trend to 1980 which was either steady or declining. Some noteworthy exceptions were neighborhoods which had changed racially.

---

[1] Pierre de Vise and Siim Soot, "Chicago in the 60's and 70's: A Study of the Chicago Area's Changing Population, 1960-1970, and a Forecast of Population Changes for Municipalities and Counties, 1970-1995," Chicago Regional Hospital Study, Working Paper V.2, January, 1970.

(2) The inner suburban ring and some older established suburbs reflected an "S"-shaped logistic curve which indicated that at a point before some given capacity, population growth was assumed to taper off in a predictable manner.

(3) The outer suburban ring forecasts demonstrated an almost linear upward trend thus reflecting the anticipated continuation of a more youthful population in these subareas.

(4) Many rural fringe areas showed a steady rate or slight decrease, but not so marked as most of the central city subareas.

For this study RERC figures were used for the City of Chicago's Community areas for 1967 and 1980 numbers. Whenever possible, NIPC figures for 1967 and 1980 were used for suburbs and the rural fringe. NIPC does not publish figures for certain smaller urban places; however, it was possible to obtain from that agency forecasts by square mile for the SMSA (excluding Chicago City). It was further possible simply to apply the square mile figures to the appropriate subareas used in this study.

Population Density was then determined for 1967 and 1980 on the basis of the previous forecasts. For the most part, current areas were used in the determination of densities; however, if the 1980 square-mile forecasts showed previously unincorporated areas taking on large population numbers by that year, these areas were added to (or subtracted from) the proper contiguous subareas.

Sources for income projections include the Hospital Planning Council for Metropolitan Chicago and the U. S. Census. For 1967, figures previously calculated by the former of the above sources were used for all subareas possible.[1] For those of the 271 subareas not accounted for, income figures from both the 1950 and 1960 U. S. Census volumes were obtained, linear trends were developed, and these trends were extended by the application of a slope from socially similar areas for which estimates in 1967 were available. Similarly, income figures for all the 271 subareas for 1950 and 1960 were combined with the 1967 estimates and projected in a straight line fashion to 1980.

Many estimates and projections are available for Per Cent Black in the Chicago area.[2] Few of these estimates attempt to look at both the central city and suburban areas, and for this reason a methodology utilizing polynomial expansions for the entire SMSA was developed. The details are to be found in Appendix C.

Obtaining age forecasts for each of the subareas presented serious problems. Although forecasts have been made for the entire SMSA and large portions of it, few if any estimates appear for small subareas. The major consideration in attempting such a task

---

[1] Pierre de Vise, "Characteristics of Chicago Area Communities," Commerce (July, 1969), pp. 1-12.

[2] Brian J. L. Berry and Katherine Smith, "Down from the Summit" (Chicago: Center for Urban Studies, 1969).

is that each of the four age groups used in this study contain relative shares of the population which at all times must add up to 100 per cent of the particular areas' population. When a linear regression method was attempted, the results did not even approach 100 per cent of the figures previously adapted for this study. The regression results either vastly underpredicted or overpredicted when shares for the four groups were totaled.

Finally, a rather conservative method was utilized, and when predictions for age groups were added up they almost always closely approximated the 1967 and 1980 figures used here. The method assumes that the rates of change within each group from 1950 to 1960 will continue to operate in 1967 and on to 1980. The following equations help explain the method in detail:

Given Δ, the rate of change for each of the K age groups determined by

$$\Delta K = 100.0 + [S_{60}(K) - S_{50}(K)], \tag{10}$$

where S_{60} and S_{50} = relative shares for each of the K age groups for 1960 and 1950 respectively, and the goal is to find $S_{67}(K)$ and $S_{80}(K)$,

$$S_{67} = \frac{[.7\,\Delta(K) * N_{60}(K)] + N_{60}(K) * 100.0}{\text{Total Population 1967}} \tag{11}$$

and

$$S_{80} = \frac{[1.3\,\Delta(K) * N_{67}(K)] + N_{67}(K) * 100.0}{\text{Total Population 1980}} \tag{12}$$

where $N_{60}(K)$ and $N_{67}(K)$ are the actual numbers within the K age groups for 1960 and 1967.

The tables in Appendix D contain the relative shares for each of the K groups over the time period under discussion. As Appendix D indicates, only 261 of the 271 areas of this study were forecasted. This is due to missing data for 1950 for ten smaller suburbs not large enough during that census to rate separate treatment. For these ten areas, relative shares for suburbs with similar life cycle characteristics were substituted.

<u>Regression results for 1967 diseases</u>

After the eight key ecological variables had been forecasted and projected to 1967, they were used as independent variables in a multiple regression analysis using known data for the eleven disease groups. The initial correlation coefficients are shown on Table 19. The overall trends for correlations between pairs of the nineteen variables showed trends similar to those of 1960; however, in many instances the correlations are even weaker than those from the previous regressions; this is not unexpected, since any ecological forecast is prone to error.

The two leading cancer groups are once more "Total Cancer" and "Other and Unspecified," but with this year the correlations are stronger than those in 1960. Con-

TABLE 19

ZERO-ORDER CORRELATION COEFFICIENTS BETWEEN DEMOGRAPHIC VARIABLES AND RMP DISEASES, 1967

Variables[a]	1	2	3	4	5	6	7	8
* 1 Population	1.000							
* 2 Density	.679	1.000						
*** 3 Income	-.047	-.118	1.000					
* 4 Per Cent Black	.392	.537	-.328	1.000				
5 % <15 Years	-.280	-.328	.016	-.079	1.000			
*** 6 % 15-45 Years	-.079	-.008	-.107	-.016	.268	1.000		
7 % 46-65 Years	.252	.238	.133	.042	-.820	-.692	1.000	
8 % >65 Years	.141	.189	-.136	.097	-.683	-.400	.480	1.000
9 Total Cancer	.107	.345	-.180	.112	-.463	-.159	.316	.553
10 Digestive Cancer	-.120	-.022	.056	-.115	-.149	-.055	.065	.271
*11 Respiratory Cancer	.117	.284	-.214	.071	-.200	-.041	.136	.220
*12 Genital Cancers	.059	.156	.077	.102	-.162	-.026	.121	.144
*13 Breast Cancer	.071	.187	.197	-.034	-.213	-.186	.197	.319
*14 Leukemia	-.169	-.129	.131	-.167	.170	.104	-.144	-.192
*15 Skin Cancer	.135	.090	-.056	.035	-.143	-.042	.100	.147
*16 Buccal Cavity	-.052	-.138	-.018	-.099	-.000	.035	-.031	.016
17 Other Cancer	.267	.483	-.368	.289	-.551	-.173	.389	.582
*18 Stroke	.053	.152	-.105	.115	-.277	-.144	.171	.444
*19 Heart Disease	.139	.479	-.133	.244	-.387	-.053	.263	.368

[a]Transformations have been made as in Table 14.

versely, the Stroke and Heart Disease correlations are lower than in 1960. This is especially true of the latter where we went from r = .626 in 1960 to r = .368 in 1967.

When put to the multiple regression model, statistical relationships which have been previewed on Table 19 show up. All of the variables which were significant in 1960 were used for the 1967 models, and the results are shown on Tables 20 to 22. The major problem at this point is that many of the variables in 1967 were not nearly so important as they were in 1960. This can be witnessed by relating the metric B coefficients to the regression errors. Nonetheless, these variables have been retained for purposes of comparison. Generally, the R^2 for Total Cancer is stronger while the coefficients of determination for Stroke and Heart Disease are weaker than in 1960.

It is worthy of mention that some of the significant variables shifted in order of importance in the models from the first to second periods. For example, Density and Per Cent >65 changed places in the Total Cancer models, and there was considerable shifting in the Heart Disease models. The Stroke models remained the most constant in spite of some shifting in the less significant variables.

TABLE 20

HEART DISEASE REGRESSION FOR CHICAGO SMSA, 1967

Dependent Variable	Multiple R	Multiple R^2	Intercept A	Standard Error of Intercept	
Heart Disease (Y_{11})	.642	.412	-3.0476	1.3180	
Independent Variables	**Partial R**	**Standardized B**	**Regression Error**	**Metric B**	**Regression Error**
Density (X_2)	0.462	0.6165	0.0731	0.2067	0.0245
Population (X_1)	-0.314	-0.3498	0.0654	-0.1745	0.0326
% > 65 Years (X_8)	0.244	0.7381	0.1813	0.0378	0.0093
% 15-45 Years (X_6)	0.197	0.8594	0.2640	0.3586	0.1102
% 46-65 Years (X_7)	0.191	1.3709	0.4343	0.0357	0.0113
% < 15 Years (X_5)	0.167	1.1160	0.4063	0.0289	0.0105
Income (X_3)	-0.099	-0.0868	0.0540	-0.0012	0.0007
% Black (X_4)	-0.006	-0.0059	0.0601	-0.0042	0.0424

TABLE 21

STROKE REGRESSION FOR CHICAGO SMSA, 1967

Dependent Variable	Multiple R	Multiple R^2	Intercept A	Standard Error of Intercept	
Stroke (Y_{10})	.461	.213	0.2052	0.1549	
Independent Variables	**Partial R**	**Standardized B**	**Regression Error**	**Metric B**	**Regression Error**
% > 65 Years (X_8)	0.348	0.4664	0.0774	0.0163	0.0027
Density (X_2)	0.092	0.1258	0.0842	0.0288	0.0193
Population (X_1)	-0.079	-0.0965	0.0754	-0.0329	0.0257
% Black (X_4)	0.035	0.0389	0.0694	0.0188	0.0335
% 46-65 Years (X_7)	-0.019	-0.0304	0.1007	-0.0005	0.0018
% < 15 Years (X_5)	0.017	0.0345	0.1218	0.0006	0.0022
Income (X_3)	-0.015	-0.0146	0.0606	-0.0001	0.0006

TABLE 22

CANCER REGRESSION FOR CHICAGO SMSA, 1967

Dependent Variable	Multiple R	Multiple R^2	Intercept A	Standard Error of Intercept	
Total Cancer (Y_1)	.641	.411	5.5604	1.3977	
Independent Variables	**Partial R**	**Standardized B**	**Regression Error**	**Metric B**	**Regression Error**
%>65 Years (X_8)	0.366	0.4260	0.0667	0.1559	0.0244
Density (X_2)	0.340	0.3891	0.0664	0.9325	0.1590
Population (X_1)	-0.234	-0.2536	0.0649	-0.9036	0.2315
Income (X_3)	-0.107	-0.0687	0.0496	-0.0086	0.0049
%<15 Years (X_5)	-0.065	-0.1104	0.1041	-0.0205	0.0193
% 46-65 Years (X_7)	0.003	0.0040	0.0867	0.0007	0.0161

Written in a form comparable to 1960, the equations for these essentially descriptive models are:

$$Y_{11} = -3.0476 + (0.2067 * X_2) - (0.1745 * X_1) + (0.0378 * X_8) + (0.3586 * X_6) + (0.0357 * X_7) + (0.0289 * X_5) - (0.0012 * X_3) - (0.0042 * X_4) \quad (13)$$

$$Y_{10} = 0.2052 + (0.0163 * X_8) + (0.0288 * X_2) - (0.0329 * X_1) + (0.0188 * X_4) - (0.0005 * X_7) + (0.0006 * X_5) - (0.0001 * X_3) \quad (14)$$

$$Y_1 = 5.5604 + (0.1559 * X_8) + (0.9325 * X_2) - (0.9036 * X_1) - (0.0086 * X_3) - (0.0205 * X_5) + (0.0007 * X_7) \quad (15)$$

Comparisons with the earlier equations ([7], [8], [9]) demonstrate that the α and β coefficients are dissimilar to the point that no single sets of coefficients from the two series of equations can possibly be used for forecasting. Furthermore, none of the disease-to-disease associations have yet been built into the models.

The 1980 forecasting models

Essentially two findings were considered when the final forecasting model was developed. First, only three of the diseases could be forecasted with any degree of confidence, but these fortunately were Heart Disease, Stroke, and Total Cancer. Even then, the stroke models were consistently weak, indicating that a substantial part of the variance cannot be accounted for by demographic and socioeconomic variables; however, there appear nowhere any really outstanding coefficients of determination, and part of this is due to the large number of observations (271). Second, the individual cancer site groups correlate much better when compared to Total Cancer within time periods than they do across time, and they can be accounted for in that manner to some extent (Table 23).

TABLE 23

REGRESSIONS FOR VARIOUS CANCER SITE GROUPS, 1967

Dependent Variable	R^2	Independent Variables[a]
Digestive Cancer (Y_2)	.104	X_8, X_1, X_7, X_2, X_5
Respiratory Cancer (Y_3)	.137	X_2, X_3, X_8, X_7, X_5
Genital Cancer (Y_4)	.028	X_5, X_8, X_7
Breast Cancer (Y_5)	.069	X_2, X_7, X_1
Leukemia (Y_6)	.067	X_5, X_4, X_6, X_3, X_7, X_2
Buccal Cavity (Y_7)	.001	X_7
Skin Cancer (Y_8)	.027	X_1, X_7, X_3, X_6
Other Cancer (Y_9)	.567	X_8, X_2, X_3, X_7, X_4

X_1 = Population (*) X_3 = Income (**) X_5 = %<15 Years X_7 = % 46-65 Years
X_2 = Density (*) X_4 = % Black (*) X_6 = % 15-45 Years X_8 = %>65 Years

Transformations have been made to approximate normal distributions: * = log; ** = $\sqrt{\ }$.

[a]In order of importance in the model.

Thus, since both the diseases and the ecological variables change over time in their spatial distribution, very different forecasting models were used to predict disease distribution to 1980. These models are of the following form:

Given $CNCR_{67}$ = Total Cancer, 1967
$CNCR_{60}$ = Total Cancer, 1960
$CNCR_{80}$ = Total Cancer, 1980
STK_{67} = Stroke, 1967
STK_{60} = Stroke, 1960
STK_{80} = Stroke, 1980
HD_{60} = Heart Disease, 1960
HD_{67} = Heart Disease, 1967
HD_{80} = Heart Disease, 1980
$\delta_1 X_1$ = Coefficient of change in Population, 1960-1967
$\delta_2 X_1$ = Coefficient of change in Population, 1967-1980
$\delta_1 X_2$ = Coefficient of change in Density, 1960-1967
$\delta_2 X_2$ = Coefficient of change in Density, 1967-1980
$\delta_1 X_3$ = Coefficient of change in Income, 1960-1967
$\delta_2 X_3$ = Coefficient of change in Income, 1967-1980
$\delta_1 X_4$ = Coefficient of change in Per Cent Black, 1960-1967
$\delta_2 X_4$ = Coefficient of change in Per Cent Black, 1967-1980
$\delta_1 X_5$ = Coefficient of change in %< 15 Years, 1960-1967
$\delta_2 X_5$ = Coefficient of change in %< 15 Years, 1967-1980
$\delta_1 X_6$ = Coefficient of change in % 15-45 Years, 1960-1967
$\delta_2 X_6$ = Coefficient of change in % 15-45 Years, 1967-1980
$\delta_1 X_7$ = Coefficient of change in % 46-65 Years, 1960-1967
$\delta_2 X_7$ = Coefficient of change in % 46-65 Years, 1967-1980
$\delta_1 X_8$ = Coefficient of change in %>65 Years, 1960-1967
$\delta_2 X_8$ = Coefficient of change in %>65 Years, 1967-1980

Then from the 1960 and 1967 data:

$$CNCR_{67} = 1.15135 + (0.6298 * CNCR_{60}) - (1.5329 * \delta_1 X_2) - (2.1711 * \delta_1 X_3) \quad (16)$$

By substituting the above δ and β coefficients to a second set of elements, one obtains:

$$CNCR_{80} = 1.15135 + (0.6298 * CNCR_{67}) - (1.5329 * \delta_2 X_2) - (2.1711 * \delta_2 X_3) \quad (17)$$

Similar applications to Heart Disease and Stroke elements give:

$$STK_{67} = 0.1050 + (0.4577 * STK_{60}) - (0.0226 * \delta_1 X_5) - (0.8290 \; (0.8290 * \delta_1 X_1) + (0.0307 * \delta_1 X_8) + (0.0843 * HD_{60}) - (0.0423 * \delta_1 X_7) \quad (18)$$

$$STK_{80} = 0.1050 + (0.4577 * STK_{67}) - (0.0226 * \delta_2 X_5) - (0.8290 * \delta_2 X_1) + (0.0307 * \delta_2 X_8) + (0.0843 * HD_{60}) - (0.0423 * \delta_2 X_7) \quad (19)$$

$$HD_{67} = 0.1923 + (0.7196 * HD_{60}) - (0.2788 * \delta_1 X_2) - (0.0448 * \delta_1 X_5) + (0.0525 * \delta_1 X_8) - (0.0678 * \delta_1 X_7) + (0.0467 * \delta_1 X_4) \quad (20)$$

$$HD_{80} = 0.1923 + (0.7196 * HD_{67}) - (0.2788 * \delta_2 X_2 - (0.0448 * \delta_2 X_5) + (0.0525 * \delta_2 X_8) - (0.0678 * \delta_2 X_7) + (0.0467 * \delta_2 X_4) \quad (21)$$

Tables 24 to 26 contain the detailed statistics for the above models. The term "coefficient of change" and the "δ" symbol were utilized because the transformations from earlier equations were retained. The resulting coefficients are thus not precisely rates of change *per se*. The table does show that the coefficients of determination for Heart Disease and Total Cancer are similar to but higher than any previous R^2's for these diseases. Stroke, however, remains about the same as with previous Stroke models.

TABLE 24

REGRESSION FOR CALIBRATING HEART DISEASE SUBMODEL

Dependent Variable	Multiple R	Multiple R^2	Intercept A	Standard Error of Intercept	
Heart Disease, 1967	.774	.599	0.1923	0.0325	
Independent Variables	**Partial R**	**Standardized B**	**Regression Error**	**Metric B**	**Regression Error**
Heart Disease, 1960	0.666	0.6135	0.0422	0.7196	0.0496
Density Δ, 1960-1967	-0.416	-0.2981	0.0401	-0.2788	0.0375
% <15 Δ, 1960-1967	-0.378	-0.2657	0.0401	-0.0448	0.0068
% >65 Δ, 1960-1967	0.143	0.1991	0.0850	0.0525	0.0224
% 46-65 Δ, 1960-1967	-0.121	-0.1682	0.0852	-0.0678	0.0344
% Black Δ, 1960-1967	0.082	0.0531	0.0398	0.0467	0.0349

TABLE 25

REGRESSION FOR CALIBRATING STROKE SUBMODEL

Dependent Variable	Multiple R	Multiple R^2	Intercept A	Standard Error of Intercept	
Stroke, 1967	.545	.297	0.1050	0.0309	
Independent Variables	**Partial R**	**Standard- ized B**	**Regression Error**	**Metric B**	**Regression Error**
Stroke, 1960	0.317	0.3665	0.0676	0.4577	0.0844
% <15 Δ, 1960-1967	-0.221	-0.1934	0.0525	-0.0226	0.0061
Population Δ, 1960-1967	0.209	-0.1833	0.0527	-0.8290	0.2382
% >65 Δ, 1960-1967	0.092	0.1686	0.1127	0.0307	0.0206
Heart Disease, 1960	0.090	0.1038	0.0708	0.0843	0.0575
% 46-65 Δ, 1960-1967	-0.082	-0.1515	0.1129	-0.0423	0.0315

TABLE 26

REGRESSION FOR CALIBRATING CANCER SUBMODEL

Dependent Variable	Multiple R	Multiple R^2	Intercept A	Standard Error of Intercept	
Total Cancer, 1967	.668	.446	1.5135	0.1974	
Independent Variables	**Partial R**	**Standard- ized B**	**Regression Error**	**Metric B**	**Regression Error**
Cancer, 1960	0.600	0.5703	0.0465	0.6298	0.0514
Density Δ, 1960-1967	-0.298	-0.2369	0.0465	-1.5329	0.3009
Income Δ, 1960-1967	-0.137	-0.1030	0.0456	-2.1711	0.9601

Equations (17), (19), and (21) were applied to the 271 subareas of this study to obtain 1980 rates. Because the Heart Disease and Stroke rates resulting initially were actually Log_{10}Stroke and Log_{10}Heart Disease, the appropriate changes were made before the final forecasts could be tabulated. All presumed 1980 disease data have been included in Appendix E. The three measures first obtained were simply Stroke mortality rates, Heart Disease mortality rates, and Cancer morbidity rates. These rates were applied to the projected 1980 populations, and actual numbers of deaths or cases were estimated. The actual hospital allocations in the last chapter of this study are made on the basis of these estimates.

The spatial distribution of RMP diseases in 1980

Although the actual hospital allocations are made from numbers indicated in Appendix E, it is also useful to generate generalized statistical surfaces for these diseases for purposes of cartographic comparisons with 1960 and 1967 as well as establishing a visual frame of reference for actual numbers of deaths and cases forecasted. The method for generating these surfaces is, once more, trend surface analysis.

Six maps (Figs. 42 to 47) show expected spatial patterns for the RMP diseases in 1980. For rates, a similar technique to the 1960 and 1967 mapping was used, i.e., the mean incidence for 1960 is taken as a reference contour and patterns ranging above and below the means are shown with differing sets of patterns. However, for the 1980 maps means for previous years have been used to improve comparisons. The actual means for 1980 are shown on Table 27 along with the previous years. It is noteworthy that, given the limitations of the forecasting models and the "predictor" variables, the 1980 distributions show an expected increase in the incidence of both heart disease and stroke, while cancer may in fact drop somewhat. However, it is suspected on the basis of previous research that the cancer model is in fact underpredicting.

TABLE 27

THE MEAN INCIDENCE PER 1,000 OF RMP DISEASES
FOR ALL THREE TIME PERIODS

Disease	1960	1967	1980
Heart disease	3.52	3.45	4.24
Stroke	.75	.83	.90
Cancer	2.71	2.78	2.53

The anticipated 1980 Heart Disease incidence (Fig. 42) follows a pattern similar to previous years. The major difference is that mortality rates are expected to be higher. As in the previous years there is an incidence above the average in McHenry County and the City of Chicago and the inner suburbs. However, on the basis of the average for 1960, a new area of high incidence is expected to start spreading from the central city area southwestward into Du Page County, northern Will County, and the Aurora area. The areas of lower incidence remain much the same as previous years. Figure 43 then shows the range of deaths expected for each of the 271 subareas, i.e., each area is expected to have a number of deaths indicated by the range between contour lines on the map.

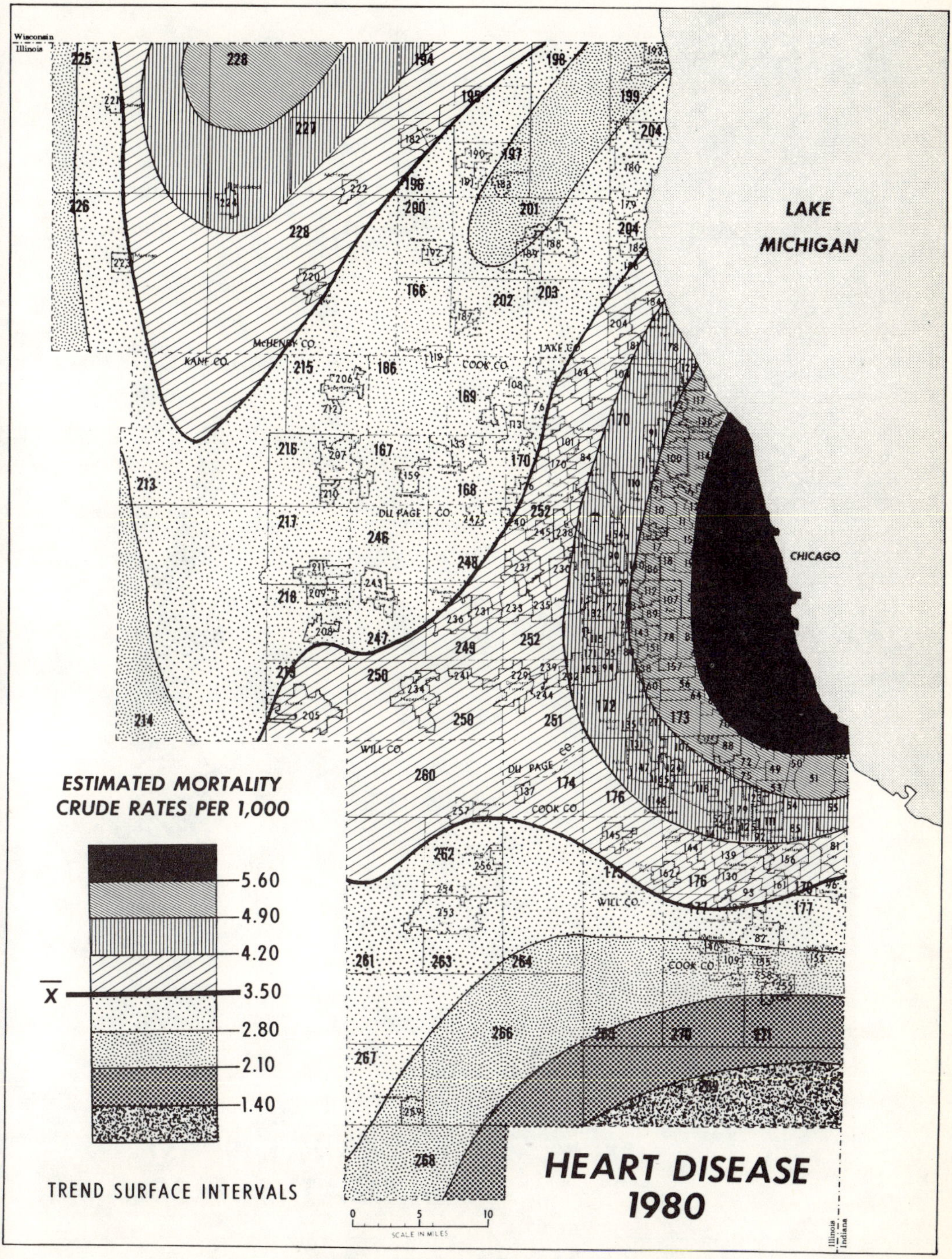

Fig. 42.--Heart disease mortality rates, 1980

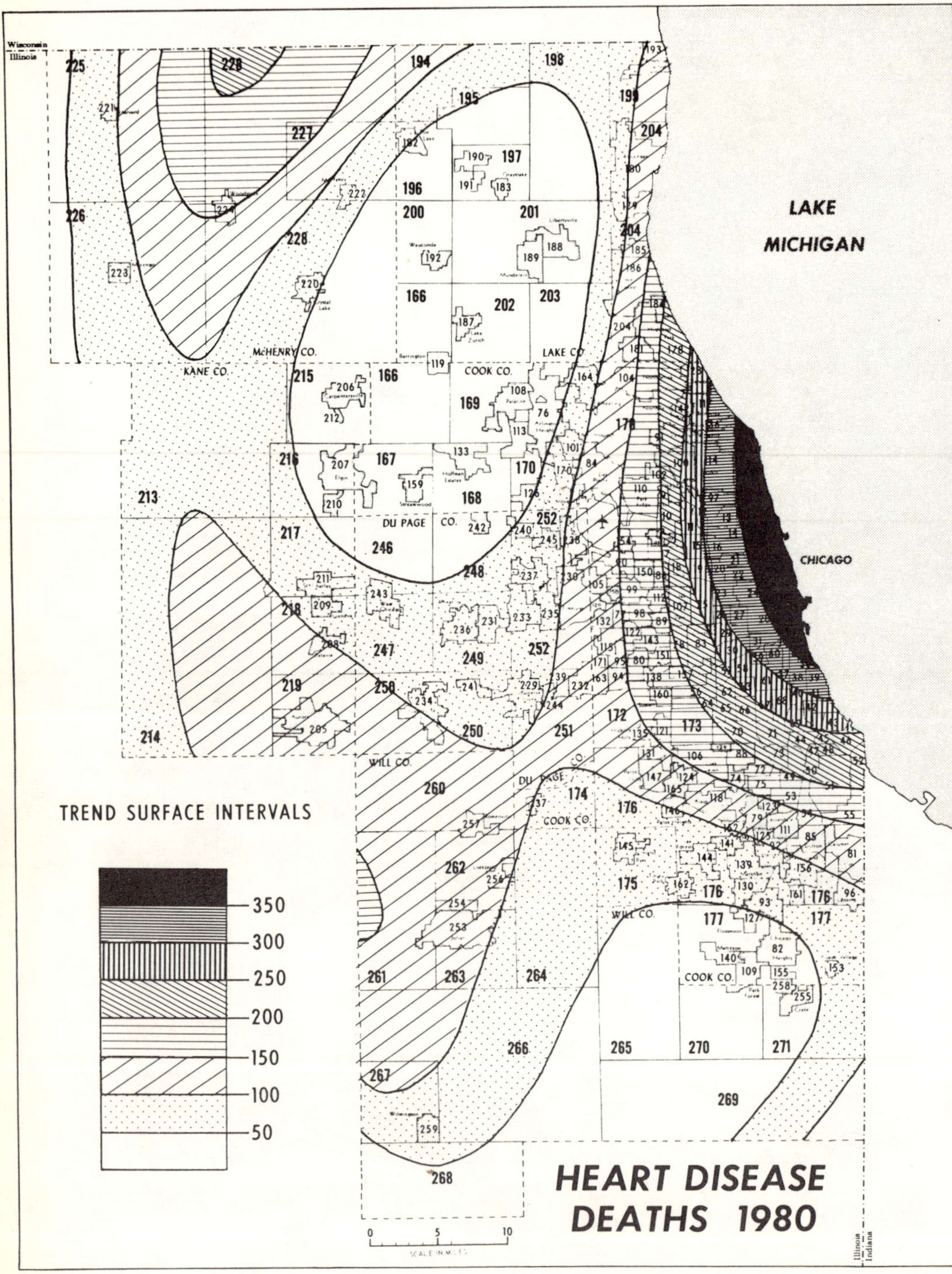

Fig. 43.--Heart disease deaths, 1980

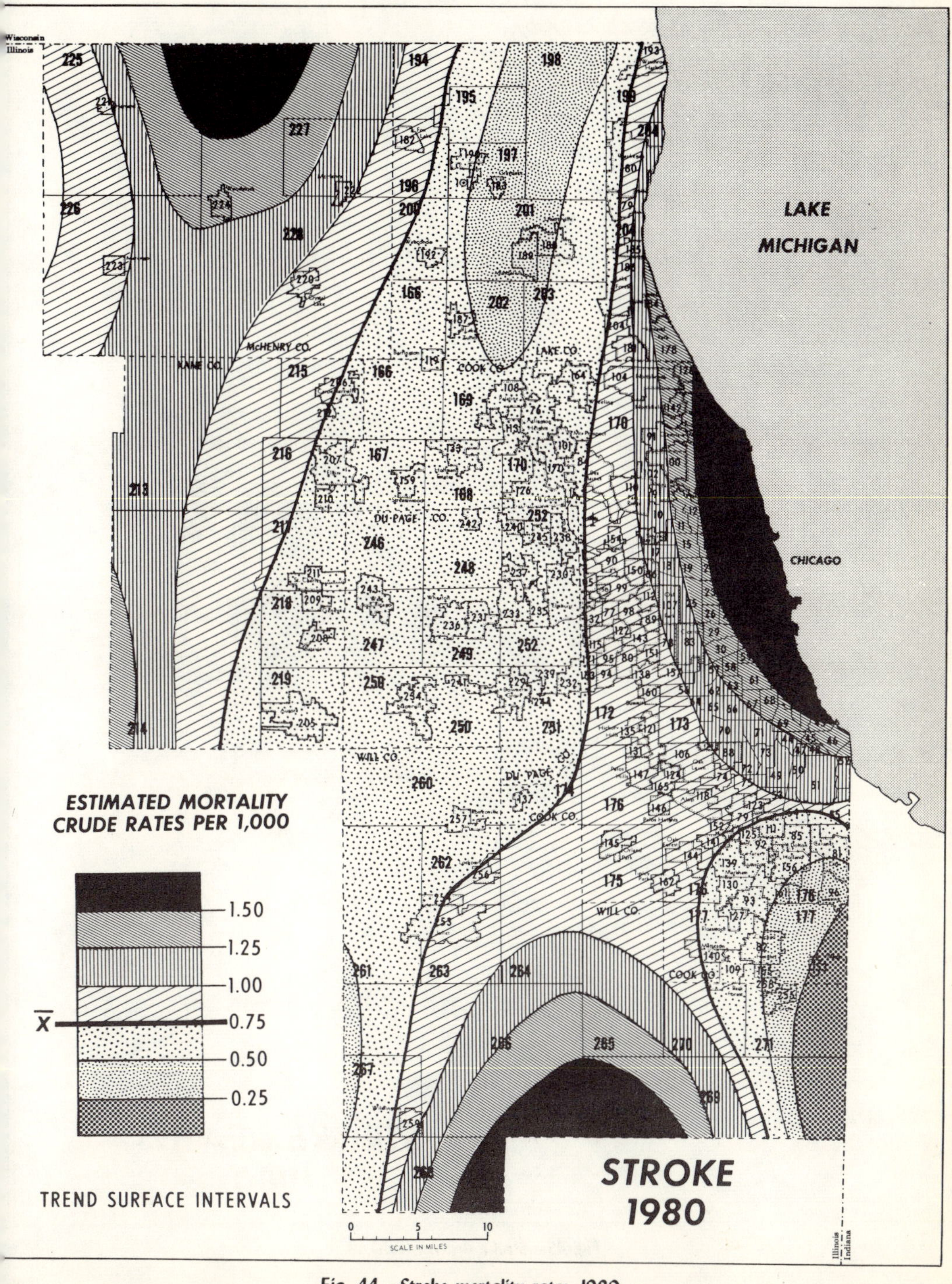

Fig. 44.--Stroke mortality rates, 1980

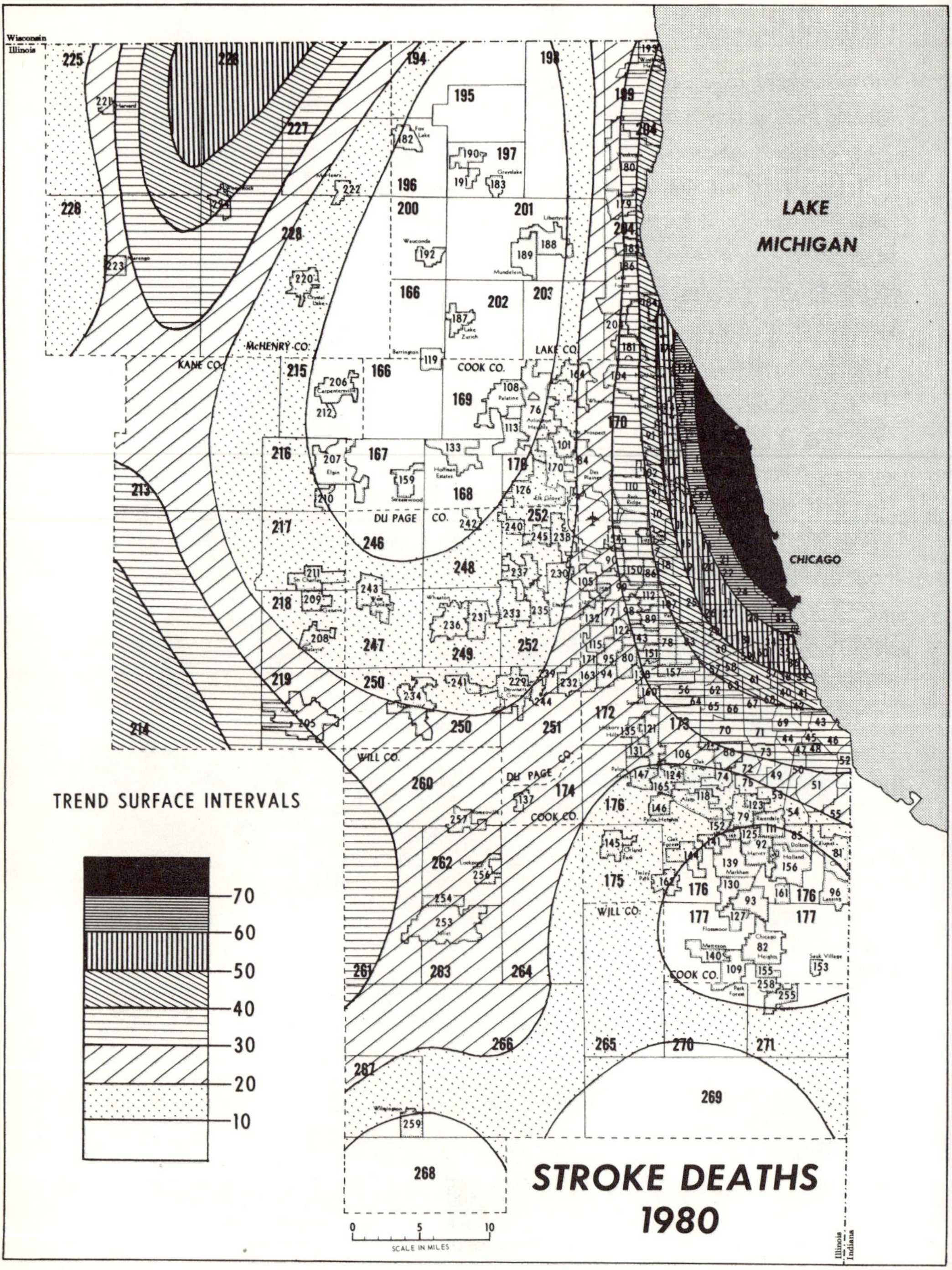

Fig. 45.--Stroke deaths, 1980

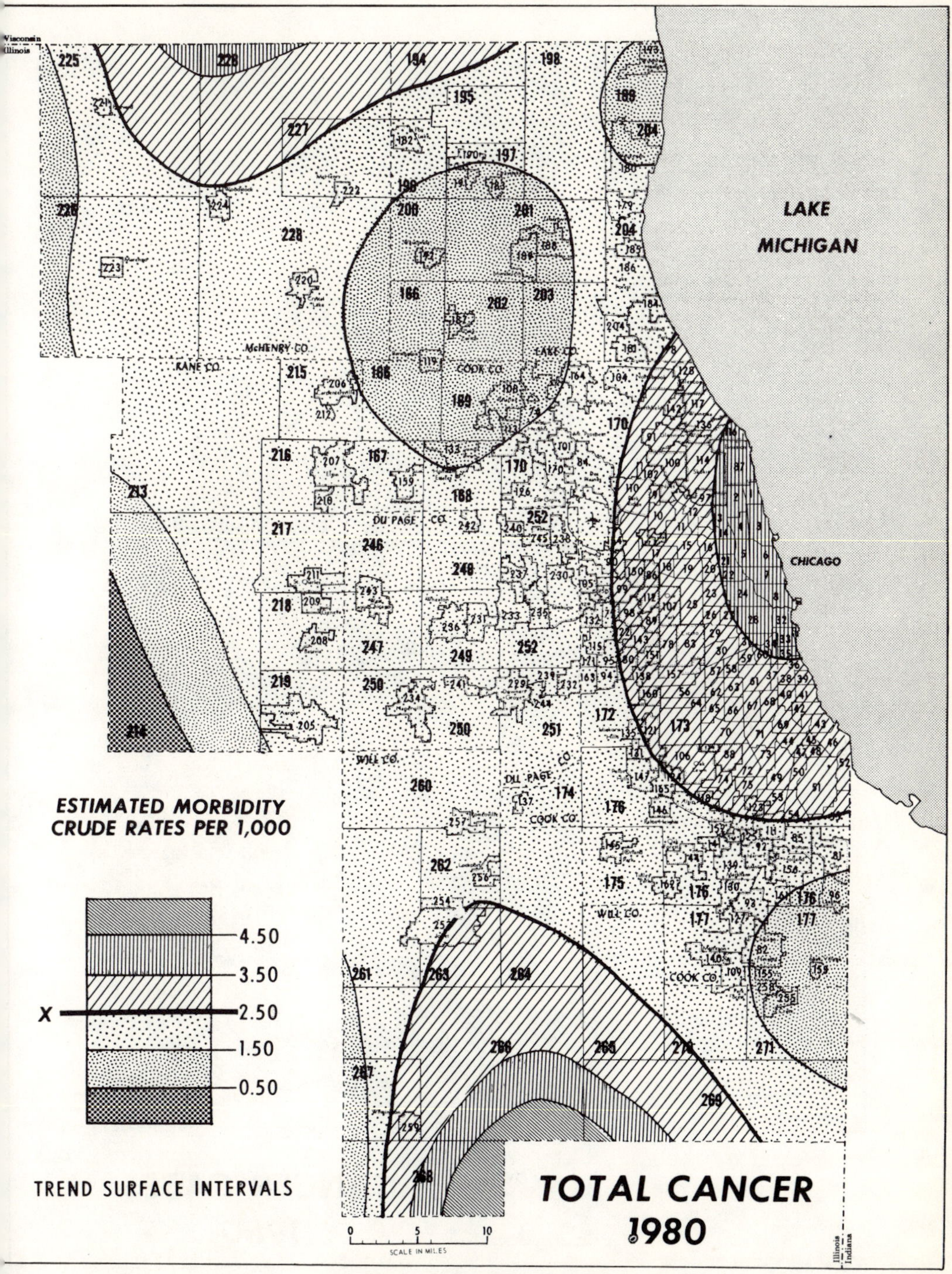

Fig. 46.--Cancer morbidity rates, 1980

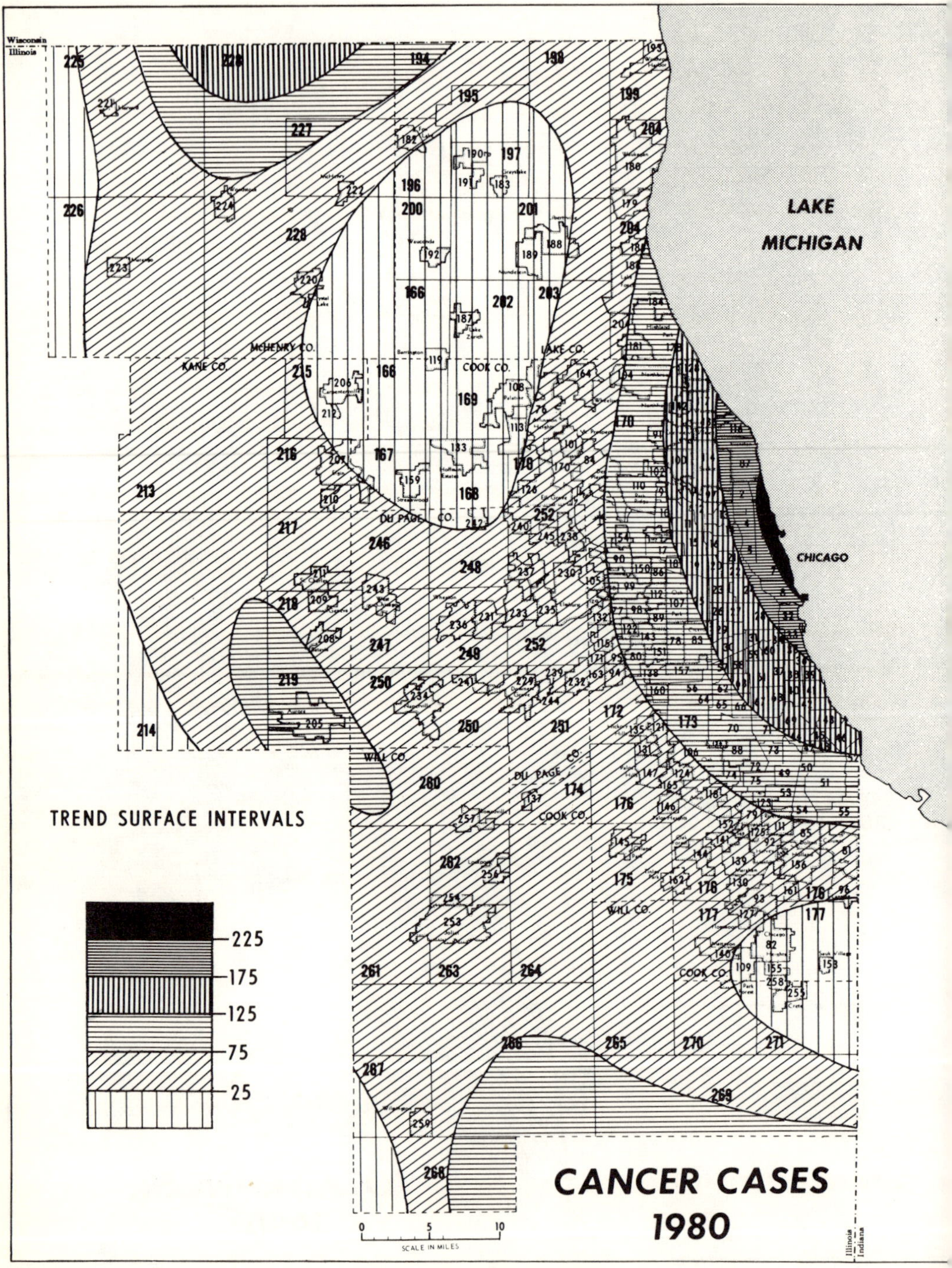

Fig. 47.--Cancer cases, 1980

The story for 1980 Stroke patterns (Fig. 44) is not unlike that for Heart Disease, as these two diseases have been consistently highly correlated at any rate. The pattern is essentially that of a more youthful outer suburban fringe showing lower rates and the central city and the rural fringe showing the higher rates. However, the outer suburban fringe for the southern part of the SMSA is expected to be "broken" by an extension of rates higher than the 1960 mean into that area. The actual number of deaths expected are shown on Figure 45. Once again, the pattern is similar to previous Heart Disease and Stroke maps.

The patterns for Total Cancer are also similar to past years; however, due to the apparent underprediction, the actual areas of higher than average (1960) have contracted (Fig. 46). The actual areas of higher and lower incidence than the mean are expected to remain about the same. Figure 47 shows the actual number of cases of cancer morbidity expected for 1980, and although this may be a rather conservative estimate, the actual areas with high cancer morbidity are probably fairly reliable.

No Heart Disease and Stroke morbidity estimates were attempted for the estimates of distributions in 1980 because of the reasons mentioned in Chapter II. When the actual allocations are made survival ratios based on hospital nursing home experiences will be used to obtain measures of morbidity. In general, the 1980 forecasts obtained should serve as fairly reliable mortality-morbidity inputs into the allocation model in Chapter VI, but it is first necessary carefully to examine the supply of treatment facilities in the Chicago SMSA and determine how these measures can serve as inputs to the allocation model. This is precisely the purpose of the next two chapters.

CHAPTER IV

CHARACTERISTICS AND DISTRIBUTION OF HOSPITALS IN CHICAGO

There are three features of the hospital system that must be understood for the supply side to be dealt with effectively in any planning model: (a) the internal effects of past growth; (b) the nature of the existing hospital hierarchy; (c) the comparative costs of differing sized hospitals. These topics are explored in this chapter.

The Dynamics of Hospital Growth and Change in Chicago

Hospitals in the Chicago area have been located in concentrations which follow urban growth along transportation lines.[1] The urban growth has moved outward from the older core of Chicago in the finger-like pattern shown on Figure 48. The crescent of industrial satellites has also experienced minor outward expansion. As shown on Figure 49, most of the supply of short-term hospitals potentially available for IRMP treatment are in areas urbanized by 1923. This means that the locations of much of the present supply were already determined 50 years ago, two decades before the beginning of area-wide health care facilities planning. Furthermore, because Public Law 89-239 specifically spells out "no new construction" for purposes of heart disease, cancer, and stroke treatment, many of the predetermined locations serve as constraints to the allocation model developed later in this study.

An additional complicating factor is that even within areas of older urbanization, the hospitals are not distributed evenly. Far more investment in hospitals has been made in neighborhoods with a higher income status over the years than those with lower status. As a result, there are many more hospitals to the north of Chicago's core than in any other single direction.[2]

---

[1]Vise, "Hospital Study Districts for Metropolitan Chicago."

[2]Richard L. Morrill, "Historical Development of the Chicago Hospital System," Chicago Regional Hospital Study, Working Paper I.2, December, 1966. Morrill came to the following more detailed conclusions about growth of the system from 1923 to 1965:

(1) The growth of new hospitals and the expansion of existing ones follows suburban and central city growth with a lag of about five years.

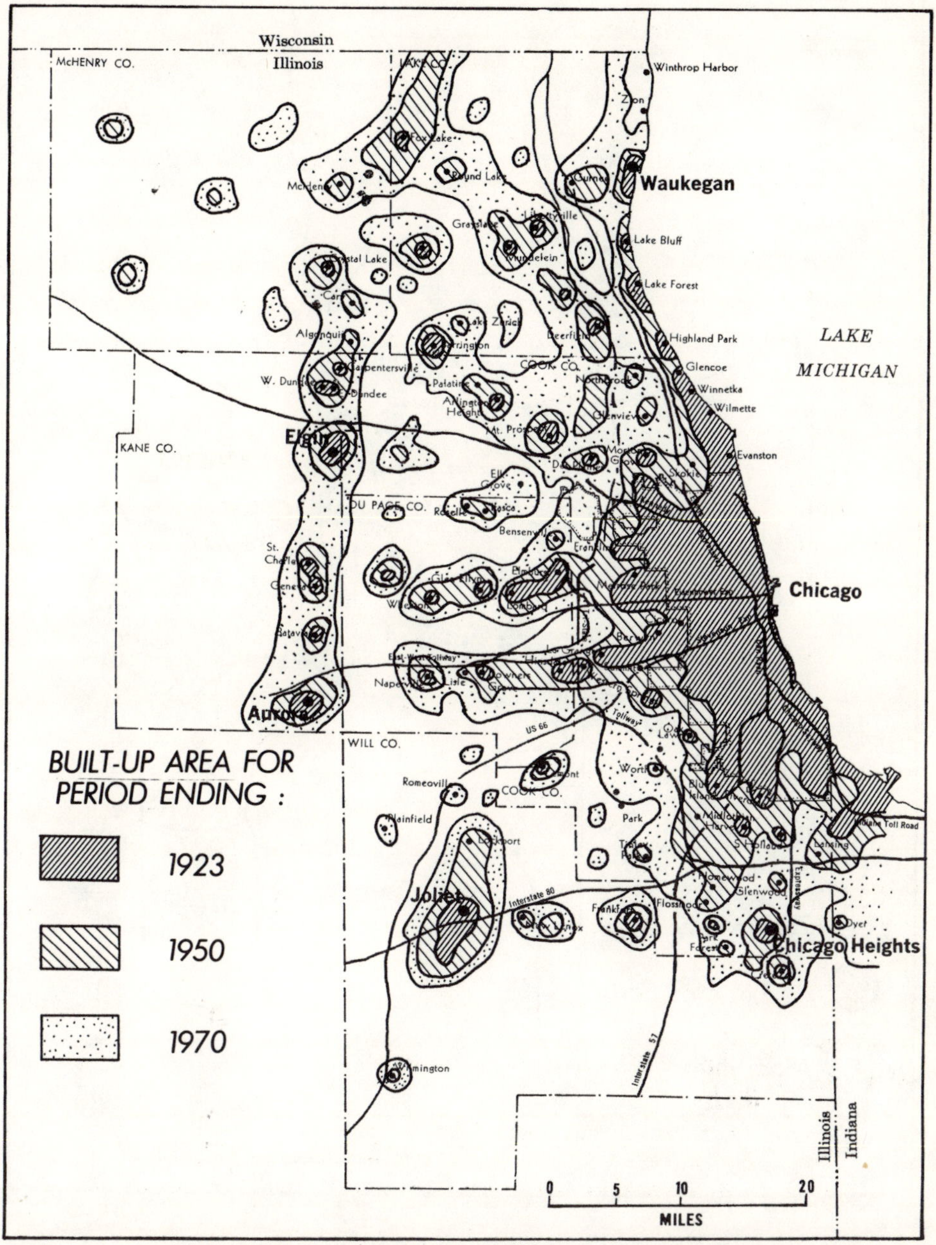

Fig. 48.--Built-up areas reflecting growth patterns in the Chicago SMSA

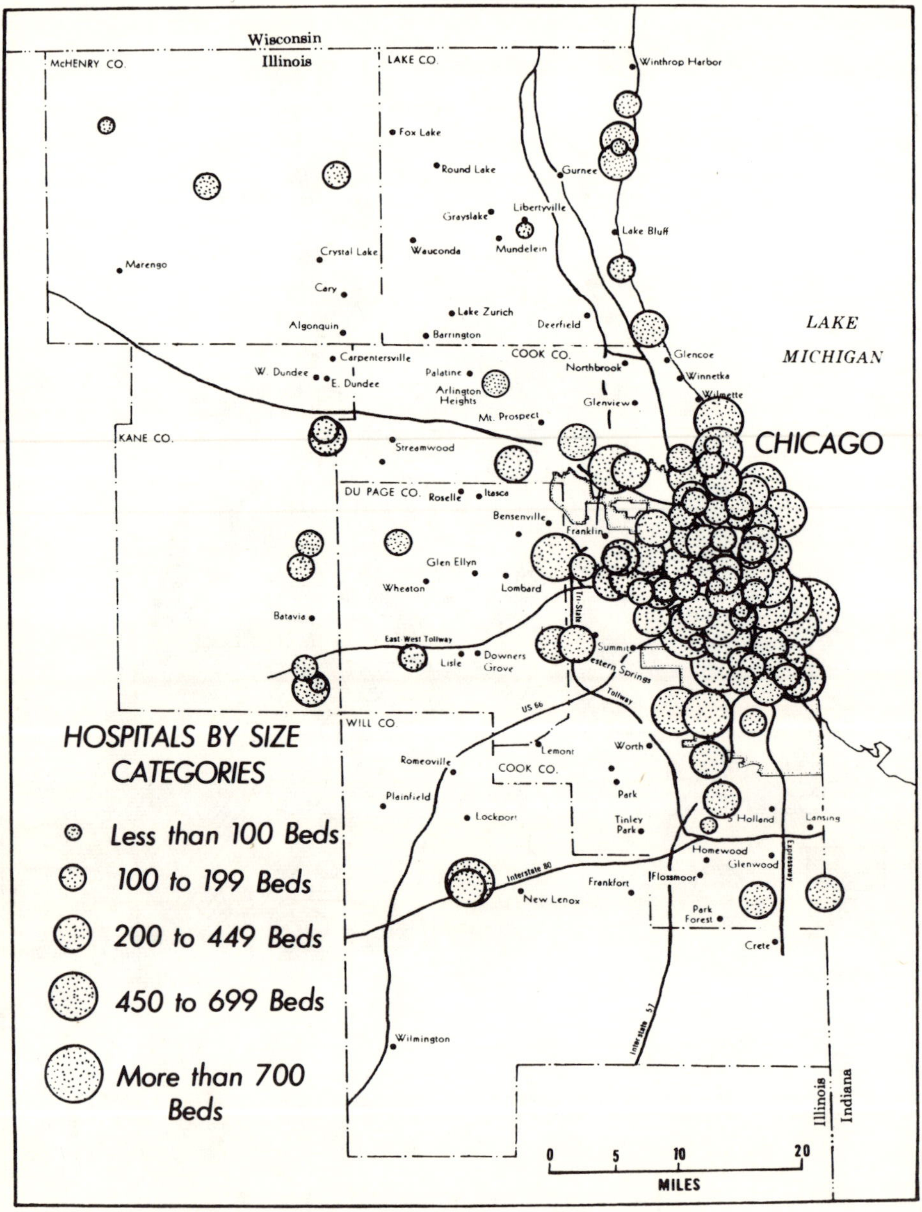

Fig. 49.--Hospitals in the Chicago SMSA classified by size

The basic nucleus of the area's hospital system was thus established by the mid-1920's, but as with the rest of the nation, growth was slowed by the Depression (Fig. 50). Within the inner city new hospital growth was to the north and south, and suburban hospital growth was concentrated in the northwest and the southeast. From 1920 to 1935 a substantial number of hospitals were actually added to the supply, but the Depression then caught up with construction. The city gained 16, and the metropolitan suburbs gained 14. The mean size at entry into the system was 83 beds, but it soon went to 98. During the same period 24 closed, and of these only 3 were in suburbs. The community population threshold was about 24,000. Also, during that period 6 hospitals, a little more than half of which were in the central city, expanded existing facilities. Clearly, considerable expansion within the system took place, but closures due to the Depression were also at an all-time high.

The period from 1935 to 1955 was one of fewer entries and fewer closures. The early part of this period was characterized by slow growth due to Depression and World War II conditions. After the war, much emphasis was placed upon expanding existing units, although there were many contractions of treatment facilities available, especially within the inner city.

From 1955 to the present time federal programs have aided the construction and expansion of hospitals in the area. Most new hospitals have been located in northern and western suburbs and on Chicago's north side. For comparative purposes Morrill divided the metropolitan area into subgroups (Inner City, Outer City, and Suburbs) and growth rates for these subareas are shown on Figure 50A. The graph indicates that since 1923 hospital growth rates for these areas have not been rising much except for suburban hospitals. However, Figure 50B shows the bed rate has been rising in keeping with national trends.

For the entire 1923 to 1965 period 71 new short-term hospitals opened and 54 closed. More entering hospitals were located in the City of Chicago than in the suburbs,

---

(2) New hospitals enter the system at a mean size of 103 beds, a figure slightly less than the 1965 average size. The threshold market for these hospitals is around 100,000 population.

(3) The total ratio of beds to population is stable, but there are subregional differences. Longer established inner city hospitals have higher bed-to-population ratios. Growing suburban areas tend to have lower but changing ratios. In general, a net shift from inner city to suburban areas is taking place.

(4) Hospitals which have closed have been smaller inner city ones.

(5) The overall mean size of hospitals has actually increased since the 1920's (a crucial period in the history of Chicago's hospitals) along with a shift in the proportion of suburban establishment. The actual number of institutions has remained fairly stable.

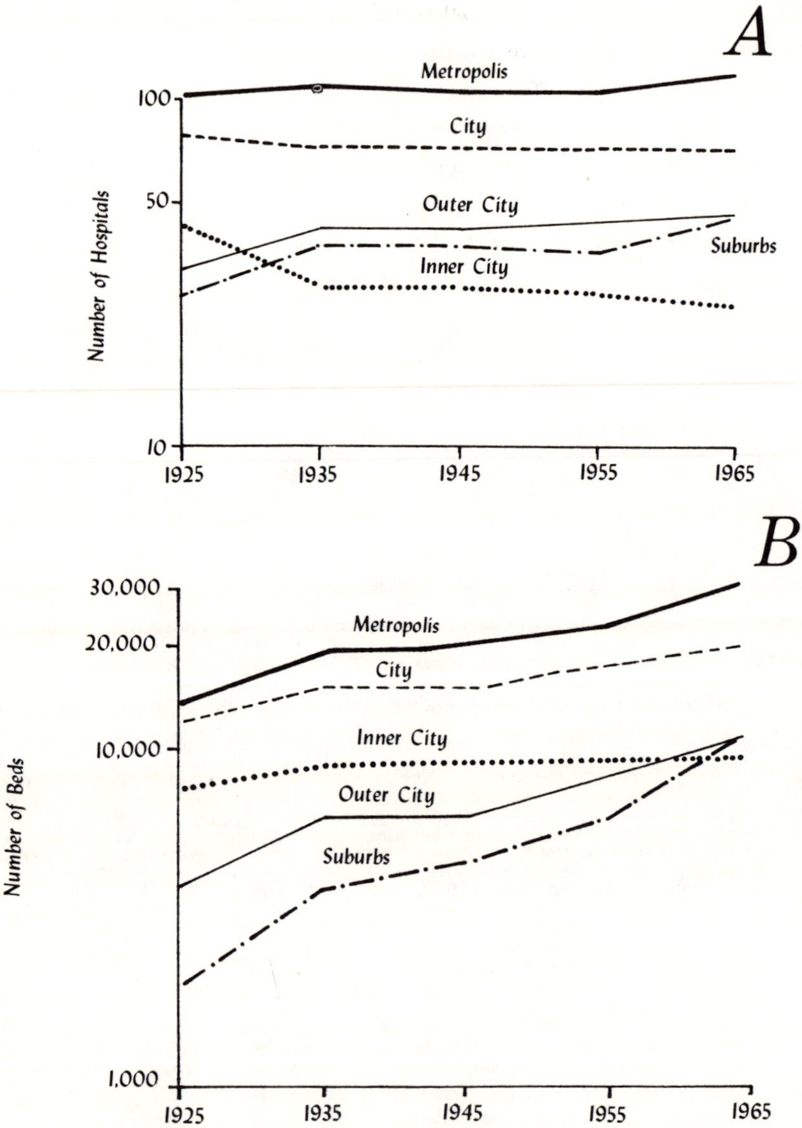

Fig. 50.--Growth of hospitals and hospital beds compared

but there were also more closures within the city. Of the new entries, 17 represent large hospitals with high level of care.

Ten were small and did not survive. In general most new entries were in growth areas. The threshold size for a community to support a hospital was 32,000 in 1965; however, the figure may be nearly double before any development takes place. There are many reasons for closure, the chief ones being small size, temporary need, over-specialization, financial failure, and obsolescence.

In many instances hospitals changed general functions and proprietorship. Also, hospitals took part in joint land acquisition efforts. The Chicago Medical Center on the west wide of the city is the best example of the above. Cook County and Presbyterian-St. Luke's were joined by the University of Illinois, Chicago State Tuberculosis, Veterans' Westside, Illinois State Pediatric, Illinois State Psychiatric, and Illinois Eye and Ear Hospitals by 1965.

The Hierarchy of Short-Term Hospitals and Their Use Patterns

One result of this growth history has been the emergence of a hospital hierarchy, the features of which also constrain future development plans.[1] The hierarchy consists of four major component groups (Table 28), and these groups can be clearly identified by measures of size and use characteristics.[2] The hierarchy was developed by Morrill when a previous study had shown the following facts:[3]

(1) Large hospitals with specialized care have wide attraction while small hospitals have strong local attraction.

(2) Physical location strongly influences patterns. Isolated or satellite hospitals generally have larger service areas than inner city ones of the same size.

It was further possible to measure these patterns of attraction by means of a selected sample of 30 hospital service areas.[4] The sample hospitals were intended to rep-

---

[1]Richard Morrill, "Hierarchy of Hospital Services: Classification of Hospitals," Chicago Regional Hospital Study, Working Paper I. 8, December, 1966.

[2]Richard Morrill and Robert Earickson, "Hospital Service Areas: General Patterns of Hospital Use," Chicago Regional Hospital Study, Working Paper I. 3, December, 1966.

[3]Richard Morrill and Robert Earickson, "Hospital Service Areas: Distance of Hospital from Patient Home," Chicago Regional Hospital Study, Working Paper I. 5, December, 1966.

[4]Richard Morrill, "Relationship Between Transportation and Hospital Location and Utilization," Chicago Regional Hospital Study, Working Paper I. 14, July, 1967.

TABLE 28

SHORT-TERM HOSPITALS MODIFIED FROM MORRILL FOR IRMP REQUIREMENTS

Hospital	Facilities*	Average Daily Census	Beds	Personnel
Group A: Major Research Hospitals				
1. University of Chicago	15	515	684	1,516
2. Michael Reese	17	779	886	2,839
3. Cook County	13	1,905	2,747	2,563
4. University of Illinois	12	403	591	1,229
5. Presbyterian-St. Luke's	16	724	838	3,775
6. Chicago Wesley Memorial	10	589	654	1,817
7. VA Research	4	498	545	1,065
8. VA Hines	10	291	360	766
9. Mount Sinai	16	320	383	1,340
10. Evanston	14	30	507	1,440
Group B1: Large Regional Hospitals, Moderate Specialization				
1. Illinois Masonic	11	456	530	1,524
2. Mercy	10	333	517	1,079
3. VA Westside	8	498	525	1,065
4. St. Joseph	11	460	488	1,065
5. Passavant Memorial	13	313	378	867
6. Columbus	9	334	408	670
7. Edgewater	13	341	389	1,117
8. Little Company of Mary	10	523	582	1,430
9. St. Francis, Evanston	10	410	505	1,107
10. MacNeal Memorial	12	384	419	939
11. West Suburban	11	339	377	810
12. Christ Community	10	469	616	1,244
Group B2: Regional Hospitals, Some Specialization				
13. Grant	11	289	339	657
14. Augustana	9	267	350	690
15. Illinois Central	5	204	299	430
16. Ravenswood	9	240	282	570
17. St. Anne's	11	329	436	798
18. Lutheran General	9	426	519	1,242
19. Norwegian-American	9	174	227	382
20. Swedish Covenant	10	204	235	585
21. Weiss, Louis A., Memorial	8	234	244	661
Group C1: Large Community - Non-specialized				
1. Memorial, Du Page	9	358	451	997
2. Victory Memorial	9	259	345	550
3. Sherman	8	300	350	793

TABLE 28--Continued

Hospital	Facilities*	Average Daily Census	Beds	Personnel
4. South Chicago Community	7	293	300	610
5. Ingalls Memorial	6	285	334	671
6. St. James	9	325	410	993
7. St. Therese	10	232	249	670
8. Silver Cross	9	270	276	714
Group C2: Community Hospitals - Some Specialization				
9. St. Joseph, Joliet	9	389	460	1,005
10. St. Mary of Nazareth	12	256	286	628
11. St. Elizabeth's	9	256	342	622
12. Hinsdale Sanitarium	10	291	360	766
13. Holy Cross	10	351	280	925
14. St. Anthony de Padua	4	170	208	446
15. Resurrection	9	225	264	564
16. American Hospital of Chicago	9	136	168	300
17. Evangelical	6	130	174	357
18. Loretto	8	137	163	377
19. Oak Park	8	196	241	576
20. Englewood	5	125	169	367
21. Loyola University	5	130	145	250
22. St. Francis (Blue Island)	10	233	336	843
Group C3: Smaller Community Hospitals				
23. Northwest	9	267	322	535
24. Provident	5	148	200	424
25. St. Bernard's	5	170	195	410
26. Walther Memorial	6	180	218	498
27. St. Alexius	8	138	225	436
28. Community Memorial, La Grange	9	190	244	463
29. Copley Memorial	4	171	200	543
30. Holy Family	6	169	248	437
31. Our Lady of Mercy	9	157	200	426
32. Belmont Community	3	120	151	273
33. Bethany Methodist	9	171	195	375
34. Louise Burg	4	92	100	209
35. Cuneo, Frank, Memorial	6	134	174	303
36. Franklin Boulevard Community	9	88	108	219
37. Garfield Park Community	4	120	141	300
38. Henrotin	6	131	192	316
39. Jackson Park	8	151	182	481
40. Roosevelt Memorial	8	133	152	244
41. Roseland Community	4	101	120	257
42. St. Frances X. Cabrini	6	154	214	389

TABLE 28--Continued

Hospital	Facilities*	Average Daily Census	Beds	Personnel
Group C3: Smaller Community Hospitals (cont.)				
43. St. George	3	91	122	206
44. South Shore	4	158	189	384
45. Mary Thompson	8	103	112	257
46. Martha Washington	6	66	108	175
47. Woodlawn	9	114	143	293
48. Central Du Page	9	100	115	197
49. Community, Geneva	9	78	115	242
50. Edward	8	100	133	239
51. Gottlieb Memorial	8	195	216	530
52. Highland Park	7	260	156	604
53. Lake Forest	10	93	137	272
54. Northwest, Arlington Heights	9	178	223	475
55. St. Charles	5	87	110	209
56. St. Joseph, Elgin	9	104	154	294
57. St. Joseph, Aurora	6	83	107	231
58. Skokie Valley Community	6	143	153	415
59. Westlake Community	6	103	132	234
60. Zion-Benton	6	61	101	151
Group D1: Small Inner City Hospitals				
1. Bethesda	7	125	151	270
2. Central Community	7	73	89	207
3. Forkosh, Syndey R., Memorial	4	135	150	250
4. Northeast Community	6	128	223	234
5. von Solbrig Memorial	6	43	88	85
6. Bethany Brethren	3	50	59	129
7. Community, Evanston	5	39	43	144
Group D2: Small Suburban Hospitals				
8. Condell Memorial	8	81	91	214
9. Memorial, McHenry	6	76	100	163
10. Delnor	6	64	105	177
11. Northlake Community	6	49	111	105
12. Lake County	4	32	49	67
13. McHenry	8	96	132	237
14. Harvard Community Memorial	2	33	40	72
15. South Suburban	8	49	56	126

Source: The hierarchical classification was modified slightly from Morrill, "Hierarchy of Hospital Services." The four columns of use data are for 1969. They were taken from Hospitals, Journal of the American Hospital Association, Vol. XLIII (August, 1969), Guide Issue for 1969, Part 2.

*Facilities include the following:

- Dental Services
- Pharmacy
- Premature Nursery
- Outpatient Department
- Emergency Department
- Post-operative Room
- Hospital Auxiliary
- Home Care Program
- Organ Bank
- Renal-dialysis, Outpatient
- Renal-dialysis, Inpatient
- Inhalation Therapy
- Volunteer Service
- Closed Circuit TV
- Intensive Care
- Self Care Unit
- Family Planning Department

represent various size groups, and as shown on Table 29, there are indeed clear-cut service-use categories. Identifying characteristics of the various hierarchical levels include:

Major research hospitals

These hospitals are all centrally located, and are the largest in the SMSA. They are all affiliated with medical schools. In addition, they possess a wide range and large number of facilities, and they have by far the largest number of employees. As indicated by Table 29 and shown by Figure 51, these hospitals show the very broad service areas and relatively shallow slopes one would expect. Cook County, however, shows a very steep slope due to extremely high demand.

Regional hospitals

All of the regional hospitals are large, have links to the area's medical schools, and have large staffs. In general, these hospitals are relatively close to the city center of Chicago, but some suburban hospitals are also included in this group. There are, in fact, two subgroups. The twelve hospitals of the B1 type have from 5 to 12 interns or residents while the twelve hospitals of the B2 type have from 2 to 4.

In general the service areas for these two types are similar. The regional hospitals with more facilities have somewhat broader slopes, but when found in clusters, the slopes steepen somewhat. Also some of these hospitals found in suburbs have steeper slopes.

Community hospitals

The community hospitals represent the norm for the Chicago SMSA. These 60 hospitals are the most ubiquitous. They are equipped to handle most health care needs. As indicated on Table 28 there are three subgroups: large community non-specialized; community with some specialization; and smaller community. The first of these subgroups

TABLE 29

POWER AND EXPONENTIAL DISTANCE DECAY FUNCTIONS COMPARED

Hospital Group	Slope	1 Mile			3 Miles			5 Miles			10 Miles			R^2	
		Pow	Exp	Act	Pow	Exp	Act	Pow	Exp	Act	Pow	Exp	Act	Pow	Exp
Special	1.47	20	12.5	14	7.1	8.3	8	3.4	5.1	5	1.2	1.6	1	.80	.95
Research	2.13	142	30	60	32	21	36	11	15	18	2.5	6	7	.87	.95
Small city	2.54	95	24	72	5.8	8.9	10	1.6	3.3	3	.3	.4	.3	.93	.86
Small suburb	2.51	75	22	42	4.8	9.5	12	1.3	4.1	5	.2	.7	.3	.90	.94
Cook County	2.61	795	334	380	129	156	170	34	73	50	5.5	16	20	.74	.89
Medium size	2.63	150	64	101	19	25	25	5	10	10	.8	1.1	1	.89	.94
Satellite	2.70	188	18	100	15	5	9	3.7	1.6	2	.6	.6	.5	.70	.66

Source: Morrill, "Relationship Between Transportation and Hospital Location and Utilization."

The first of these functions were determined using the gravity or "power" type model:

$$F_{ij} = A/D_{ij}^{b} \qquad (22)$$

where F_{ij} = number of patients from area i to hospital j
D_{ij} = distance between
b = slope

Here the model was used to describe the frequency with which hospital use decreases with increasing distance.

The second, or exponential, function utilized the model:

$$F_{ij} = Ae^{-bD_{ij}} \qquad (23)$$

The exponential functions proved to have a slightly better fit.

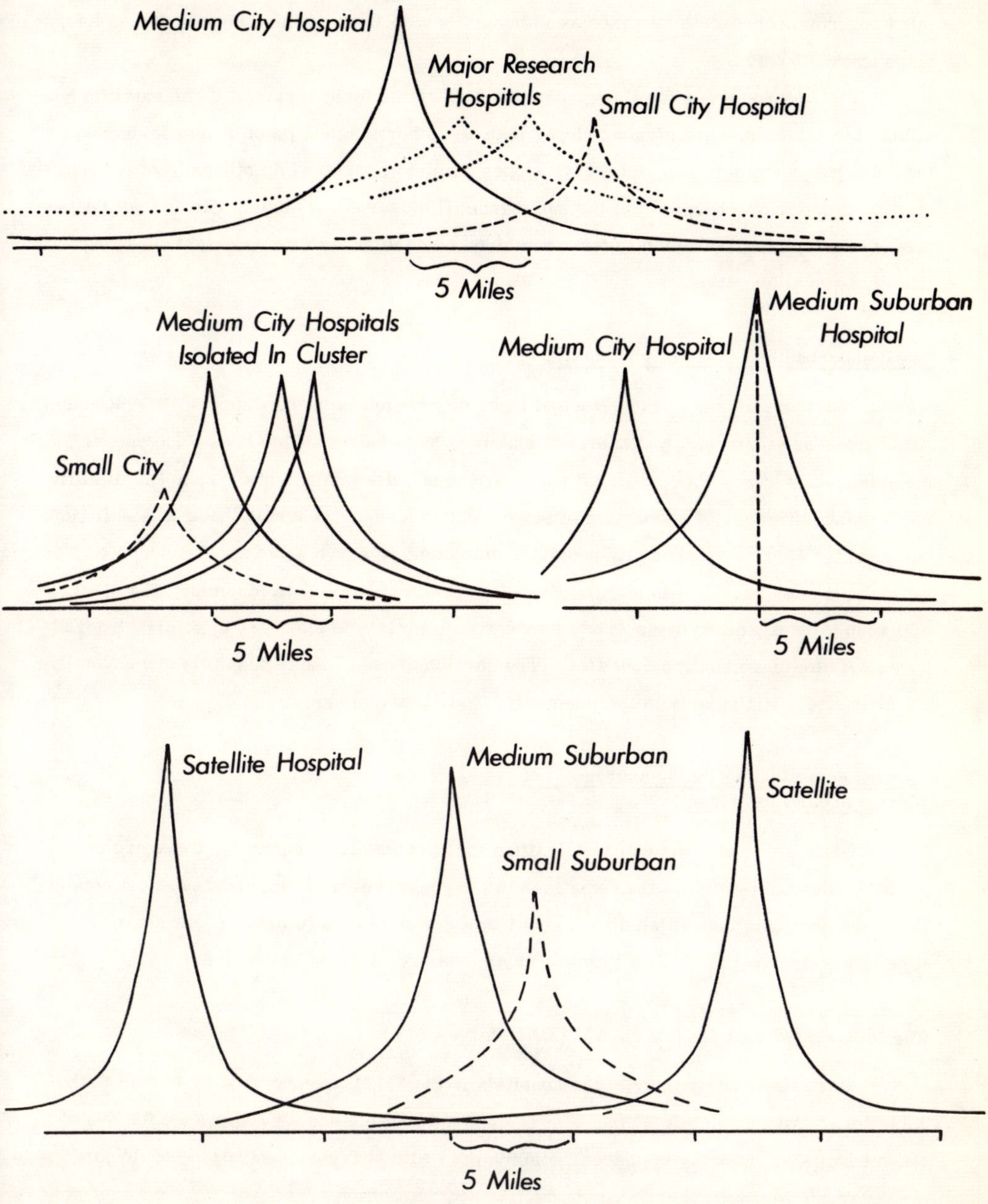

Fig. 51.--Distance decay 'demand cones' for classes of hospitals

contains the largest mean bed figure, 369 in 1969, but has fewer interns and residents. The second subgroup has more residents and interns and hence more specialization. The third subgroup represents 39 widespread hospitals with from 100 to 300 beds and no internships or residencies.

The service areas for this group also display the most variance. The satellite hospitals, for example, have steeper slopes than any other single type of hospital. Some of the suburban community hospitals have slopes almost as steep while others have slopes similar to inner city hospitals of the same general hierarchical class. Clusters of hospitals of this type in the inner city form combined service areas with an extent equalling that of regional hospitals.

Small suburban and inner city hospitals

There are 15 small suburban and inner city hospitals in the Chicago SMSA (Group D). All of these are quite widely dispersed, and most have less than 100 beds. In general these hospitals have a more difficult time attracting staff and patients. They find it difficult to take advantage of economies of scale, and as a result generally have less sufficient equipment. There are inner city hospitals which tend to serve some special purpose. For example, some specialize in serving the health needs of black patients only. The other subgroup is represented by suburban fringe area hospitals which cater to semi-urbanized areas with lower population densities. The service areas of these hospitals are normally not extensive, particularly in the inner city. Slopes are moderate.

Factors complicating the measurement of service areas in Chicago

While service areas can be identified for various class hospitals, there are complicating elements which cause variations in the general spatial alignments. Most notably, there are complications related to cultural patterns and those related to changes over time in service areas. In fact these two elements are at times interrelated.

The influence of religion and race[1]

More than one-quarter of the hospitals in the SMSA are operated by Roman Catholic orders. Approximately 60 per cent of Roman Catholics show a preference for one of these hospitals. In many instances, communities with heavy concentrations of Roman

---

[1]Robert Earickson, The Spatial Behavior of Hospital Patients: A Behavioral Approach to Spatial Interaction in Metropolitan Chicago, Department of Geography Research Paper No. 124 (Chicago: University of Chicago, 1970).

Catholics also house Roman Catholic hospitals. In other instances, Catholic hospitals in residential areas which have undergone changes from predominantly white Catholic to Negro continue to attract white Roman Catholics now living in other neighborhoods, e.g., Mercy Hospital.

There is apparently some mild preference amongst Protestants to utilize hospitals with no particular religious affiliation. Some 70 such hospitals are located in the metropolitan area. There are only 17 hospitals with a pronounced Protestant nature, and most are to be found in areas predominantly of German or Scandinavian Lutheran origin.

Secondly, cultural preferences can be related to health care units under Jewish direction or with large numbers of Jewish physicians. Four such hospitals (Edgewater, Michael Reese, Weiss, and Mount Sinai) draw heavily from such communities as West Ridge, Rogers Park, Skokie, Wilmette, and Morton Grove. Lutheran General and Skokie Valley hospitals also attract many Jewish patients because of community proximity. The capacity of the first four hospitals alone far exceeds the Jewish population, so that even with these examples the patient population is normally less than half Jewish.

The area's poverty neighborhoods are limited by the dual system to Cook County and a few other hospitals.[1] Nearly one half of all black patients are forced by poverty circumstances to either Cook County, VA Westside or Hines. The incredibly high demand for health treatment met by Cook County could easily be reallocated to other hospitals.

Changes in service areas

Morrill and Earickson have shown that patterns of hospital allegiance do not necessarily hold constant.[2] It was possible to compare data from 1961 and 1965 hospital patient discharge surveys to glean some notions about shifts in service area coverage. Five causes for change have been suggested.

Construction of new hospitals often causes transformation in the shape of service areas. New hospitals can apparently form service areas quickly. At times the new area may simply compress others; however, it can upon occasion seriously "act into" another hospital's former area of attraction. If sheer population growth in an area, particularly suburban, is the reason for a new hospital, there is an improvement in the composite pattern of service areas.

Change in the number of beds certainly alters the service area. If hospitals increase their bed complement, it could easily increase the size of their service areas.

---

[1] Vise et al., Slum Medicine.

[2] Richard Morrill and Robert Earickson, "Hospital Service Areas: Changes in Service Patterns Between 1961 and 1965," Chicago Regional Hospital Study, Working Paper I.6, December, 1966.

Conversely, if a hospital moves to another location, the communities of origin and destination will both display new patterns of use.

Racial and ethnic changes have affected the service areas of several hospitals. In many instances, the people who move out of neighborhoods still utilize the same hospitals, thus elongating service areas. If hospitals move out of communities due to racial change, this also obviously changes service areas.

Major transportation changes have caused modifications. New expressways contribute to a more dispersed population, and hence possibly larger service areas. Also, as people disperse they often want to change their hospital affiliation.

The spatial structure of use patterns

In spite of change in use, overall patterns for the SMSA can be effectively determined. The hierarchy of hospitals is clearly reflected in Figure 52, where Average Daily Census in 1969 is plotted against mean service areas in square miles in 1965. The slope of the relationship is nearly a perfect straight line fit. The major research and regional hospitals show obviously much smaller areas. This hierarchical relationship becomes very important when planning for new locations for RMP disease treatment, especially cancer facilities (Chapter VI).

Furthermore, these hierarchical relationships become very important in the allocation model-building process. As explained by Earickson:

> These distance relations demonstrate a meaningful, consistent, and significant behavior. They support the notion of an hierarchical spatial structure of hospital distribution in the Chicago area. The distance relations described were so homogeneous within a hospital type, and so consistently different between groups, that such findings can be safely incorporated into models of hospital use.

Hospital Cost Curves

Unit costs of hospital operation vary with hospital size as well as type of service performed. It is to be expected that the more intricate or demanding the service, the more sophisticated the hospital must be. Thus, the better equipped hospitals are usually the larger major research hospitals which tend to experience increasing returns to scale and, simultaneously, increasing costs of more complex facilities, but they do have available a greater range of services.

---

[1]Earickson, Spatial Behavior . . . , p. 58.

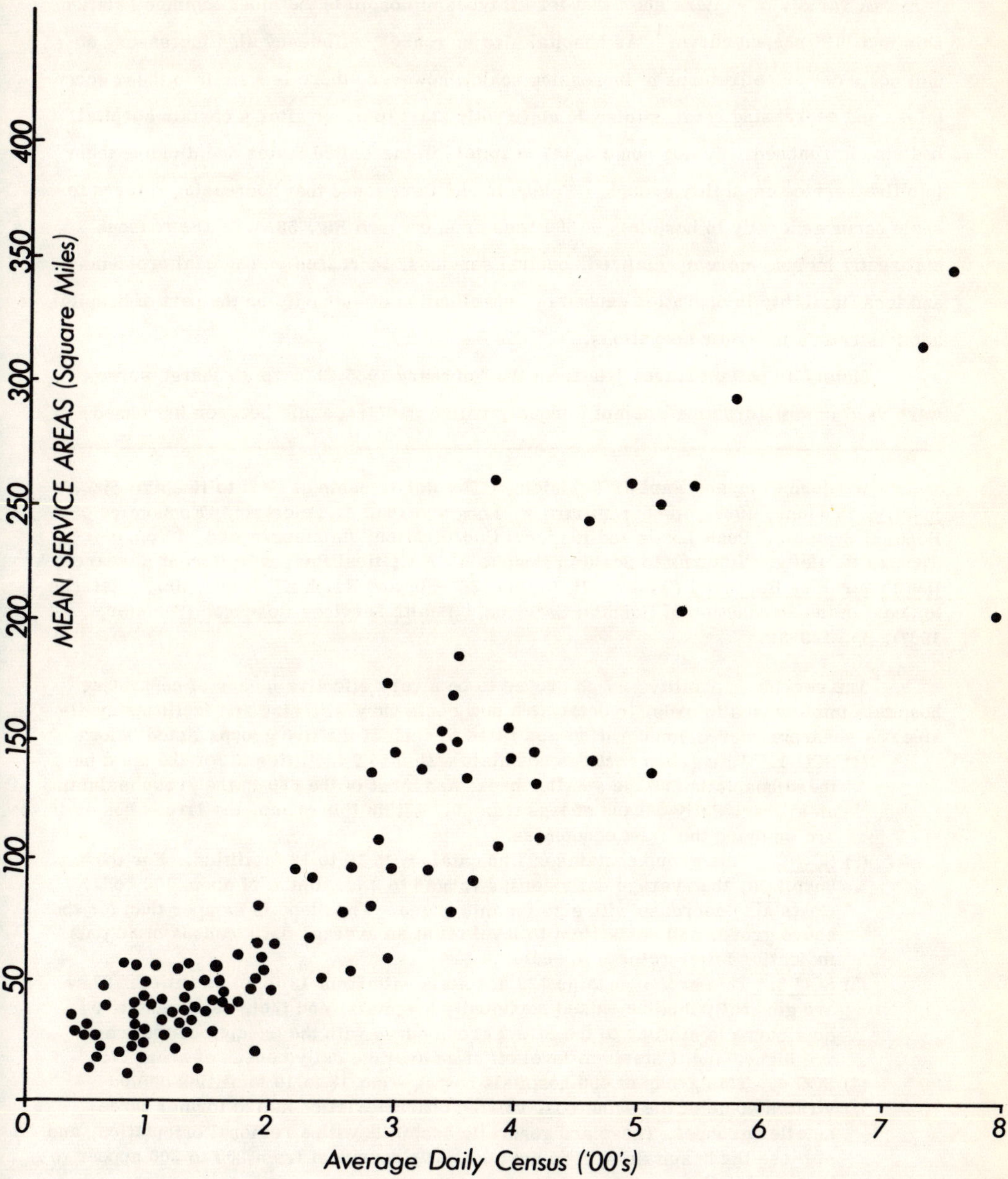

Fig. 52.--The hierarchy of hospital service areas

General contributions

A variety of writers show that for all types of hospitals the most common relationship is a "U" shaped curve.[1] As hospital size increases, efficiency also increases, so unit costs decrease (returns to increasing scale); however, there is a limit to these economies, and decreasing returns to scale apparently start to occur after a certain hospital bed size is reached. Taking some 3,147 hospitals in the United States and dividing them into five service capability groups,[2] Feldstein and Carr found that decreasing returns to scale occur generally in hospitals of 500 beds or more (see Fig. 53A). The reasons apparently include more specialized, central services, increased managerial problems, and less flexibility in operation caused by consolidation of authority on the part of hospital administrators in larger operations.

Maternity patient travel data from the February 1965 Chicago discharge survey were used in an interesting attempt to conceptualize the "trade off" between increased

---

[1] W. John Carr and Paul J. Feldstein, "The Relationship of Cost to Hospital Size," Inquiry, IV (June, 1967), 45-65; Millard F. Long and Paul J. Feldstein, "Economics of Hospital Systems: Peak Loads and Regional Coordination" (mimeographed, 17 pp.); Thomas R. Hefty, "Returns to Scale in Hospitals: A Critical Review of Recent Research," Health Services Research (Winter, 1969), pp. 267-80; and Ralph E. Berry, Jr., "Returns to Scale in the Production of Hospital Services," Health Services Research (Summer, 1967), pp. 123-39.

[2] The service capability groups proved to be a very effective means of separating hospitals into classes in order to determine how costs vary with size and facilities available. A separate regression equation was fitted to each of the five groups listed below:

(1) SCG 1. This group contains hospitals with 0 to 9 facilities. For the most part these hospitals are the smaller ones, and most of the 680 in the group maintain an average daily census of less than 60. Within this group, the larger hospitals are enjoying the most economies.

(2) SCG 2. This group contains 693 hospitals with 10 to 12 facilities. For these hospitals, the average daily census ranges to a maximum of about 100 beds. Costs also decrease with size for this group. The slope is steeper than for the above group, and costs start to level off at an average daily census of 80 thus indicating fewer returns to scale.

(3) SCG 3. This group contains 729 hospitals with from 13 to 16 facilities. They are generally medium-sized community hospitals, and their representative cost curve is similar to the SCG 2 group curve with the exceptions that costs are higher and it starts to level off at an average daily census of about 175.

(4) SCG 4. This group of 490 hospitals having from 17 to 19 facilities demonstrates some of the same cost-related characteristics as the former three smaller groups. These are generally hospitals with a regional orientation, and of these the hospitals with an average daily census of from 200 to 300 appear to be enjoying the most economies within the group.

(5) SCG 5. This group contains 555 hospitals with from 20 to 28 facilities. They are large regional and major research hospitals. It is with this group that diseconomies start to set in. Hospitals with an average daily census of more than 400 (about 500 beds) start to demonstrate a marked pattern of decreasing returns to scale. Herein lies the paradox, for these hospitals are generally capable of producing more and better health care than smaller ones.

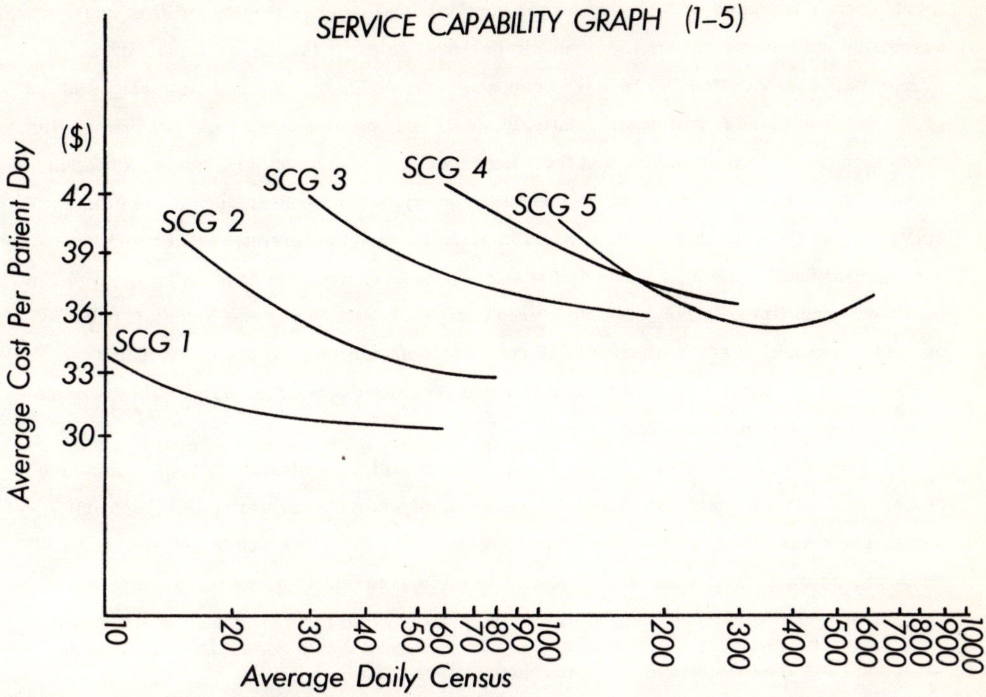

Fig. 53A.--The cost curves of various classes of hospitals

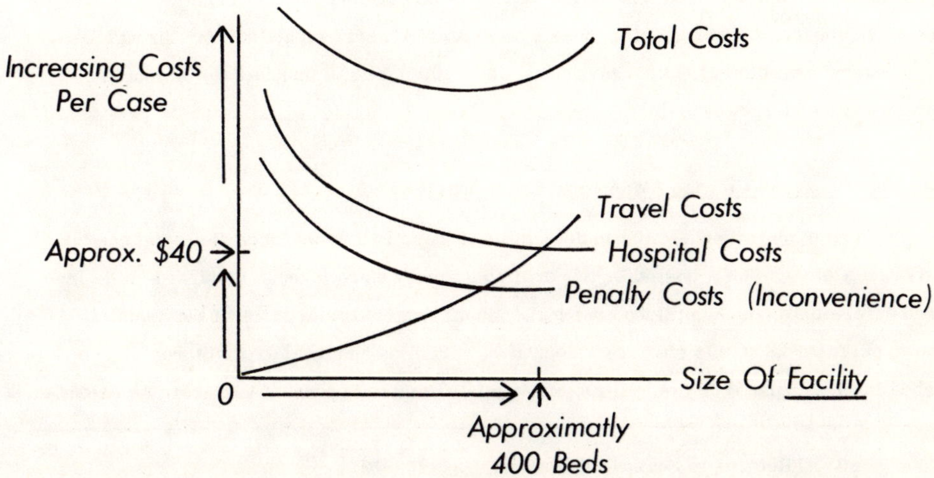

Fig. 53B.--The U-shaped hospital cost curve

travel costs associated with fewer, larger hospitals and the loss of economies of scale associated with more, but smaller, hospitals closer to patients. There is, of course, a well-documented relationship between occupancy rate and hospital size. Maternity and pediatric departments, with their relatively small bed complements, their predominantly random, non-elective clientele, and their high fixed costs, are prime examples of the high financial costs of empty beds, on the one hand, and the high inconvenience costs of unavailable beds, on the other hand. Many small maternity wards will reduce travel cost but will also increase empty bed costs and penalty costs of unavailable beds. Fewer large wards will reduce the latter costs but increase travel costs. Long and Feldstein have offered an optimal solution whereby maternity costs should be minimized, including the costs of hospital care, travel and inconvenience (Penalty Costs, Fig. 53B). This relationship is illustrated in Figure 53B.

According to Hefty in a review of recent research, the most recurrent explanation of long-run average costs for short term general hospitals appears to be the U shaped curve, and costs slowly rise beyond some optimal point within the 200 to 300 bed range. However, he warns that such studies should be applied carefully by planners:[1]

> Planning agencies should recognize the strong evidence for a U-shaped average cost curve for short-term hospitals, and should incorporate this knowledge into their decisions, but the evidence must be considered advisedly.

One reason for the higher costs incurred by larger hospitals is simply that they are providing much more in the way of services. Furthermore, cost, level of service, and hospital size are highly interdependent. Berry warns that in many instances costs of specific services are indeed less to the patient in larger short-term hospitals. The major obstacles appear to be identifying these less expensive services and cutting through sometimes excessive reimbursement programs which often tend to inundate the accounting departments of larger hospitals.

Aspects of cost for Chicago SMSA short-term hospitals

In an exploratory attempt to determine if there is a pronounced U shaped cost curve for Chicago SMSA hospitals, several approaches were taken. First, a simple linear regression was accomplished using the identifying characteristics of the hospitals shown on Table 28 of this study as independent variables and total expenditures as published in the August 1969 Guide Issue of Hospitals[2] as the dependent variable. As expected,

---

[1] Hefty, "Returns to Scale in Hospitals," pp. 278-79.

[2] Hospitals, Journal of the American Hospital Association, XLIII (August, 1969), Guide Issue for 1969, Part 2.

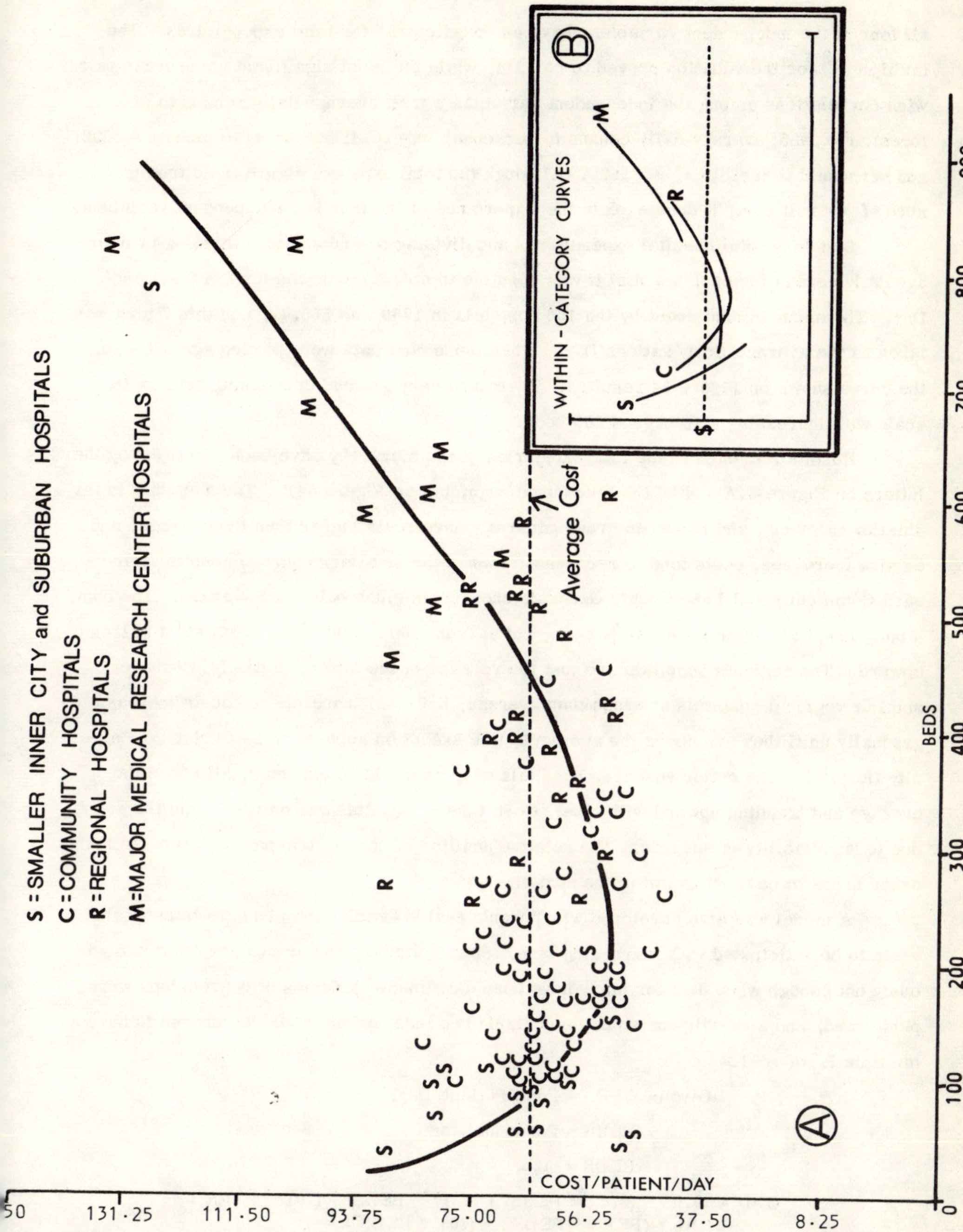

Fig. 54.--The Chicago hospital cost curve

all four of the independent variables serve as "predictors" for total expenditures. The multiple R^2 for the equation proved to be .914, while the most significant zero-order pairwise correlations among the independent variables were: average daily census to size (beds), r = .935; average daily census to personnel, r = .824; personnel to size, r = .692; and personnel to facilities, r = .625. Although the total expenses figure is no true measure of per unit cost, it does explain the importance of the four key independent variables.

By taking total hospital expenditures and dividing by 365 and then dividing by average daily census for each hospital it was possible to obtain measures for Cost/Patient/Day. The mean amount spent by the 106 hospitals in 1969 was $66.47, and this figure was taken as the average Cost/Patient/Day. When these cost data were plotted against size, the curve shown on Figure 54 resulted. There are very gradual decreasing returns to scale with increasing size beyond 200 beds.

Hospitals in each of the four categories of the hierarchy have been identified by the letters on Figure 54A and by the four curve segments on Figure 54B. The hospitals in the smaller inner city and suburban group generally have costs higher than the average, and as size increases, costs tend to decrease. Two of the smaller suburban hospitals, Harvard Community and Lake County General, show costs much below the average. The community hospitals show a similar pattern, but at from 250 to 300 beds, costs start to trend upward. The regional hospitals are just the reverse of the latter. Initially, costs for smaller regional hospitals are less than average, but as size increases, costs increase gradually until they are above the average. One exception appears to be Christ Community Hospital. The major research hospitals are, as would be expected, all above the average and trending upward with size. Cook County Hospital was omitted from the graph due to unreliability of records. The relative position of each of the groups within the hierarchy prove to be most useful in the next chapter.

A model was also developed which would enable health care planners to estimate costs to be anticipated with increasing size. Simply viewing one or two hospitals is obviously not enough when data for many have been examined. A series of regressions were performed, and a curvilinear equation utilizing two independent variables proved to have a multiple R^2 of .691:

Given: CPD = Cost/Patient/Day,

PERS = Personnel, and

BEDS = Size.

$$CPD = 59.05 - (0.41 * PERS) + (0.17 * BEDS) + (.01 * PERS^2) - (.01 * (PERS * BEDS)) - (.01 * BEDS^2) \qquad (24)$$

CHAPTER V

THE SPATIAL DISTRIBUTION OF MAJOR HOSPITAL TREATMENT FACILITIES FOR CANCER, HEART DISEASE, AND STROKE

In the previous chapter, it was possible to identify 106 hospitals within particular levels of a hierarchy in the SMSA. This chapter now takes a look at which hospitals within the various levels contain major treatment facilities for cancer, heart disease, and stroke. This inventory is utilized for the first in a series of allocations in the next chapter. Included with general counts of facilities are actual use data. These data can be projected to determine approximately how many additional facilities will be needed, since the patients expected by 1980 will exceed existing capacities if no new facilities are added.

Cancer Treatment

Major teletherapy units

Traditionally, surgery has been the primary method used in cancer treatment.[1] It has, in fact, increased in importance over the past two decades for many sites.[2] However, the method has now met limits in terms of the amount of tissue which can be removed and timeliness of operations. Figure 55 indicates the possible relative shares of surgery, radiation therapy, and other more common methods of treatment. When putting forth a plan for coordinating methods of treatment, Denoix points out the fact that some of the time there are no clear-cut divisions between type of cancer and method of treatment, and that often the method of treatment is dictated by the particular specialty of the physician first visited.[3] It should also be pointed out that various combinations of methods of treatment are increasing in number with advances in medical knowledge, and combining

---

[1] Shimkin, Science and Cancer; Sidney J. Cutler, "Trends in the Management of Cancer," Cancer Journal for Clinicians, XVIII (July and August, 1968), 189-204; R. J. C. Harris, Cancer (Baltimore: Pelican Books, 1962).

[2] L. Mannilla, S. Moles, P. Rentchnick, New Trends in the Treatment of Cancer (New York, 1967).

[3] Pierre Denoix, "The Organization of Cancer Treatment," in New Trends in the Treatment of Cancer, by Mannilla et al., pp. 165-72.

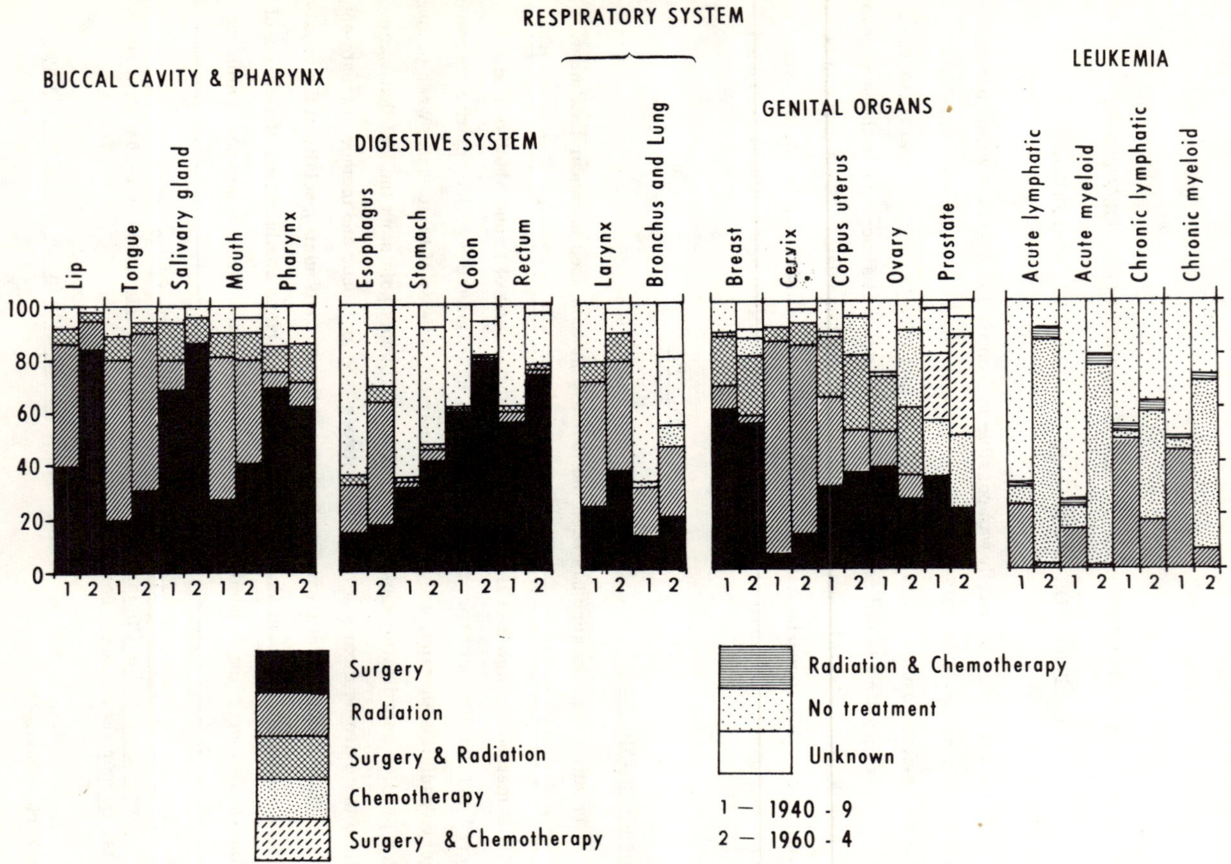

Fig. 55.--Types of treatment for various cancer sites in Connecticut

surgery and radiation therapy has become quite common. It has been estimated that from 50 to 60 per cent of all persons with cancer will probably have radiation therapy, either with or without surgery.[1]

Included within the categories of sites generally suitable for irradiation are three main groups of patients: the first is made up of those whose carcinoma has been detected early and is in a particular site suited to irradiation; the second is made up of those with a favorable site for irradiation and moderately early detection; the third contains those with surgery and radiation therapy. Usually there is hope of cure for these people. The second major type of treatment is considered palliative. Included within this category are patients for whom, either through late detection or a particularly difficult carcinoma, there is no cure presently possible. However, radiation therapy can do much to extend the lives of the latter persons, thus contributing greatly to the psychological need of the patients and their loved ones. Furthermore, it is sometimes simply not known if radiation therapy is a cure until it has been administered.

Schultz explains essentially three sources of radiation for cancer treatment.[2] The first are low energy x-ray units primarily used for the superficial treatment of tumors such as skin cancer. The second are medium voltage (previously called orthovoltage) units which were quite popular during the 1950's and before. They are now commonly used for moderately deep tumors and to obtain palliation. The third kind, now considered the most useful, are x-ray machines of one million volts or more. Better than 85 per cent of all of these so-called supervoltage machines in the United States utilize the artificially produced elements, Cesium 127 and Cobalt 60. Known to most hospitals as teletherapy units, these machines have to their advantage much greater versatility than any of the others mentioned.

In a recent contribution to Cancer, Stein has listed several advantages resulting from using teletherapy units:[3]

(1) Doses of radiation can be delivered at greater depths with little damage to overlying structures.

(2) Unlike with some of the lower voltage machines, severe skin damage can be avoided.

---

[1] "A Prospect for Radiation Therapy in the United States," Final Report, Subcommittee on Regional Medical Programs, October 24, 1968, 32 pp.

[2] Milford D. Schultz, "Radiation Therapy in the Clinical Management of Cancer," Cancer, XIX (January and February, 1969), 18-26.

[3] J. J. Stein, "Some Observations on the Logistics of Radiation Therapy for Cancer in the U.S.," Cancer, XIX (March and April, 1969) 96-97.

(3) Since control at depth is greater, there is less scattering of rays, thus preventing damage to surrounding healthy tissue.

(4) Cancer sites close to bone can be treated easily, because absorption per gram in the bone, unlike the other machines, is about the same as for soft tissue.

(5) Maintenance costs are relatively low.

(6) Teletherapy units can treat from 8 to 10 patients per hour.

The Cesium 127 and Cobalt 60 gamma ray sources are used in essentially two ways. One method involves the placement of small needles or tubes directly into tumors with subsequent delivery of a high dose of radiation. Another makes use of bombs, primarily Cobalt 60. Large amounts of Cobalt 60 are usually used as gamma ray beam sources, thus functioning as supervoltage x-ray machines. A cobalt bomb is considered essentially the same as a supervoltage x-ray machine, and these constitute most of the Chicago SMSA supply.

The Chicago SMSA supply of teletherapy units

In the spring of 1970, the Illinois Regional Medical Program made a survey of teletherapy units in the state. Some of the results of the survey are shown on Table 30. There are twenty-four major teletherapy installations in the Chicago SMSA. One is a free-standing installation (see discussion below), and the remainder are located in hospitals of relatively significant size. Twelve units are located in eight major research hospitals, and only two of the hospitals in this category did not report a teletherapy unit. None of these hospitals enjoy returns to scale (Fig. 54); however, the large numbers of professionals on the staffs compensate for this somewhat, and these are the places where most of the more difficult cases are treated. Eight regional hospitals account for nine units, and most of these hospitals also do not generally enjoy scale economies, but costs are somewhat lower than in the major research hospitals. Only seven community hospitals out of a possible 65 have units, and of these, the last three are the smallest and all have costs higher than the average for area hospitals.

Clearly, this numerical distribution of installations and patients represents a generally unplanned and uncoordinated situation. Although larger hospitals are carrying the heaviest loads, there is no equal distribution of units down the hierarchy to some reasonable size limit (see Chapter VI). In addition, some sort of upper limit would be expected as well for treatment. Cook County Hospital, long called a "dumping-ground,"[1] would appear to reflect this situation once more with cancer patients by carrying nearly three times the average number of patients with its two units.

---

[1] Vise et al., Slum Medicine.

TABLE 30

MAJOR TELETHERAPY INSTALLATIONS IN THE CHICAGO SMSA

Hospital	Teletherapy Patients, 1967	Level in Hospital Hierarchy[a]
Cook County	1210[b]	M
University of Chicago	720[b]	M
Michael Reese	243[c]	M
University of Illinois	210	M
Presbyterian St. Lukes	415[b, c]	M
Chicago Wesley Memorial	486[b, c]	M
VA Research	220	M
Evanston	224	M
Mercy	124	R
St. Joseph (Chicago)	198	R
Christ Community	250	R
Columbus	243[c]	R
Edgewater	194	R
Little Company of Mary	177	R
St. Francis (Evanston)	142	R
Lutheran General	535[b]	R
Memorial Du Page	187	C
Silver Cross	109	C
St. Joseph (Joliet)	79	C
Hinsdale Sanitarium and Hospital	245	C
Roseland Community	102	C
Lake Forest	250	C
Northwest Community	225	C
Eugene F. Lutterbeck[d]	326	–

Source: Survey made by the Illinois Regional Medical Program in the Spring of 1970.

[a]M = Major Research Hospital; R = Regional Hospital; C = Community Hospital; and S = Small Inner City and Suburban Hospital.

[b]Two installations.

[c]Average use on the basis of Chicago SMSA and surrounding area installations.

[d]Free-standing, privately-owned unit.

Other aspects of the hospital system which have been identified by the Chicago Regional Hospital Study and others are also reflected in the supply of teletherapy units. The University of Chicago installations are taxed to slightly beyond both the average use for the area and suggested numbers of patients made by the national Regional Medical Program.[1] There is duplication. In Joliet, for example, each of the two units is treating

[1]"Prospect for Radiation Therapy in the United States."

about half the average number of patients. One of the two Joliet hospitals has a Roman Catholic affiliation, and it would be expected according to Earickson's findings mentioned in the last chapter that this religious preference is reflected in the use of cancer treatment facilities. Roseland Community Hospital, with a known reputation for turning away charity patients is also treating about half the patients possible without exceeding the average number. Also, the three smallest hospitals with units do not enjoy returns to scale but are in higher status residential communities and can thus presumably better afford to have teletherapy units if they so choose or are perhaps endowed with one by a wealthy benefactor.

The spatial distribution of these installations is shown on Figure 56. Once again, the somewhat unplanned nature of the hospital system is reflected. There is only one installation in the Lake-McHenry County area, confirming the "medical wasteland" label recently applied by de Vise. The entire Fox River Valley settled area has no installation at all (compare Figs. 48 and 56). The entire south suburban area of Cook County is without an installation, and because of the selective nature of many hospitals, patients may have to make regular visits to hospitals 20 to 30 miles distant. The real test of the adequacy of the system of installations, however, comes in the next chapter where it is possible to compare the distribution of cancer and unmet need after initial allocations to the supply of treatment units.

Approximate costs of teletherapy installations

Recent concerns in communities over the adequacy of cancer treatment facilities have resulted in numerous studies related to the feasibility of establishing installations and specialized treatment centers. The major issue, once the need for new facilities is apparently recognized, is whether the proposed new units be connected to a hospital or free-standing. This concern is of no little import, for it may mean a difference of from $100,000 for a hospital unit to $1,000,000 for a free-standing unit.

Immediately a major exception comes to mind, but it is probably a one-of-a-kind operation--at least in the Chicago area. Two radiologists were able to invest in a Cesium 137 unit and have it installed in a Chicago Loop office for an investment of a little more than $100,000. The major advantages were that the physicians were able to obtain unusual financing, they did not have to buy land or build a structure, and the unit they purchased was somewhat less expensive than a linear accelerator.[1]

A study recently done in the Fox River Valley for the nine hospital association there showed that it would cost better than $825,000 for a free-standing unit and about

---

[1]Personal interview with Eugene F. Lutterbeck, April, 1970.

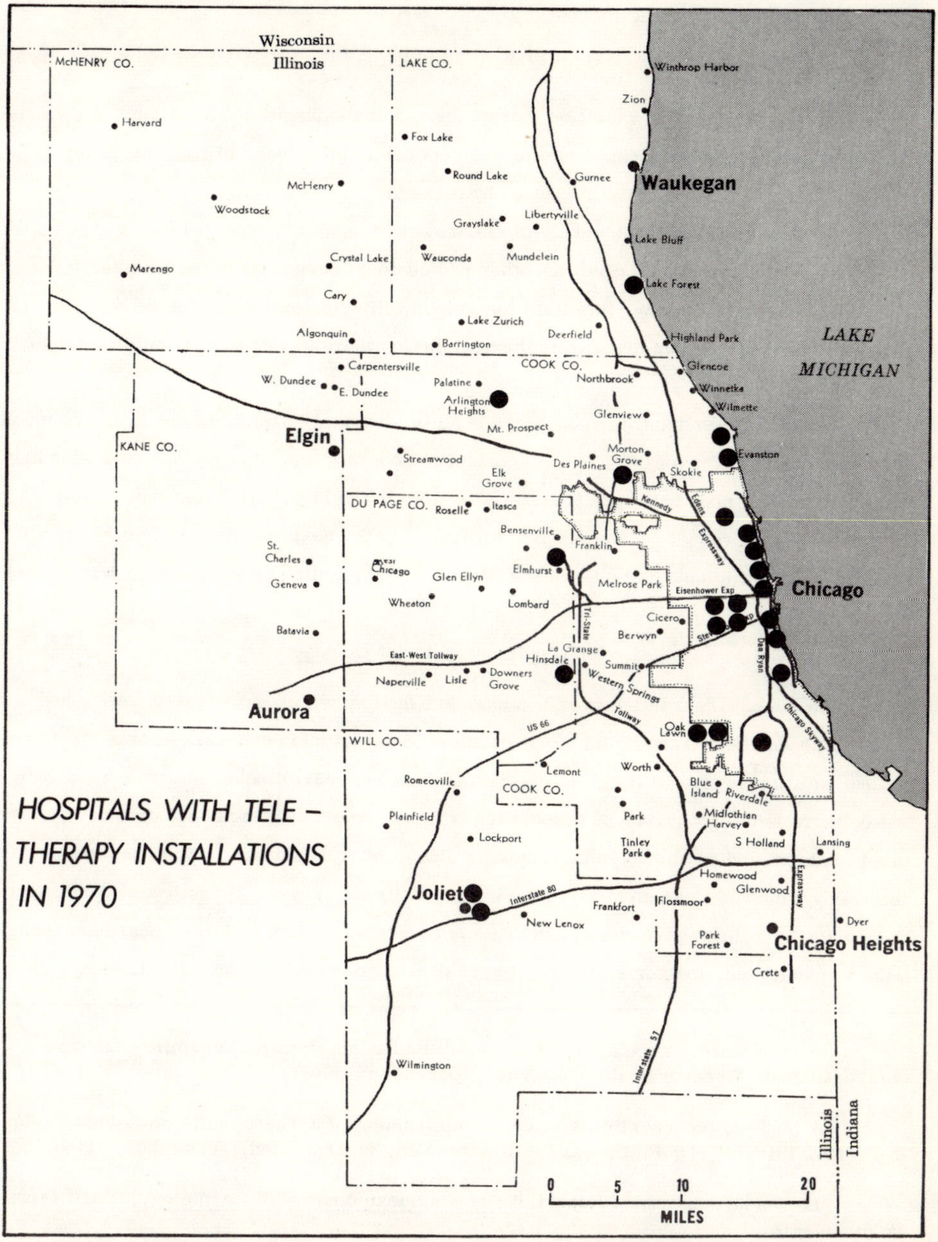

Fig. 56.--The distribution of teletherapy installations in the Chicago SMSA in 1960

$250,000 for a hospital-based installation.[1] Most radiologists appear to favor free-standing units. Conversely, a consumer orientation favors a hospital-based unit for several reasons. Some of these include:

(1) Access to medical and surgical treatment or any other combinations with little or no delay,

(2) Direct access of radiation therapy by any of the hospital's inpatients,

(3) Lower unit operating costs (e.g., general maintenance, billing, records),

(4) Use of other hospital facilities by patients,

(5) Maximization of the supply of medical and technical personnel,

(6) Direct communication with other professional personnel in the hospital.

Another recent study, this time for Peoria, Illinois, called for the construction of a very elaborate free-standing megavoltage radiation therapy unit which would cost a little more than $1,000,000.[2]

It would appear from the consumer point of view that hospital-based units are much more reasonable. Once again, it is important to note that there is only one free-standing unit in the SMSA, and it appears to be an exception to the high initial cost rule. New installations are needed. Locations are discussed in the next chapter with morbidity allocations. It is sufficient to mention here that all the new units proposed are in-hospital ones.

The Treatment of Heart Disease

The disease data in the previous chapters dealing with heart disease were concerned with mortality from most of the cardiovascular-related causes. As was mentioned in Chapter II, it is often difficult to distinguish between heart disease subgroups. Furthermore, there is a high degree of association between the general incidence of heart disease in a population and cardiovascular problems diagnosed in hospitals.[3] The phenomenon commonly referred to as an "heart attack" is usually a Coronary Thrombosis, a blockage of arteries by a thrombosis (clot) causing a coronary occlusion.[4] The myocardium (heart muscle) cannot function normally, and tissue degenerates and becomes functionally

---

[1] Herman Smith Associates, "Fox Valley Radiation Therapy Feasibility Study, Illinois" (Chicago: Herman Smith Associates, December, 1969).

[2] "A Study of the Feasibility of the Establishment of a Therapeutic Radiology Center in Peoria, Illinois" (La Jolla, Calif.: Enviro-Med, Incorporated, September, 1969).

[3] "Bethesda Conference Report," *The American Journal of Cardiology*, XXIII (April, 1969), 603-18.

[4] Gerald Falk *et al.*, "Hospital Treatment for Cancer, Heart Disease, and Stroke," Chicago Regional Hospital Study, Working Paper VII.3, 1970.

impaired. This condition is known as an infarct, and hence the term Myocardial Infarction is normally used as a synonym for "heart attack." There are, of course, related and other conditions as well as a variety of symptoms involved in a coronary thrombosis.

The delivery of hospital care for myocardial infarction and related conditions

It has been estimated that in the United States about 800,000 myocardial infarctions occur annually.[1] Half of these can result in death, and as many as 250,000 deaths could occur before a hospital is even reached. Kowal, et al., have explained this problem in the following manner:[2]

> The literature on cardiac arrests repeatedly has emphasized that success depends on rapid recognition of the arrest followed immediately by resuscitative efforts. The sooner the resuscitative procedure is started, the sooner the circulation is restarted and the greater the chance of success.

One problem is in the recognition of symptoms.[3] Another is in failure to attempt either to contact or to reach a doctor. Still another serious problem results when emergency service units are not fully equipped to deal with myocardial infarction.

Within a hospital, myocardial infarction means intensive care. This care may take place in separate intensive cardiac care units, combined general intensive and cardiac care units, or in general intensive care units in smaller hospitals. After initial attention, the primary care given is in various forms of intensive observation, intensive therapy, and heavy-duty nursing.[4] In cases where there are no complications, general therapy includes:

(1) Reassurance and Sedation. The psychological impact of what has happened to a patient requires high degrees of reassurance. The period of prolonged rest required often calls for sedation.

(2) Bed Rest. Usually a period of from two to three weeks bed rest is required with gradual exercise of unused muscles.

(3) Diet and Cigarettes. A specialized diet is started immediately, and cigarettes are forbidden permanently.

(4) Bowel Care. Straining is kept to a minimum.

---

[1] "Bethesda Report."

[2] John S. Kowal, Lawrence M. White, and Stanley A. Forward, "Cardiac Resuscitation Program," Hospitals, XLIV (May 16, 1970), 77-80.

[3] James K. Cooper, Knight Steel, and James P. Christodoulou, "Mobile Coronary Care - A Controversial Innovation," New England Journal of Medicine, CCLXXXI (1969), 906-7.

[4] "Guidelines for Coronary Care Units," Public Health Service Publication No. 1824, (Washington, D.C.: U.S. Department of Health, Education, and Welfare, July, 1968), pp. 19-22.

(5) Oxygen Therapy. Even with uncomplicated cases, oxygen is used in some hospitals for particular symptoms.

(6) Deep Breathing Routines. Periodic deep breath therapy aids some patients.

(7) Drugs. Several types of drugs are commonly used for control of blood flow.

(8) Monitoring. Several types of cardiac monitoring units must be employed.

The above measures are intended to prevent complications, but often complications already are present when treatment starts. Furthermore, some complications can develop even with good general treatment.

Coordination and use of personnel is another important aspect of cardiac care, and the amount and type of talent available for those purposes is heavily dependent upon hospital size (a commonly-used efficient threshold size is 200 beds).[1] Under optimum operational conditions, the following kinds of personnel would be required. A planning committee consisting of representatives of most hospital departments would decide policy matters pertaining to rapid emergency access to treatment, a referral system, and related matters. The medical staff should consist of a director of activities and staff physicians on call around the clock. In larger hospitals, the nursing staff would include especially trained registered nurses, backup nurses, well trained licensed practical nurses, and some nurses aids. In some of the smaller hospitals with intensive cardiac care facilities, a great deal of responsibility rests with all kinds of nurses, and most of them should be trained in using the equipment.

The physical design of intensive cardiac care units is also heavily dependent on hospital size. Normally, ICC installations are measured in numbers of beds. General hospitals of 200 beds or more would be expected to support at least one separate ICC installation. The ideal size of a unit is 6 beds, and if larger hospitals have or are planning more beds, groups of 6 ICC beds are the most efficient in terms of nursing stations. Provisions must be made for easy access to and constant visual observation of patients. ICC installations are best located close to emergency rooms and other kinds of intensive treatment facilities. The latter is critically important in larger hospitals without separate ICC units or in moderately-sized (100 to 200 beds) hospitals with smaller units of from 4 to 6 beds. Although it appears to be less economical to support units (separate or otherwise) of less than 4 beds in hospitals of less than 100 beds, the benefits of providing emergency care to people stricken with a myocardial infarction far outshadows any economies to be realized. It is possible and not uncommon to have 1 bed units in hospitals of the 50 bed range.

---

[1] Ibid., pp. 3-10.

An inventory of Intensive Cardiac Care units in the Chicago SMSA

Early in 1970, the Illinois Regional Medical Program made an extensive survey of all ICC units in the State of Illinois. The results of the survey include the actual number of ICC beds and the total number of patients treated for the calendar year, 1969. Data for the above measures for the Chicago SMSA are shown on Table 31. Also included on the table are actual ratios of ICC beds to total beds for the Chicago area hospitals. The average ratio for the 76 hospitals with ICC units is .024 ICC beds for each hospital bed. The 26 hospitals which have a ratio higher than the average are of all sizes except the smallest, and they are not concentrated in any one part of the SMSA.

There appears to be no particularly logical reason explaining either the ratios or their locations (see Fig. 57). The hospitals with the largest units are not necessarily the largest hospitals in the SMSA, and some of the smaller community hospitals have more beds than would be expected. However, the factors which appear to control the economic efficiency of ICC units are present. Only 13 of the units have fewer than 4 ICC beds. On the other hand, 34 units have from 4 to 6 beds, and 20 have from 6 to 9. It seems that if a hospital is to start a program for intensive cardiac care, a minimum of four beds is the most economical. Once again, however, this guideline may not always operate in favor of the consumer of health care who requires immediate attention.

Stroke Care Facilities

During the 1960's about 200,000 persons died annually from causes diagnosed commonly as vascular lesions affecting the central nervous system (ICDA 330-334).[1] Furthermore, the mortality rate of around 100 per 100,000 was highly seasonal, with more deaths during cold weather than warm.[2] Since a high proportion of stroke deaths are from persons over 65 with possible other complications, many users of mortality data have been somewhat skeptical of the efficacy of reporting stroke via death certificates. Fortunately, a recent study accomplished by 15 public health physicians helps to destroy any serious notions about artifacts of certification on any large scale.[3] Kuller et al. found in the

---

[1]D. M. Berkson and J. Stamler, "Epidemiological Findings on Cerebrovascular Diseases and Their Implications," Journal of Arteriosclerosis Research, V (1965), 192-202.

[2]Nemat O. Borhani and John S. Meyer, Medical Basis for Comprehensive Community Stroke Programs (Washington, D.C.: National Heart Institute and National Institute of Neurological Diseases and Blindness, June, 1968).

[3]Lewis Kuller et al., "Nationwide Cerebrovascular Disease Study," Stroke, I (March-April, 1970), 86-99.

TABLE 31

INTENSIVE CARDIAC CARE USE DATA FOR CHICAGO SMSA HOSPITALS, 1969

Hospital	Intensive Cardiac Care Beds	Intensive Cardiac Care Patients	Ratio: ICC Beds/ Total Beds
Cook County	8	(464)	.003
University of Chicago	7	400	.010
Michael Reese	8	(464)	.008
University of Illinois	10	(580)	.018
Presbyterian St. Lukes	5	700	.006
Chicago Wesley Memorial	8	270	.012
VA Hines	3	150	.002
Mount Sinai	8	365	.021
Evanston	8	630	.017
Illinois Masonic	10	(580)	.019
Mercy	8	(464)	.022
VA Westside	3	150	.002
St. Joseph (Chicago)	6	(348)	.021
Christ Community	12	440	.029
Passavant	5	275	.014
Columbus	7	(406)	.017
Edgewater	11	(638)	.028
Little Company of Mary	8	(464)	.014
St. Francis (Evanston)	4	240	.008
MacNeal Memorial	12	300	.028
Augustana	5	211	.014
Illinois Central	6	(348)	.020
Ravenswood	6	(348)	.021
St. Anne	4	(232)	.009
Lutheran General	8	450	.017
Norwegian-American	4	140	.021
Swedish Covenant	12	(696)	.051
Weiss	20	(1160)	.080
Memorial Du Page	9	561	.019
Victory Memorial	4	149	.011
Sherman	10	(580)	.029
Ingalls	8	494	.024
St. James	6	443	.014
St. Therese	5	(290)	.013
Silver Cross	3	75	.011
St. Joseph (Joliet)	4	302	.009
St. Mary of Nazareth	4	168	.008
St. Elizabeth	4	(232)	.019
Hinsdale Sanitarium	5	290	.014
Holy Cross	6	561	.016
Resurrection	6	459	.023
American	8	(464)	.047
Oak Park	4	343	.017
Englewood	5	(290)	.038
Northwest Hospital	4	(232)	.014
St. Bernard	2	(116)	.010

TABLE 31--Continued

Hospital	Intensive Cardiac Care Beds	Intensive Cardiac Care Patients	Ratio: ICC Beds/ Total Beds
Walther Memorial	8	210	.036
St. Alexius	4	(232)	.020
Community General (La Grange)	6	(348)	.027
Copley Memorial	2	120	.010
Holy Family	2	275	.008
Belmont Community	7	(406)	.046
Bethany Methodist	1	(58)	.006
Henrotin	4	(232)	.038
Jackson Park	3	(174)	.018
Roosevelt Memorial	11	(638)	.088
St. Frances X. Cabrini	4	(232)	.019
South Shore	9	(522)	.048
Woodlawn	4	(232)	.027
Central Du Page	3	150	.026
Geneva Community	4	110	.035
Grant	4	(232)	.012
Gottlieb	5	(290)	.023
Highland Park	6	375	.031
Lake Forest	6	159	.053
Northwest Community	4	(232)	.018
St. Francis (Blue Island)	1	(58)	.004
St. Joseph (Elgin)	4	(232)	.026
St. Joseph (Aurora)	3	140	.028
Zion-Benton	2	(116)	.019
Bethesda	4	(232)	.028
Central Community	4	(232)	.043
Condell Memorial	4	157	.044
Memorial McHenry	2	(116)	.020
Delnor	4	121	.038
South Suburban	5	(290)	.089

Source: Survey made in 1970 by the Illinois Regional Medical Program. The ICC patients shown in parentheses are estimates made due to nonreporting of numbers. The multiplicative constant used was the Chicago SMSA average of 58 patients per ICC bed treated annually.

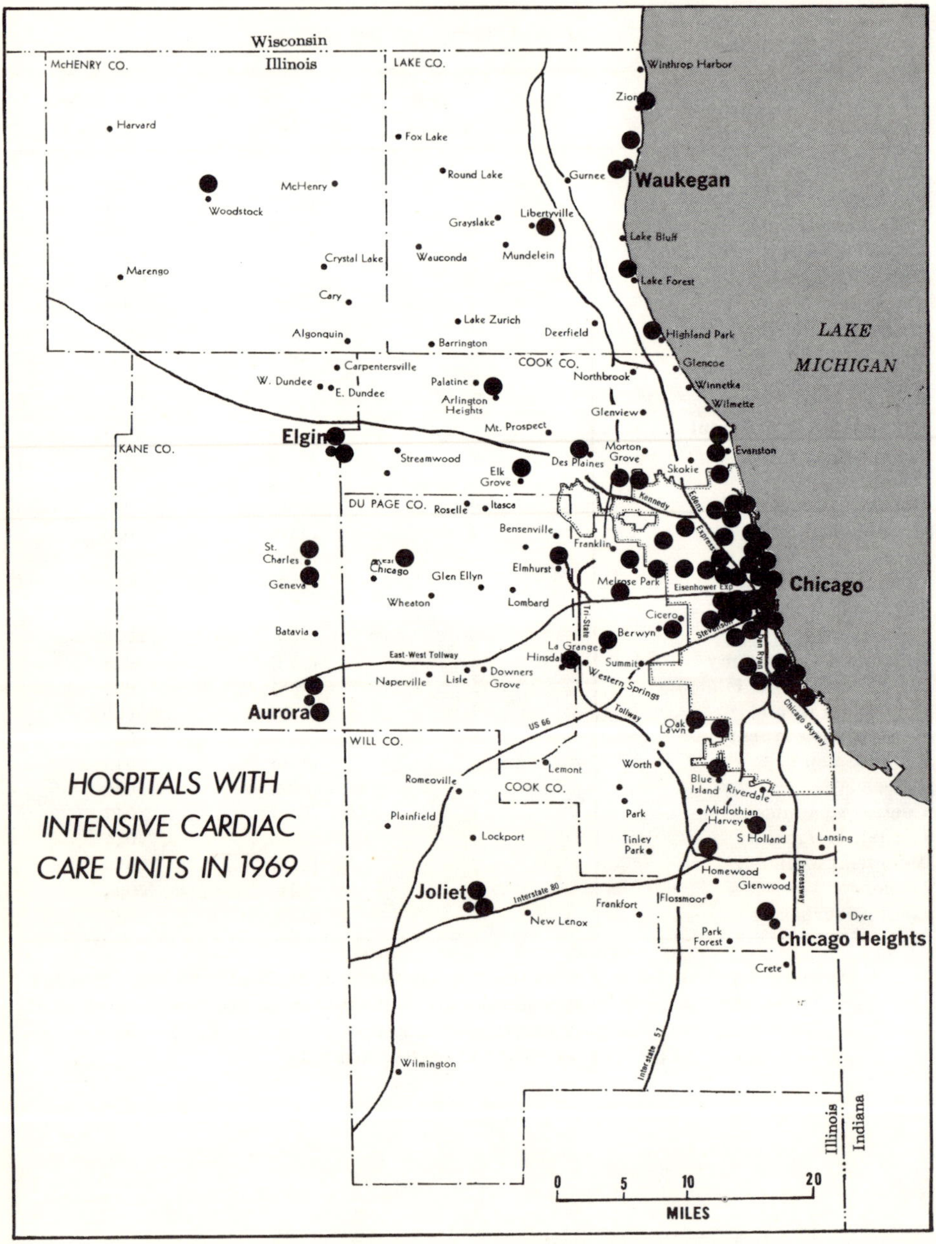

Fig. 57.--Intensive cardiac care units in the Chicago SMSA in 1970

study mentioned above that in areas with higher stroke mortality rates reported there were also higher stroke case loads in hospitals. In addition, deaths tended to occur earlier in the hospitalization process in high stroke areas.

In general, chances of recovery from the initial stroke are better than are chances with cancer and myocardial infarction.[1] The term stroke need not carry the implication of permanent disability. There is a wide range of neurophysiological impairment associated with stroke. Furthermore there are varying levels of recovery, many of which mean sufficient recovery to function in meaningful ways.

Hospital treatment and rehabilitation

Stroke patients are normally evaluated individually in order to determine severity of the disease process and recommend treatment. Often this treatment depends upon the hospital facilities available. Stroke patients can in fact be treated relatively close to their home community provided the treatment is close. Even with the severe cases, the key to treatment is activity. This activity should be instituted as soon as possible. The main purpose of physical therapy is to control the disability and when possible start rehabilitation.

In 1969, Gelperin spelled out in detail the sorts of hospital facilities required for efficient rehabilitation programs.[2] Gelperin's findings were based largely on a survey of 31 hospitals in the Chicago area providing major rehabilitation services. The following guidelines were established:

(1) Organization. The stroke center medical staff should consist of a full-time medical director (a physiatrist or qualified physician), one or more trained RN's, trained LPN's, physical and occupational therapists, services of a speech pathologist, a social worker, psychological services, and vocational counseling.

(2) Facilities. Training areas for motor relearning (e.g., gymnasium, occupational therapy area), speech training facilities, specialized areas for psychological, social worker, etc., assistance, prevocational and homemaking areas (included with occupational therapy).

(3) Types of Patients. Any patients who can be "functionally upgraded" are included.

(4) Education. Educational facilities include in-service training for professional staff and general facilities for patients.

(5) Post-Hospital Followup. This aspect of treatment includes home visits by nurses, occupational and physical therapists, outpatient visits to the hospital,

---

[1] Charles M. Wylie, "Death Statistics for Cerebrovascular Disease: A Review of Recent Findings," Stroke, I (May-June, 1970), 184-93.

[2] Abraham Gelperin, "Rehabilitation," Chicago Medicine, LXXII (November, 1969), 859-62.

visits to the patient's private physician and any of the above stroke personnel required.

In addition to hospitals with rehabilitation units Gelperin studied three others with stroke programs. Since the above study, the Chicago Heart Association has conducted a survey, and results from this survey could be combined with the efforts of the Hospital Planning Council for Metropolitan Chicago to make an inventory of stroke care facilities in the Chicago area with estimates of the number of patients treated in 1969.

Physical medicine and rehabilitation centers in the Chicago area

In addition to the 31 centers and three other hospitals with facilities in the Chicago area mentioned by Gelperin, there are 17 other hospitals with the facilities for stroke rehabilitation.[1] Table 32 lists these 51 hospitals with estimates of completed strokes for 1970. The estimates were necessary because the priority scheduling of the Illinois Regional Medical Program has not yet permitted a comprehensive survey. Fortunately the Chicago Heart Association made a 12-hospital sample survey in April of 1970, and the results from this can be used to complete a fair estimate. The "completed stroke" figures on Table 32 represent calculations based upon an average ratio of .31 completed strokes per general hospital bed in hospitals with rehabilitation facilities. The result is a sliding scale wherein the number of stroke cases presumed to be handled is actually a function of total beds.

The locations of the stroke treatment hospitals appear to be generally closer to concentrations of the incidence of stroke than do the cancer and heart disease treatment hospitals to their respective disease concentrations. Figure 58 shows the stroke hospital locations, and when Figures 15 and 16 are compared to the distribution of hospitals, the similarities of concentration are obvious. For example, there is a string of treatment facilities along the Lake County lakeshore no doubt responding to the incidence there. Also, there are two facilities in McHenry County where there are also heavy concentrations of stroke patients. Neithers of the above counties have traditionally had a superabundance of any sort of medical facility. Also, hospitals in Elgin and Joliet are equipped to serve the rural fringe areas with their higher stroke incidence.

Conclusions about the Locations of Treatment Facilities

The purpose of this chapter is primarily to inventory existing treatment facilities for the major cases of cancer, heart disease, and stroke. This inventory in turn serves

---

[1] Hospital Planning Council for Metropolitan Chicago, "Survey of Unusual and Highly Specialized Services in Hospitals," Research Report No. 10, June, 1969.

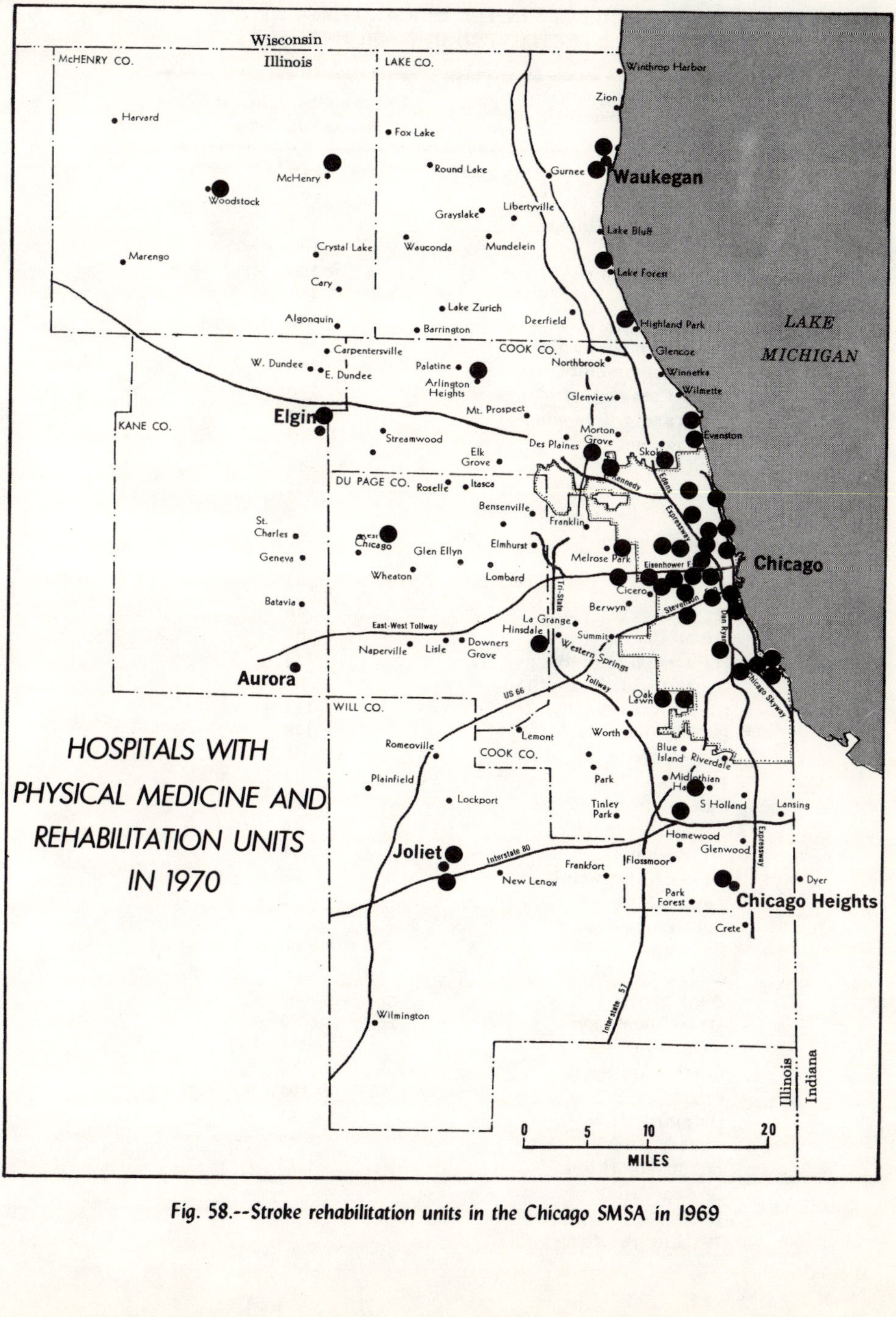

Fig. 58.--Stroke rehabilitation units in the Chicago SMSA in 1969

TABLE 32

PHYSICAL MEDICINE AND REHABILITATION FACILITIES IN THE CHICAGO SMSA WITH ESTIMATED USE FOR 1970

Hospital	Estimated Completed Strokes in 1970[a]
Cook County	310[b]
Michael Reese	275
University of Illinois	183
Evanston	157
Illinois Masonic	164
Mercy	160
VA Westside	169
St. Joseph (Chicago)	151
Christ Community	200
Little Company of Mary	180
St. Francis (Evanston)	157
Ravenswood	87
St. Anne	135
Lutheran General	161
Swedish Covenant	73
South Chicago	93
Ingalls	103
St. James	127
St. Therese	15
Silver Cross	86
St. Joseph (Joliet)	143
St. Mary of Nazareth	21
Hinsdale Sanitarium	111
Holy Cross	118
Resurrection	82
Loretto	51
Oak Park	75
Loyola University	46
St. Bernard	61
Walther Memorial	68
Louise Burg	31
Cuneo Memorial	52
Henrotin	60
Jackson Park	56
South Shore	59
Mary Thompson	35
Woodlawn	44
Central Du Page	35
Grant	104
Highland Park	81
Lake Forest	42
St. Joseph (Elgin)	48
Skokie Valley	47
Northeast Community	69
Bethany Brethren	18

TABLE 32--Continued

Hospital	Estimated Completed Strokes in 1970[a]
McHenry Memorial	31
Lake County General	15
McHenry	41
South Suburban	17

Source: Hospital Planning Council for Metropolitan Chicago, "Survey of Unusual and Highly Specialized Services in Hospitals."

[a]Estimates are based on a 12-hospital survey for the year 1969 made by the Chicago Heart Association in April, 1970. The average ratio for the sample hospitals in 1969 was .31 completed strokes per general hospital bed.

[b]Cook County is estimated to have 1000 effective beds.

as an aid to the first in a series of allocations in the next chapter. There are, however, some characteristics particular to each of the kinds of treatment facilities which in turn serve for the equally important additional allocations of need otherwise unmet. Cancer treatment facilities, for example, are heavily dependent upon certain economies of scale in terms of hospital sizes, and with few exceptions, only hospitals with certain specified prerequisites would normally warrant new facilities. Although the emergency aspects of myocardial infarction treatment are of primary importance, there are some subtle economic aspects pertaining to groups of treatment beds. Stroke treatment facilities have apparently "grown" with demand for physical rehabilitation on the part of persons in particular communities, and the real question here (indeed, the question with all the above facilities) is whether or not there are communities of persons not being adequately served.

CHAPTER VI

THE LOCATIONAL EFFICIENCY MODEL OF THE ILLINOIS REGIONAL MEDICAL PROGRAM (IRMP): ALLOCATIONS AND SUGGESTIONS FOR NEW FACILITIES

The previous analyses of the incidence of the IRMP diseases, taken as the need for treatment, and the supply of treatment facilities both serve as inputs to the locational efficiency model developed here. The model differs from the Morrill-Earickson Chicago Regional Hospital Study model in several important ways. The model assumes distance has been minimized, and distance measures are used in the selection of locations of new facilities rather than as constraints to travel. Religious behavioral constraints have been used, but racial constraints have been completely relaxed. The latter is the case because regardless of the outright segregation which exists presently in Chicago, it is assumed that by 1980 this problem will have been eliminated. Even if the problem is not totally eliminated it is assumed sufficient progress will have been made for the assumption to be changed. Furthermore, segregation cannot be perpetuated by the addition of racial constraints into a planning model. The third major difference is that patients are allocated to the closest hospital with treatment facilities for each particular disease until reasonable capacities are reached. In this way the need aspect of treatment replaces previous measures of revealed demand.

The Allocation Model

The allocation model, developed for the University of Chicago's IBM 360/65 system but obviously easily adaptable to other systems, contains essentially eight major separate operational steps. Shown on Figure 59, these steps are discussed in sequence below.

Step (1): input data

Several arrays of input data are required. The first of these (la) consists of the morbidity data. For cancer cases the morbidity data are based on the actual 1980 forecasts with proper modifications for teletherapy treatment. With the heart disease and stroke data, it was necessary to develop scalars from reported hospital survival rates and

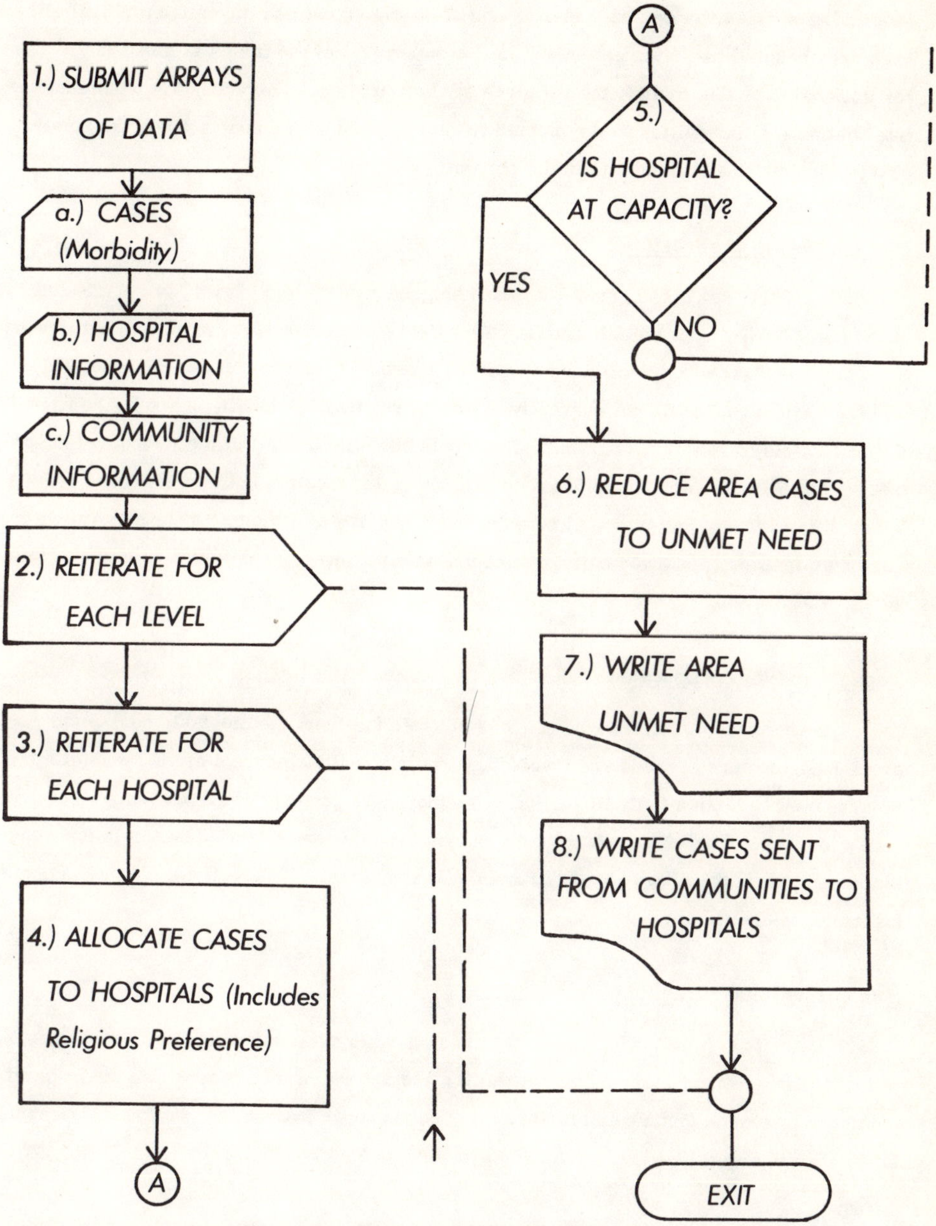

Fig. 59.--A simplified flowchart of the allocation model

apply these scalars to the forecasted mortality data for 1980. The hospital information (1b) includes capacities for each major kind of disease treatment taken from actual Chicago area hospital use information and shown on several of the tables in this study. The institutional data also include the religious affiliation of each hospital. The community information (1c) in addition to the morbidity data already mentioned includes the relative shares for Jewish and Roman Catholic populations.

Step (2): levels of allocation

Each hospital in the array (1b) was assigned a particular "level" of service. Those of the highest level represent hospitals with existing facilities. Those of the next (lower) level are hospitals with the capacity to render treatment for a particular disease, but which for some reason do not currently offer that service. Allocations are to the first level hospitals on the first iteration. If patients remain after all of the first level hospitals have reached capacity, the "do loop" allows reiterations to both the first and second levels of facility. If patients still remain, all cases are allocated on a third iteration to all hospitals after capacities have been completely removed. There are, in effect, three levels of allocation.

Steps (3) and (4): patient flows

In these steps, each hospital seeks out patients from the most adjacent communities. Religious preferences are involved, however, and 60 per cent of all Roman Catholics are sent to Roman Catholic affiliated hospitals; 70 per cent of all Jewish patients are sent to Jewish affiliated hospitals; and a 30 per cent random selection factor influences the remainder of the above populations and all other groups.[1] The flows stop when hospital facilities are filled up.

Step (5): hospital capacities

Patients are thus allocated in the above manner until capacities are reached. This step involves a major decision. If capacities are not reached for hospitals, the hospital continues to search farther and farther away until enough patients can be found. Once all hospitals have been filled up the residual patients are stored.

---

[1]These percentages were taken from the findings of Morrill and Earickson for the Chicago Regional Hospital Study.

Steps (6) and (7): unmet need

The residual patients stored above are the most important ingredients in this study. They represent the probable numbers of persons who will have difficulty in receiving treatment or will not receive it at all if no new facilities are added. These steps first arrange an array of unmet need and then prepare it for the three maps of that subject which appear in this chapter. The unmet need thus recorded serves as one of several inputs to the decision-making process regarding new facilities. The large "do loop" in step (2) is not accomplished completely without first consulting the results of these steps.

Step (8): final flows

In this step final flows of patients to hospitals are printed out, and it is thus possible to determine the numbers of patients expected at each institution in 1980 if the hospital has the recommended treatment facilities.

There were, of course, minor alterations to the basic model to fit the requirements of each disease. Each of the separate allocations is discussed in the remainder of this chapter.

Allocations for Cancer Treatment

Initially the allocation model calls for the 24 locations[1] with teletherapy units to "seek out" patients for treatment from 60 per cent[2] of the total cancer patients forecasted for 1980. After these allocations have been made, there will be a surplus of patients over teletherapy unit capacities--the unmet need. Nineteen new installations are then recommended on the basis of particular hospital characteristics explained in Chapter IV, and the supply of patients is reallocated to the 43 units. The results for the cancer model allocations are highly successful on the second iteration, and there are only minor concentrations on unmet need in a few areas.

The first iteration

On the first pass, each hospital is assigned a reasonable capacity. Most reports completed for Regional Medical Programs suggest the treatment of about 250 patients

---

[1]Existing units. See Chapter V.

[2]We have assumed 60 per cent for two reasons. The findings in Chapter V indicate that from 50 to 60 per cent of most cancer patients will probably have radiation therapy. Furthermore, it was indicated in Chapter III that the cancer estimate was on the conservative side. It is thus possible to slightly compensate for the lower forecast by taking the higher figure for teletherapy treatment.

annually for teletherapy units. This is obviously with the assumption that the machines will be used on a 40-hour weekly basis with each patient averaging about 15 minutes per visit. As we have seen in Chapter V, some machines are taxed to their limits while others are used only half the time. This problem was solved by assigning to each unit a "capacity" of 243 patients annually. This figure is, in fact, the average number per teletherapy unit for the Chicago area for 1969. Cook County Hospital, then, receives a capacity of 486 instead of the 1210 patients actually treated last year. Conversely, St. Joseph Hospital in Joliet is assigned 243 instead of the 79 patients shown on Table 29.

After the forecasted patients (60 per cent) for 1980 have been allocated to the 24 existing facilities, the resultant unmet need is shown on Figure 60. The distributions on that map represent 60 per cent of the remainder of the cancer population eligible for treatment but with no place to go <u>without overtaxing any one hospital's facilities</u>. The areas within the contour lines are actually the same 271 control points used for forecasting. The base map used is intended to match the hospital supply maps for purposes of cartographic comparison. The ranges indicated by different contour lines represent possible values for each point rather than numbers for entire areas. Also the cartographic method in this case is SYMAP[1] rather than the more general trend surface maps used previously in this study. For the earlier maps general trends were sufficient, but for these maps which contribute more to decisions about new locations more detail (albeit unexponentiated) for smaller areas is required.

The unmet need forms some interesting patterns. There are large areas of unmet need in Lake and McHenry Counties, and this was certainly not unexpected. Somewhat more surprising is the small high concentration in northern Cook County along Lake Michigan. There is a very high concentration in the Aurora area and another in the southeastern part of Chicago. Southern Cook County also has heavy concentrations which are not unexpected.

<u>Locations for additional teletherapy installations</u>

Four major considerations were given to the selection of the nineteen hospitals shown on Figure 61. All are important, and if any one reason has more importance than the others, it is probably economies of scale.

Scale economies and size

The economies of scale discussed in Chapter IV have been brought into play in a manner as indicated by Figure 62. Several larger hospitals with higher costs were

---

[1] The method was developed by the Harvard University Laboratory for Computer Graphics and Spatial Analysis.

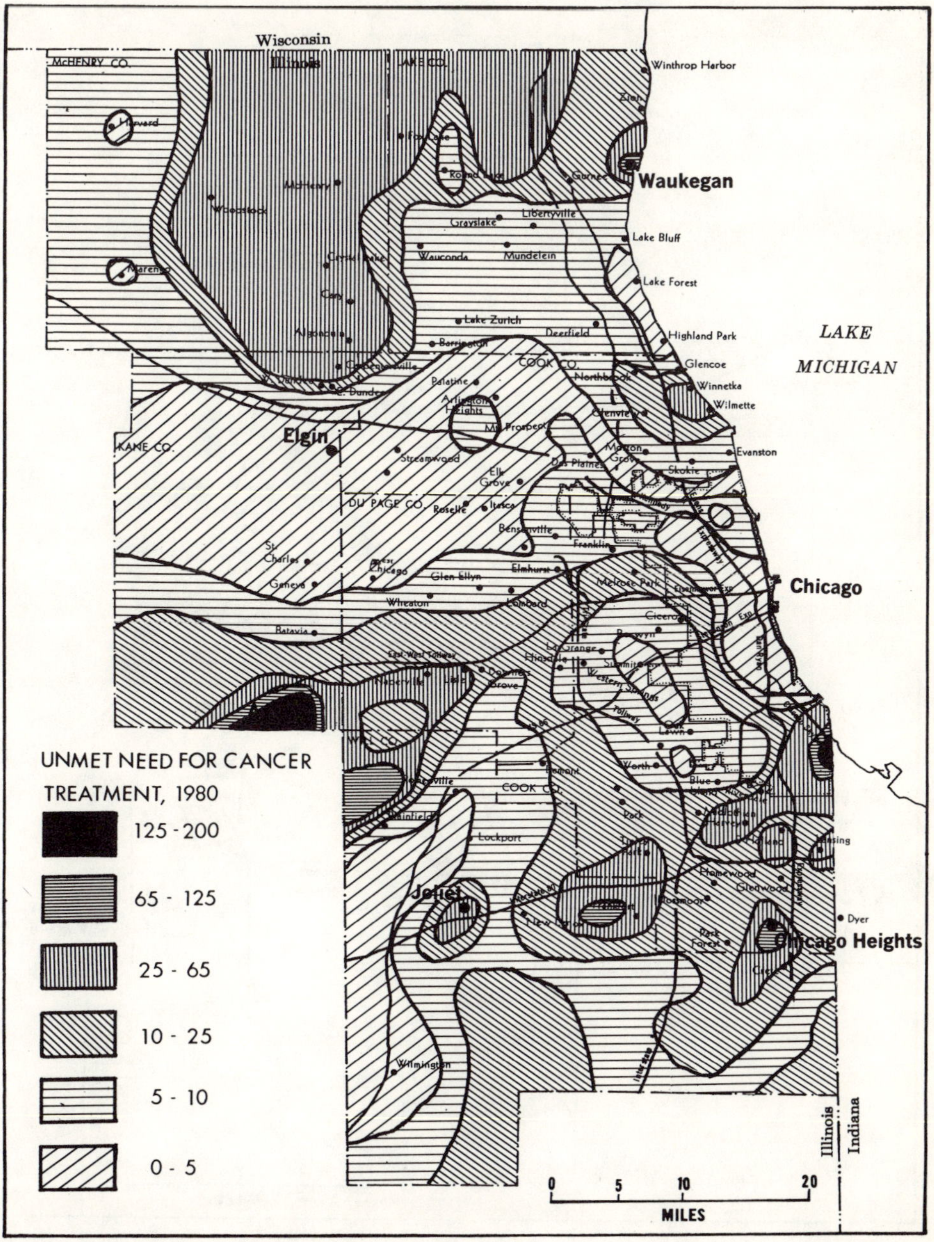

Fig. 60.--Unmet need for cancer treatment in 1980

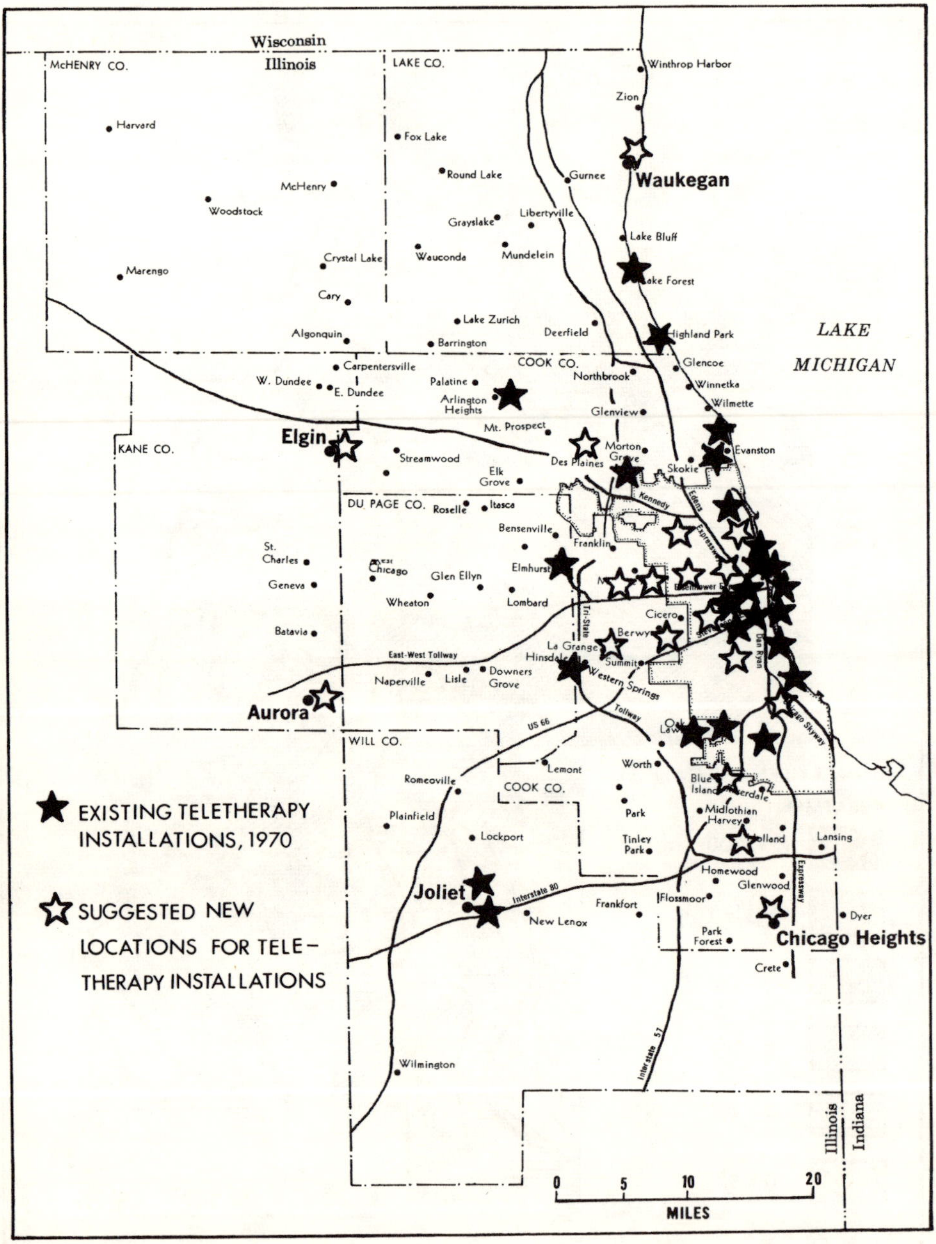

Fig. 61.--Existing and suggested new locations for teletherapy installations

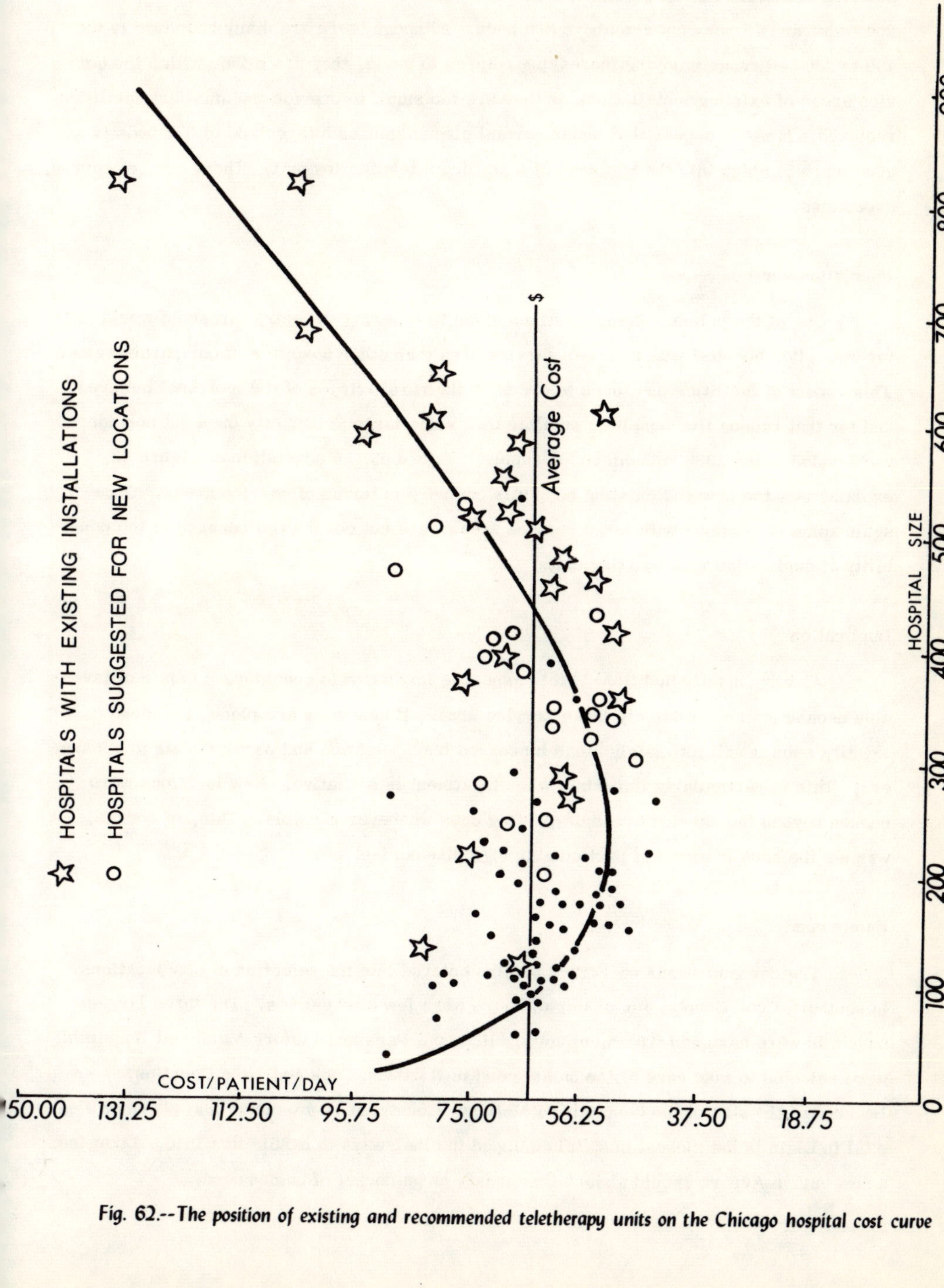

Fig. 62.--The position of existing and recommended teletherapy units on the Chicago hospital cost curve

selected because of the availability of staff. Most of the remainder of the hospitals selected are around or below the average cost figure. All the hospitals selected are above 200 beds, and 75 per cent are above 300 beds. Although there are many hospitals in the 150 to 250 bed range enjoying increasing returns to scale, they are either within the service areas of existing installations or they are too small to provide the ancillary facilities required. It would appear that under normal circumstances a threshold of 250 beds is a good place to enter into the business of installing a teletherapy unit. There are, of course, exceptions.

Population served

One of the primary considerations given to lowering the entry threshold would be for a smaller hospital with a larger service area than other hospitals of comparable size. This aspect of facilities use tends to occur on the rural fringes of the metropolitan area, and for that reason five hospitals smaller than some larger inner city ones not considered were added to the 1980 recommended supply. Figure 63, an adaptation of Figure 52, explains how the new and existing hospitals compare in terms of service areas. Once again some of the ones with large service areas were not considered because of the possibility of duplication with existing units.

Duplication

Already briefly mentioned, this aspect is important to consider. In spite of favorable economies and relatively large service areas, if new units are placed too close to existing ones it will ultimately mean increased transportation and penalty costs to consumers. This is particularly important when treatment is palliative. New locations were chosen beyond the service areas of existing ones whenever possible. This, of course, was not the case in areas of particularly high disease incidence.

Unmet need

The concentrations on Figure 60 also entered into the selection of new locations. In southern Cook County, for example, there were few alternatives. The three largest hospitals were assigned treatment units. Highland Park and Victory Memorial Hospitals were selected to take care of the unmet need in Northern Cook and Lake Counties. Because of the size of the hospitals in McHenry County, it is presumed that Sherman Hospital in Elgin is the closest hospital equipped in other ways to handle that load. Likewise, a new unit in Aurora should absorb that area's large pocket of unmet need.

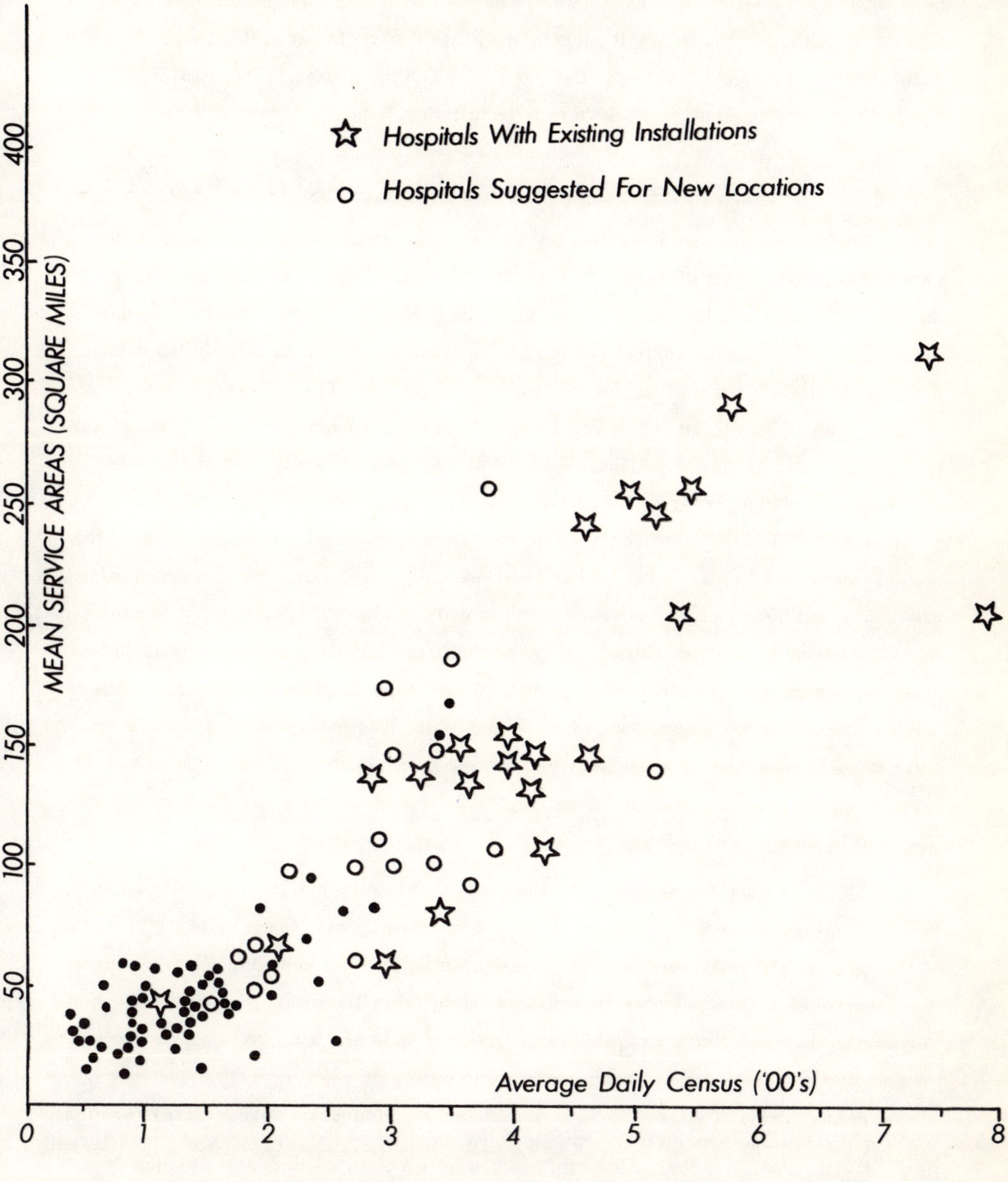

Fig. 63.--Existing and recommended teletherapy units in relation to area served

The second iteration

The second allocation proved to be most satisfactory. Most of the 43 units would be expected to treat comfortably from 225 to 250 patients in 1980. Most of the unmet need is accounted for (95 per cent if patients are served) with only a slight additional surplus number of patients. These small pockets are all to the southwest of the Loop. Two are in the central city, and the other is the Palos area. None of these concentrations are sufficient to call for an additional teletherapy installation.

Allocations for Myocardial Infarction and Related Problems

The disease data we have thus far been dealing with represent mortality from all forms of coronary heart disease. It is a difficult but not impossible task to estimate from the 1980 forecasts just how many persons are likely to suffer from a myocardial infarction, possible myocardial infarction, angina, or a more difficult to identify but related problem (at times a form of stroke, for example). Studies of morbidity/mortality ratios have been made, and these can be combined with various reported survival rates to estimate the supply of possible patients.[1] There are several elements, age and past history of coronary problems being the two most commonly mentioned examples, which cause a great deal of variability between persons; two ratios were developed on the basis of the studies mentioned above. First, it has been assumed that the forecasted mortality figures represent 35 per cent of persons with coronary problems. Secondly, it is assumed that 85 per cent of persons with coronary problems can be allocated to hospitals on the assumption that, if facilities exist, this will be the probable proportion in 1980. The above assumptions were developed into a scalar which was in turn applied to the mortality estimates, and the results were taken as need for treatment.

The first iteration

The first iteration was made on the basis of facilities existing in 1970. Table 31 shows actual use in 1969 on the basis of the survey already mentioned by IRMP, but many of the existing ICC units were not serving as many patients as they actually might have. The capacities on Table 33 were therefore constructed on the assumption that those hospitals serving less than the average of 58 patients per year per ICC bed would be brought up

---

[1]See for example Albert S. Most and Donald R. Peterson, "Myocardial Infarction Surveillance in a Metropolitan Community," The Journal of the American Medical Association, CCVIII (June 30, 1969), 2433-38; and Sam Shapiro, Eve Weinblatt, Charles W. Frank, and Robert V. Sager, "Incidence of Coronary Heart Disease in a Population Insured for Medical Care," American Journal of Public Health, LIX (June, 1969), 1-101.

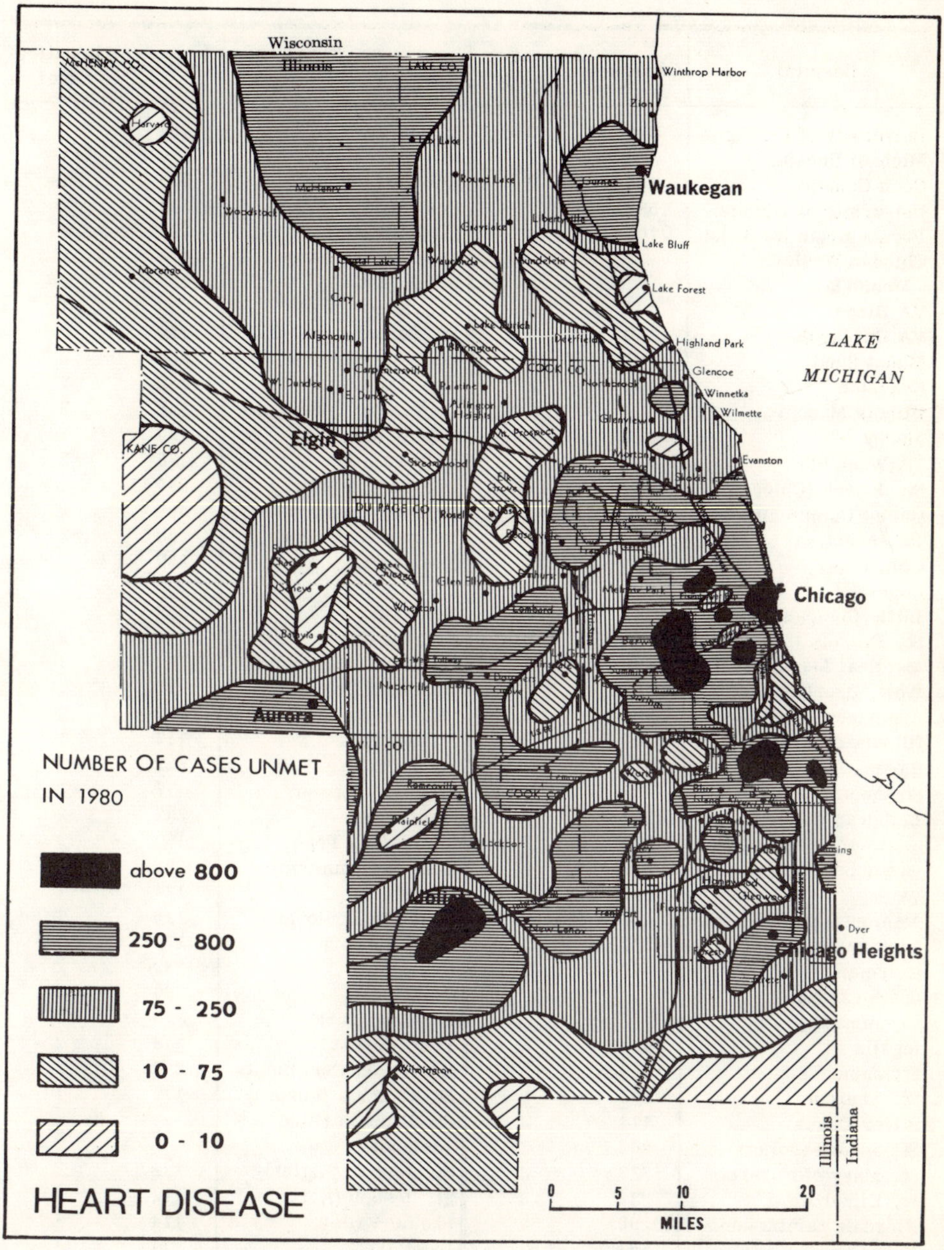

Fig. 64.--Unmet need for cardiac care in 1980

TABLE 33

CAPACITIES FOR TWO LEVELS OF CARDIAC CARE FACILITIES

Hospital	Capacity	Allocation Level
University of Chicago	406	2
Michael Reese	464	2
Cook County	464	2
University of Illinois	580	2
Presbyterian St. Lukes	700	2
Chicago Wesley Memorial	464	2
VA Hines	464	2
VA Research	150	1
Mount Sinai	464	2
Evanston	630	2
Illinois Masonic	580	2
Mercy	464	2
VA Westside	350	2
St. Joseph (Chicago)	348	2
Christ Community	696	2
Passavant	290	2
Columbus	406	2
Edgewater	638	2
Little Company of Mary	464	2
St. Francis (Evanston)	240	2
MacNeal Memorial	696	2
West Suburban	464	1
Augustana	290	2
Illinois Central	348	2
Ravenswood	348	2
St. Anne	232	2
Lutheran General	464	2
Norwegian-American	232	2
Swedish Covenant	696	2
Weiss	1160	2
Memorial Du Page	561	2
Victory Memorial	232	2
Sherman	580	2
South Chicago Community	406	1
Ingalls	494	2
St. James	443	2
St. Therese	290	2
Silver Cross	174	2
St. Joseph (Joliet)	302	2
St. Mary of Nazareth	232	2
St. Elizabeth	232	2
Hinsdale Sanitarium	290	2
Holy Cross	561	2
St. Anthony de Padua	290	1
Resurrection	459	2
American	464	2
Evangelical	174	1
Loretto	174	1
Oak Park	343	2
Englewood	290	2
Loyola University	174	1
Northwest	232	2
Provident	290	1
St. Bernard	116	2
Walther Memorial	464	2
St. Alexius	232	2
Community Memorial	348	2
Copley Memorial	120	2
Holy Family	275	2
Our Lady of Mercy	290	1
Belmont Community	406	2
Bethany Methodist	58	2
Louise Burg	232	2
Frank Cuneo	232	1
Henrotin	232	2
Jackson Park	174	2
Roosevelt Memorial	174	1
Roseland Community	117	1
St. Frances X. Cabrini	232	2
St. George	117	1
South Shore	522	2
Mary Thompson	117	1
Woodlawn	232	2
Central Du Page	150	2
Geneva Community	232	2
Edward	174	1
Franklin Boulevard	116	1
Garfield Park	174	1
Grant	232	2
Gottlieb	290	2
Highland Park	375	2
Lake Forest	348	2
Northwest Community	232	2
St. Charles (Aurora)	117	1
St. Francis (Blue Island)	58	2
St. Joseph (Elgin)	232	2
St. Joseph (Aurora)	174	2
Skokie Valley	174	1
Westlake	174	1
Zion-Benton	116	2
Bethesda	232	2

TABLE 33--Continued

Hospital	Capacity	Allocation Level	Hospital	Capacity	Allocation Level
Central Community	232	2	Delnor	232	2
Forkosh	174	1	Northlake Community	117	1
Northeast Community	290	1	Lake County	58	1
Von Solbrig	117	1	McHenry	174	1
Bethany Brethren	58	1	Harvard	58	1
Community (Evanston)	58	1	South Suburban	290	2
Condell Memorial	232	2	Martha Washington	117	1
McHenry Memorial	116	2			

to that average. The emergency nature of cardiac care calls for a different sort of redistribution than was accomplished for the teletherapy units, and the hospitals with more than average ICC patients were maintained at their higher patient load levels. There are two levels of allocation for this disease, and they are labeled "2" and "1." The "2" category indicates existing facilities, and the "1" category indicates hospitals which do not now have ICC care. The capacities for the latter hospitals are all determined on the average use basis.

On the first allocation, patients were sent only to category "2" hospitals. After all allocations had been made, the unmet need shown on Figure 64 resulted. Comparisons of Figures 42 and 43 show how in many communities the predicted need is substantially reduced but not eliminated. But other communities have hardly been changed. The implication is that if no new ICC beds are added, many persons will go without proper care. Beds must obviously be added. The purpose of this locational efficiency model in this case is to determine the best possible new locations for these beds.

The second iteration

For the second iteration, allocations were made to hospitals in levels "2" and "1." Some of the unmet need was absorbed, but the supply of facilities remained essentially inadequate. Clearly, something had to be done to adjust capacities to meet the need.

The third iteration

Several considerations were given to adjusting hospital capacities in order to meet the forecasted need for treatment:

(1) Hospitals with a history of treating more than the average number of patients would be expected to continue to operate in this manner.

TABLE 34

ALLOCATIONS OF ALL 1980 UNMET NEED TO HOSPITALS AND SUGGESTED LEVELS IN A NEW HIERARCHY OF ICC TREATMENT FACILITIES

Hospital	1980 Patients[a]	New Hierarchy Level[b]	Hospital	1980 Patients[a]	New Hierarchy Level[b]
University of Chicago	1140	D	St. Joseph (Joliet)	850	E
Michael Reese	1300	C	St. Mary of Nazareth	650	F
Cook County	1300	C	St. Elizabeth	650	F
University of Illinois	1630	C	Hinsdale Sanitarium	820	E
Presbyterian St. Lukes	1970	B	Holy Cross	1580	C
Chicago Wesley Memorial	1300	C	St. Anthony de Padua	820	E
VA Hines	1300	C	Resurrection	1290	C
VA Research	420	F	American	1300	C
Mount Sinai	1300	C	Evangelical	490	F
Evanston	1770	B	Loretto	490	F
Illinois Masonic	1630	C	Oak Park	970	D
Mercy	1300	C	Englewood	820	E
VA Westside	990	D	Loyola University	490	F
St. Joseph (Chicago)	980	D	Northwest	650	E
Christ Community	1960	B	Provident	820	E
Passavant	820	E	St. Bernard	330	G
Columbus	1150	D	Walther Memorial	1300	C
Edgewater	1790	B	St. Alexius	650	E
Little Company of Mary	1300	C	Community Memorial	980	D
St. Francis (Evanston)	680	E	Copley Memorial	340	G
MacNeal Memorial	1960	B	Holy Family	770	E
West Suburban	1300	C	Our Lady of Mercy	820	E
Augustana	820	E	Belmont Community	1140	D
Illinois Central	980	D	Bethany Methodist	160	H
Ravenswood	980	D	Louise Burg	160	H
St. Anne	650	E	Frank Cuneo	650	E
Lutheran General	1300	C	Henrotin	650	E
Norwegian-American	650	E	Jackson Park	490	F
Swedish Covenant	1960	B	Roosevelt Memorial	490	F
Weiss	3260	A	Roseland Community	330	G
Memorial Du Page	1580	C	St. Frances X. Cabrini	650	E
Victory Memorial	650	E	St. George	320	G
Sherman	1630	C	South Shore	1470	C
South Chicago Community	1140	D	Mary Thompson	330	G
Ingalls	1390	C	Woodlawn	650	E
St. James	1250	C	Central Du Page	420	F
St. Therese	820	E	Geneva Community	650	E
Silver Cross	490	F	Edward	490	F
			Franklin Boulevard	330	G
			Garfield Park	490	F
			Grant	650	E

TABLE 34--Continued

Hospital	1980 Patients[a]	New Hierarchy Level[b]	Hospital	1980 Patients[a]	New Hierarchy Level[b]
Gottlieb	820	E	Northeast Community	820	E
Highland Park	1050	D	Von Solbrig	330	G
Lake Forest	980	D	Bethany Brethren	160	H
Northwest Community	650	E	Community (Evanston)	160	H
St. Charles (Aurora)	330	G	Condell Memorial	650	E
St. Francis (Blue Island)	160	H	McHenry Memorial	330	G
St. Joseph (Elgin)	650	E	Delnor	650	E
St. Joseph (Aurora)	490	F	Northlake Community	330	G
Skokie Valley	490	F	Lake County	160	H
Westlake	490	F	McHenry	490	F
Zion-Benton	190	G	Harvard	160	H
Bethesda	650	E	South Suburban	820	E
Central Community	650	E	Martha Washington	330	G
Forkosh	490	F			

[a]Estimates to the nearest 10 patients.

[b]ICC Bed Levels: A = 36; B = 30; C = 24; D = 18; E = 12; F = 6; G = 4 to 6; H = 2.

(2) Capacities had to be raised to levels where need would be met.

(3) Existing capacities should be used as lower limits. This would prevent the "removal" of facilities which already exist.

(4) The economies realized by grouping ICC units should be kept in mind.

Capacities were then taken as lower limits, and upper limits were relaxed. All cases were thus allocated to the 106 hospitals. The resultant numbers of patients are shown on Table 34. In some instances the case load has increased by a factor of three, while in others it is unchanged. Economies realized from groups of 6 ICC beds and groups of at least 4 beds have been taken into account. The following hierarchy of new ICC treatment centers was developed on the basis of the third iteration. The letters on Table 34 indicate the following classes of ICC units:

A = 6 Groups of 6 Beds
B = 5 Groups of 6 Beds
C = 4 Groups of 6 Beds
D = 3 Groups of 6 Beds
E = 2 Groups of 6 Beds
F = 1 Group of 6 Beds
G = A Unit of 4 to 6 Beds
H = A Set of 2 Beds

This scheme allows hospitals specializing in intensive cardiac care to continue to do so while, at the same time, it calls for other hospitals to participate actively in producing such treatment.

Allocations for Stroke Rehabilitation

As mentioned in Chapter VI, survival rates for stroke are generally better than for myocardial infarction and much better than for those of cancer. Some reports indicate all but about 20 per cent of stroke victims can be saved in hospitals. Other reports range from 60 to 70 per cent of strokes surviving,[1] particularly when all age groups are considered. The above mentioned studies have at their disposal detailed hospital morbidity data which enable researchers to separate cases into various age and sex groups. When dealing with the ecological data in this study it is necessary to consider entire community populations, and because of this a rate of 65 per cent surviving has been assigned to all 1980 mortality forecasts. A scalar of 2.87 was therefore applied to the disease data to obtain expected cases. The cases were in turn allocated to various hospitals in a series of three iterations.

The first iteration

For this first pass, stroke cases were allocated to all those treatment facilities shown on Figure 58. Capacities were given as those shown on Table 32. The use data on Table 32 were not altered because they actually represent estimates based on about a 25 per cent sample of hospitals in 1969. The predicted 1980 cases overflowed the facilities more than the cancer allocations on the first pass and substantially less than the first heart disease iteration. The resultant predicted stroke treatment overflow if no new facilities are added in the next ten years is shown as unmet need on Figure 65.

The distribution of unmet need is not unexpected. There are still heavy concentrations of stroke cases in Lake and McHenry Counties. There are also heavy concentrations around the other industrial satellites and the rural fringe areas beyond these cities. There are also several areas of high incidence in the inner city and in some of the inner western suburbs. In fact, the pattern of unmet need for treatment of stroke is generally lighter than but quite similar to that of unmet need for heart disease treatment. This similarity is no doubt related to the distribution of the diseases rather than to facilities, because the types of treatment are quite different and facilities for the two types of treatment are presently allocated in very different ways.

---

[1] Wylie, "Death Statistics for Cerebrovascular Disease," pp. 184-93.

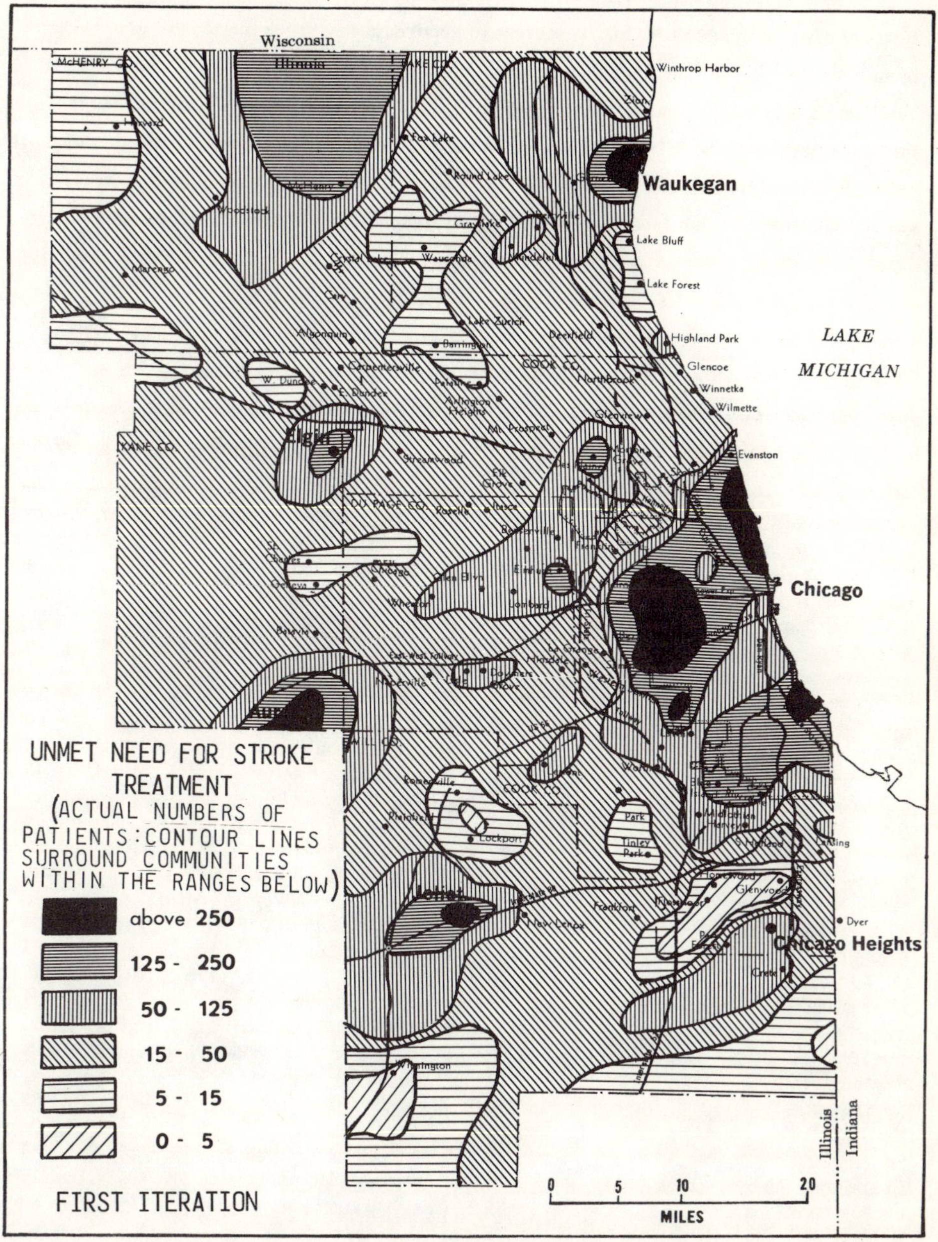

Fig. 65.--Unmet need for stroke treatment in 1980: first iteration

The second iteration

On the second allocation, all hospitals presently without stroke rehabilitation facilities are assigned capacities for treatment in accordance with the number of general treatment beds they had in 1969. These hospitals are then added to the supply and the total 106 hospitals are allocated patients in accordance with the supply. The actual numbers of facilities necessary to bring the remainder of the supply up to par with hospitals currently active in treatment are shown on Table 35. Even with the added supply of facilities, it is not enough to handle the forecasted 1980 supply (Fig. 66). However the facilities shown

TABLE 35

STROKE TREATMENT CAPACITIES REQUIRED OF HOSPITALS WITHOUT FACILITIES TO MATCH THOSE WITH FACILITIES

Hospital	Stroke Capacity[a]	Hospital	Stroke Capacity[a]
University of Chicago	212	Our Lady of Mercy	32
Presbyterian St. Lukes	260	Belmont Community	47
Chicago Wesley Memorial	201	Bethany Methodist	60
VA Hines	112	Roosevelt Memorial	47
VA Research	169	Roseland Community	37
Mount Sinai	119	St. Frances X. Cabrini	66
Passavant Memorial	120	St. George	38
Columbus	126	Community, Geneva	35
Edgewater	120	Edward	40
MacNeal Memorial	130	Franklin Boulevard	32
West Suburban	117	Garfield Park Community	45
Augustana	109	Gottlieb Memorial	104
Illinois Central	93	Northwest Community	69
Norwegian-American	70	St. Charles (Aurora)	34
Weiss, Louis A.	76	St. Francis (Blue Island)	104
Memorial Du Page	150	St. Joseph's Mercy (Aurora)	48
Victory Memorial	107	Westlake Community	41
Sherman	108	Zion-Benton	31
St. Elizabeth's	106	Bethesda	47
St. Anthony de Padua	65	Central Community	27
American	52	Forkosh	47
Evangelical	53	Von Solbrig Memorial	27
Englewood	51	Community (Evanston)	13
Northwest	75	Condell Memorial	28
Provident	32	Delnor	33
St. Alexius	70	Northlake Community	34
Community Memorial General	75	Harvard Community	12
Copley Memorial	62	Martha Washington	33
Holy Family	77		

[a]If facilities added in proportion to total beds. Numbers are patients. The patient capacity is the potential number of persons who could be treated.

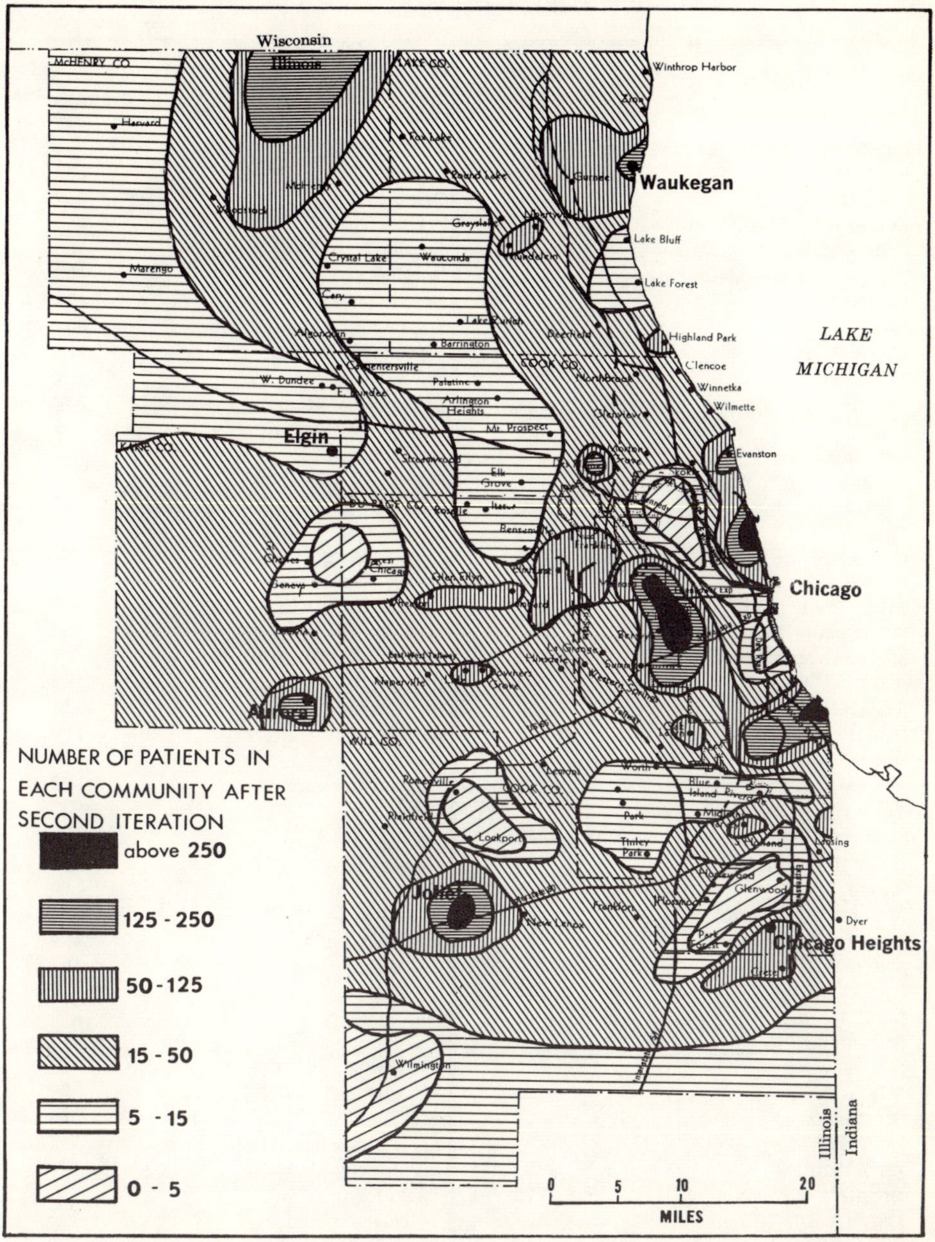

Fig. 66.--Unmet need for stroke treatment in 1980: second iteration

TABLE 36

PROBABLE PATIENT LOADS FOR STROKE TREATMENT IF SUFFICIENT FACILITIES ARE ADDED BY 1980

Hospital	Expected Patients, 1980	Hospital	Expected Patients, 1980
University of Chicago	385	Evangelical	71
Michael Reese	343	Loretto	725
Cook County	554	Oak Park	270
University of Illinois	240	Englewood	378
Presbyterian St. Lukes	357	Loyola University	180
Chicago Wesley Memorial	251	Northwest	253
VA Hines	189	Provident	114
VA Research	186	St. Bernard	314
Mount Sinai	136	Walther Memorial	102
Evanston	294	St. Alexius	160
Illinois Masonic	214	Community Memorial	333
Mercy	194	Copley Memorial	99
VA Westside	213	Holy Family	213
St. Joseph (Chicago)	201	Our Lady of Mercy	47
Christ Community	470	Belmont Community	95
Passavant	186	Bethany Methodist	110
Columbus	176	Louise Burg	237
Edgewater	170	Cuneo Memorial	102
Little Company of Mary	515	Henrotin	110
St. Francis (Evanston)	238	Jackson Park	238
MacNeal Memorial	1173	Roosevelt Memorial	87
West Suburban	223	Roseland Community	172
Augustana	159	St. Frances X. Cabrini	116
Illinois Central	194	St. George	199
Ravenswood	137	South Shore	516
St. Anne	182	Mary Thompson	59
Lutheran General	307	Woodlawn	332
Norwegian-American	215	Central Du Page	126
Swedish Covenant	120	Geneva Community	88
Weiss	126	Edward	265
Memorial Du Page	200	Franklin Boulevard	148
Victory Memorial	157	Garfield Park	158
Sherman	252	Grant	154
South Chicago Community	323	Gottlieb	175
Ingalls	573	Highland Park	273
St. James	465	Lake Forest	77
St. Therese	224	Northwest Community	177
Silver Cross	518	St. Charles (Aurora)	280
St. Joseph (Joliet)	366	St. Francis (Blue Island)	154
St. Mary of Nazareth	81	St. Joseph (Elgin)	148
St. Elizabeth	194	St. Joseph (Aurora)	79
Hinsdale Sanitarium	275	Skokie Valley	200
Holy Cross	133	Westlake	105
St. Anthony de Padua	115	Zion-Benton	200
Resurrection	302	Bethesda	97
American	167	Central Community	105

TABLE 36--Continued

Hospital	Expected Patients, 1980	Hospital	Expected Patients, 1980
Forkosh	97	Delnor	57
Northeast Community	104	Northlake Community	220
Von Solbrig	383	Lake County	92
Bethany Brethren	118	McHenry	198
Community (Evanston)	28	Harvard	40
Condell Memorial	206	South Suburban	36
McHenry Memorial	295	Martha Washington	70

on Tables 32 and 35 can be taken as the minimum number needed before 1980, because in some communities the unmet need was completely eliminated on this second pass. Unfortunately, there were still very high concentrations in particular areas.

The third iteration

In order to take care of the need still unmet after two iterations, all upper limits on hospital capacities were relaxed when previous capacities were reached. The results in terms of total expected patients for stroke treatment for all 106 hospitals in 1980 are shown on Table 36. In some instances the figures are very close to capacities previously suggested, but in other hospitals the numbers of expected patients are high. They may in fact be considered staggering by hospitals not now having facilities. For hospitals with facilities, it will be easier to add capacities, but for others it will be harder.

Manpower needs

The results of the stroke allocations are particularly appropriate to Regional Medical Programs because this example spells out one of the more important themes of the program--that of insufficient manpower. It may be somewhat unrealistic, for example, to expect a hospital with absolutely no plans to add a physical medicine and rehabilitation facility suddenly or gradually to start treating several hundred stroke patients per year. This possibility becomes even more remote if the personnel are not available to operate the facility. With stroke treatment, there should, however, be a great deal of optimism regarding new manpower if for no other reason than the fact that it does not require nearly the large investment in time to train many of the paramedicals required in the treatment. The need can be forecasted, and the locations of new facilities can be determined, but these efforts must be augmented with parallel manpower training programs if we are indeed to take care of otherwise unmet need.

Conclusions about the Allocation Model

The allocation model works best for cancer treatment. There are several reasons for this. Cancer is often easier to identify. More precise diagnoses thus enable more accurate morbidity estimates. The methods of treatment and the economic aspects of their location have been documented in such a way as to make the selection of new locations more precise. For these reasons, we were able to take care of nearly all unmet need on the second iteration. The morbidity estimates for heart disease and stroke were less precise, and in many instances they overlapped strongly. Use data for myocardial infarction and related ailments were based on a very accurate survey, but stroke incidents were estimated. In spite of the pitfalls of the above calculations, the bare fact is that there is such a current lag in treatment for heart disease and stroke that it may take a superhuman effort merely to take care of the 1970 unmet need. If many new facilities are not added for all three of the RMP ailments there is little doubt that 1980 unmet needs will be even higher than those forecasted. Conversely, if treatment is added, the rates could be lower, and this is certainly a goal to work toward. Unfortunately, as Morrill has pointed out, for general treatment it often takes nearly three times a community population threshold actually required to support a hospital before a hospital is built.[1] Must we be faced with the same problem here? The allocation model can meanwhile serve as a means of presenting an optimum solution to the problem of how many new facilities are needed and where they might best be located.

---

[1]Morrill, "Historical Development of the Chicago Hospital System."

CHAPTER VII

GENERAL CONCLUSIONS

The problem presented to the Illinois Regional Medical Program for this study was to develop a locational efficiency model for treatment of the 1980 incidence of heart disease, cancer, and stroke. It was necessary to accomplish several other important tasks in order to address properly the problem of allocating patients from communities of residence to particular treatment facilities. These tasks, in effect, constitute a portion of the overall investigation.

The approach to the problem has several important steps which offer contributions to urban geography and health care planning. In Chapter I it was possible through a review of the geographic aspects of health care planning to establish a rationale for building a model of allocation within the context of the Regional Medical Programs. Chapter II explains how it is possible to firmly establish patterns of spatial variability among the diseases of the Regional Medical Programs. Next, it was possible to make use of methods of analysis from previously defined Urban Medical Geography to build a calibrated submodel capable of forecasting disease patterns in the Chicago area (Chapter III). Such forecasting is of particular concern because it has applications to many problems beyond the scope of this study. Existing facilities were inventoried, and the hospitals housing these facilities were placed in a previously established system of orderly classification (Chapters IV and V). These tasks constituted the identification of the facilities supply side of the analysis. Finally in Chapter VI numbers of the forecasted disease cases were allocated to the nearest possible hospitals, given certain behavioral constraints, until capacities were reached. The result was the identification of unmet need, and this need was eventually met by adding sufficient elements of equipment and personnel to the supply of treatment facilities.

The determination of optimal locations of new treatment facilities was the major accomplishment of this study. Concentrations of surplus patients if no new facilities are added by 1980 could be estimated with a fair degree of accuracy. Obviously, facilities will need to be added. Knowledge of where these facilities are needed should influence where the new facilities will be added over the next decade. The suggested additional facilities represent the most efficient locations to meet estimated need with least travel on the part of the patient. Some hospitals do not "specialize" in particular kinds of treatment, stroke being the best example. But if the need for such treatment is consistently high near such hospitals, perhaps the hospitals should be offering the treatment. It is not expected that the new facilities will all be added as recommended (if at all). Hopefully, however, some hospitals will add sufficient facilities to make up for those not adding any.

The magnitude of hospital supply needs by 1980 is incredible. For example, if no new teletherapy units are added by 1980, we can expect effectively to treat only about 7000 cancer patients out of a possible 12,500 who will probably require high intensity radiation therapy by 1980. We can expect perhaps 90,000 heart patients by 1980, but our current supply of facilities can comfortably handle at the most only 30,000. Thus, unmet need for heart disease treatment could be as high as 60,000 patients if nothing is done about increasing the supply of treatment facilities. Of an anticipated 24,000 stroke patients in 1980, as many as 16,000 may not find proper treatment if the facilities are not brought up to necessary requirements.

The magnitude of costs is large. It will take from $7 million to $9 million to add the suggested new cancer treatment facilities (see Chapter VI for locations). It will take at today's costs $175 thousand for each 6-bed cardiac care unit. For stroke treatment personnel is the key; training hundreds of nurses should be underway right now. The costs of such training are constantly going up.

It is clear where new facilities for the treatment of each disease are needed. Most of the new teletherapy units should be built along expressways in suburban areas (see Fig. 61, p. 182). However, several inner city hospitals should consider the acquisition of units also. Needs for new heart disease treatment facilities are particularly acute in the southwest suburbs and Lake and McHenry Counties. New heart disease treatment facilities are needed also in the inner city on the west and south sides. New facilities for stroke treatment should be built in much the same geographic locations as those for heart disease. In addition, many new stroke facilities are going to be needed for Chicago's North Shore area.

APPENDIX A

SOURCES OF HEALTH INFORMATION IN CHICAGO

SOURCES OF HEALTH INFORMATION IN CHICAGO

In late 1969, the Hospital Planning Council for Metropolitan Chicago completed an inventory of sources of health data for the Chicago area.[1] This study was the short term result of intensive efforts on the part of a half-dozen health care facilities researchers, including the author of this study. Some of the more salient items of that document have been combined with other aspects of health information collection to produce this appendix. It is possible to place sources of health data into three broad categories dependent upon the purpose of the research and geographical areas covered. These categories, as itemized below, include:

(1) General Bibliographic and Methodological Aids;
(2) Primary sources of Health Data; and
(3) Sources of Ancillary Health Data for the Chicago area.

General bibliographic and methodological aids

A comparison with national trends in health is one extremely useful way to establish a frame of reference for any urban area. There are several such references published by the federal government. The Department of Health, Education, and Welfare annually publishes causes of death by state,[2] but such data are of limited utility when any refinement of detail is sought. The U. S. Public Health Service periodically publishes methodological studies for health purposes, and a 1964 report pertaining to the generation of data from previous reports is of much use.[3] Also, the National Center for Health Statistics publishes a series of bulletins treating health data analysis and interpretation.[4] Also of particular value are the weekly morbidity and mortality reports released by the

---

[1]Unpublished survey developed by the Hospital Planning Council for Metropolitan Chicago, October, 1969.

[2]See U. S. Department of Health, Education, and Welfare, Vital Statistics of the United States, 1967 (Washington: National Vital Statistics Division, 1969).

[3]National Committee on Vital and Health Statistics, Medical Economics: Present Status and Recommendations for Additional Data, U. S. Public Health Service Publication 1125 (Washington: U. S. Government Printing Office, 1964).

[4]National Center for Health Statistics, Vital and Health Statistics Listing: Series 2, U. S. Public Health Service Publication 1000 (Washington: U. S. Government Printing Office [occasional]).

Communicable Disease Center in Atlanta, Georgia.[1] In general morbidity data are the charge of the Public Health Service, and many divisions and bureaus publish data through the latter agency.

There are two recent publications of a bibliographic and methodological nature that no health study would be complete without consulting. The first of these is an extremely useful bibliography of health statistics prepared by Holleb.[2] In a compendium of information sources for social and economic planning, Holleb itemizes no less than 81 possible places to find some sort of health data. Of the above number nearly two-thirds of the references contain data directly related to potential or actual studies of Chicago while the remainder could be used for comparative analyses.

The second study to be considered is the monograph by Anderson and Kravits mentioned in Chapter I.[3] The authors explain limitations and uses of health data as well as some key sources. The data available are divided into six categories which indicate sources:

(1) Vital Statistics (Includes Mortality and Morbidity),
(2) Facilities,
(3) Personnel,
(4) Public Medical Care,
(5) Facilities Use, and
(6) Expenditures.

In spite of the several perspectives listed and the list developed by Holleb, few of these sources meet the needs of this RMP study as previously spelled out.

Primary sources of health data

When dealing with the geographical nature of health data the actual number of presently useful sources on a primary level is quickly reduced to a limited few. Of these, only the Department of Public Health collects statistics by small subareas for the entire SMSA. For many communicable diseases, morbidity data are gathered. Registries for heart disease, cancer, and stroke do not exist, and the health departments of Chicago and Illinois release only data for mortality. It is necessary to contact these departments

---

[1] U. S. Department of Health, Education, and Welfare, Morbidity and Mortality Weekly Report (Atlanta: Communicable Disease Center, Public Health Service).

[2] Doris E. Holleb, Social and Economic Information for Urban Planners, Vol. II: A Directory of Data Sources, Center for Urban Studies (Chicago: University of Chicago Press, 1969).

[3] Odin W. Anderson and Joanna Kravits, Health Services in the Chicago Area - A Framework for Data, University of Chicago Center for Health Administration Studies, Research Series No. 26 (Chicago: University of Chicago Press, 1968).

separately to obtain detailed data other than those reported in general reports.

Illinois Department of Public Health

The State of Illinois regularly publishes health data pertaining to cities and counties. The most recent of these reports, for example, demonstrates the scope of the data.[1] Basically, there are three kinds of health information tabulated.

The first group of information relates to live births and infant and maternal mortality. The data are separated in several ways, including by racial breakdown. Geographical subunits include counties and cities of 10,000 or more people.

The second type of data consists of breakdowns of leading causes of deaths in the state. Once again, the geographic subunits are counties and more important cities. The following table has been extracted from the vital statistics report. When comparing white and nonwhite populations, the three leading causes of death in 1967 (Heart Disease, Cancer, and Stroke) were the same. Diseases of early infancy took a greater toll of nonwhite than white infants. Also, homicide was the seventh cause for nonwhite mortality, but it did not show up in the white tabulation.

The third group of health statistics reported are the Notifiable Diseases, i.e., morbidity required to be reported to the Illinois Department of Public Health. These data are published only as state totals, Chicago totals and "Downstate" (remainder of Illinois) totals, but upon contact more detailed geographical breakdowns are available.

The major problem is whether or not there exist aggregations by areas small enough to fit particular purposes. Figure 67 shows what happens from the time death occurs until the final statistics are published in Illinois.[2]

Deaths are recorded either by private physicians or coroners. In accordance with 1957 Illinois legislation, a coroner must either be a physician or have a physician (hopefully a pathologist) as an assistant. The major pitfall here is that confusion can result from possible multiple causes of death. Bridger has pointed out how quite often some physicians have failed to fill out death certificates completely enough to meet the requirements of the statistical tabulation methods. Many certificates are returned for more complete information. Furthermore, it is often difficult for physicians to pinpoint only one cause of death in many instances.

---

[1]Illinois Department of Public Health, "Vital Statistics, Illinois" (Springfield, February, 1969).

[2]Interview with Clyde Bridger, Chief Statistician, Illinois Department of Public Health, November, 1969.

TABLE 37

TEN LEADING CAUSES OF DEATH, ILLINOIS RESIDENTS: 1967
(Rates Are per 100,000 Estimated Population as of July 1, 1967)

Cause	Number	Rate	Per Cent
White			
ALL CAUSES	97,065	1,014.3	100.0
1. Heart disease	43,453	454.1	44.8
2. Malignant neoplasms	16,562	173.1	17.1
3. Vascular lesions affecting central nervous system	10,036	104.9	10.3
4. Accidents	4,844	50.6	5.0
5. Influenza and pneumonia	2,705	28.3	2.8
6. Diseases of early infancy	1,987	20.8	2.0
7. General arteriosclerosis	1,945	20.3	2.0
8. Diabetes mellitus	1,774	18.5	1.8
9. Cirrhosis of liver	1,428	14.9	1.5
10. Other circulatory diseases	1,361	14.2	1.4
Nonwhite			
ALL CAUSES	12,965	1,012.9	100.0
1. Heart disease	4,570	357.0	35.2
2. Malignant neoplasms	1,877	146.6	14.5
3. Vascular lesions affecting central nervous system	1,172	91.6	9.0
4. Diseases of early infancy	896	70.0	6.9
5. Accidents	735	57.4	5.7
6. Influenza and pneumonia	733	57.3	5.7
7. Homicide	496	38.8	3.8
8. Cirrhosis of liver	270	21.1	2.1
9. Diabetes mellitus	257	20.1	2.0
10. Other circulatory diseases	161	12.6	1.2

Source: Tabulations in Illinois Bureau of Statistics.

The Chicago Board of Health

Near the end of the nineteenth century and during the first part of the twentieth, the City of Chicago published many technical reports about the health of its citizens. In more recent decades the annual reports of the Chicago Board of Health have taken on the nature of public relations documents which would appear at first glance to contain little hard data. The most recent of these reports contains information with the following characteristics:[1]

[1] Chicago Board of Health, "Annual Report for 1967" (Chicago, 1969).

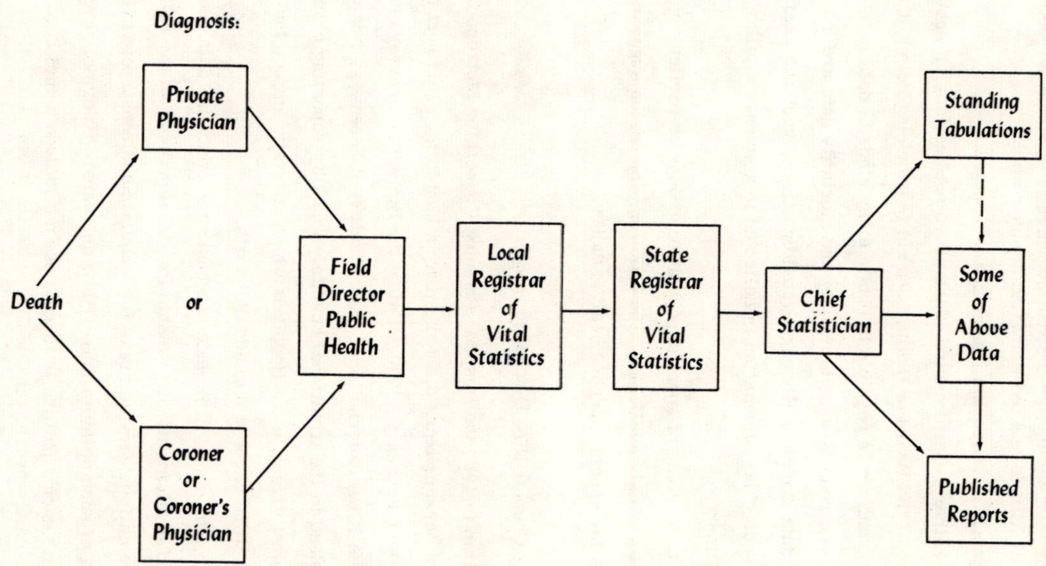

Fig. 67.--The flow of health data in Illinois

(1) Report about programs which are specific to the nature of an urban environment, e.g., rodent control, venereal disease control and lead poisoning detection.

(2) City-wide totals for leading causes of mortality are given and in these totals the very different nature of Chicago's health problems can be seen. For example, influenza and pneumonia and diseases of early infancy are the causes of more deaths than accidents--a situation which is different for both the white population of Illinois and the United States as a whole.

(3) City-wide totals for reported illnesses are published.

In spite of the rather general nature of the above publications, it should be remembered that one purpose of the Board of Health is to aid in providing help to Chicago's sick-poor when they are in need. It is possible to obtain many kinds of data for subareas of the city. Under normal circumstances morbidity and mortality data are made available upon request. These data are normally aggregated by census tract and Community Area before they are released. The information is collected in a manner similar to that used in the remainder of Illinois.

If studies are to be made of specific population groups or particular neighborhoods there are other sources of data available. The following discussion suggests four possible additional sources for special purpose health studies.

The Hospital Planning Council 1970 Discharge Study

In 1961 and again in 1965 the Hospital Planning Council for Metropolitan Chicago carried out surveys of persons being discharged from hospitals. This sort of survey took place during the month of February, 1970. Unlike the two earlier surveys, the most recent one included the ICDA (International Classification of Diseases, Adapted) classification system as opposed to the traditional hospital morbidity reporting of medical-surgical, pediatric, obstetrical, etc. Hospitals which normally employ the Standard Nomenclature system were requested to add diagnosis.

When released, the data will include diagnosis and other use data coded by census tracts for Chicago and municipality or township for the remainder of the SMSA. It will be possible once more to delimit service areas for hospitals and construct various demand surfaces. The result of such delimitations will be an overall pattern of revealed demand. The basic problem with such a pattern is that it does not include unmet needs for hospital care.

The Illinois Department of Public Aid

One method of accounting for what has above been termed unmet needs is to examine information provided by the Illinois Department of Public Aid about health care utilization of public aid recipients. This source is one of the better ones when dealing with health conditions in poverty areas. Data available include: (1) cases hospitalized; (2) physician visits; (3) prescriptions filled; (4) nursing home care; and (5) dental care. All information includes either length of stay or number of visits and average costs. The above data are available on an annual basis. Also useful is a daily report of all payments made by the Cook County Department of Public Aid for health services. The reports include the locations of both the "consumers" and "producers" of medical care.

The Chicago Board of Education

Yet another relatively untapped source of health status is to be found in a rather elaborate system of records kept by the Chicago Board of Education. Illinois law requires that all school age children have a complete physical and dental examination upon entry into school, in the fifth grade, and again in the ninth. Also, innoculations for polio, measles, diphtheria, tetanus, and smallpox must be obtained.

There are in addition special circumstances such as the identification of a handicap or a school accident which require recording. The resultant system of records includes about thirty-five separate forms. The most important of these forms (about half) are kept in a Cumulative Health Record Folder (CHRF) for each student.

The Welfare Council of Metropolitan Chicago

As indicated in the Chapter I discussion, the Welfare Council of Metropolitan Chicago has long been concerned with the health of Chicago's citizens, particularly the poor. During the 1960's this agency has been engaged in many projects related to health care. Two of these are of particular value as primary data sources. The first of these is the well-known four-part Maternal, Infant, and Preschool Child Survey supported by the United States Children's Bureau and the Illinois Department of Public Health. The references in Holleb and Anderson and Kravits spell out the value of that project in detail.

A more recent study was started in October, 1968. The Welfare Council has undertaken for the Chicago Housing Authority (CHA) an inventory of availability and use of health and welfare facilities. The data generated are sufficient to represent Chicago's public housing population. The sample includes six sites with nearly half of all Chicago CHA units. The racial composition is 95 per cent nonwhite and 7 per cent white. The actual survey was conducted in two parts. The first part consists of the results of a questionnaire sent to agencies providing services and the second part contains the results of questionnaires sent to tenants of CHA units. There are many kinds of information about attitudes toward and use of health care facilities.

Sources of ancillary health data

Several additional sources of supporting health data exist in Chicago. Although the data categorized here may not warrant separate studies, they should be considered for possible inclusion in larger research projects.

Health status of long-term care patients

The Hospital Planning Council for Metropolitan Chicago recently completed a survey of long-term care facilities in the Chicago SMSA. Many of the data in the final reports generated from the survey include aspects of the health status of inhabitants of these institutions. The survey included most licensed nursing homes, homes for the aged and sheltered care facilities in the metropolitan area. Health data include a 12.5 per cent sample of diagnosed maladies and services required. One important aspect of this study is that it includes the last non-institutional address of patients coded either by Chicago community areas or suburban municipalities.

Mental health data

The Illinois Department of Mental Health keeps records of admissions to state mental institutions by twenty-one diagnostic categories. The data are listed by place of residence, but aggregations are by mental health planning areas which do not correspond to existing demographic data collection units. The data are available by race, sex, and age, but there is a two to three year lag. Another source, the *Chicago Community Area Factbook*, published in 1962 a tabulation of patients admitted to 44 public and private psychiatric hospitals. Five diagnostic categories were included, and of particular interest to the Regional Medical Program research is the category "chronic brain disorders associated with senility or arteriosclerosis." Psychiatric admissions to general hospitals were included in the 1965 and 1970 discharge surveys by the Hospital Planning Council.

Conclusions

Although the specific data sources mentioned in this appendix are hardly exhaustive, they point out two major considerations in health data collection: (1) for accurate tabulations by small geographic subareas it is often necessary and perhaps desirable to establish interpersonal contacts to obtain data; (2) for many health studies one single kind of information may prove to be inadequate, and it could be useful to augment specific studies with comparisons of data from other primary and ancillary studies.

APPENDIX B

REPORTED MORTALITY AND MORBIDITY ESTIMATES

REPORTED MORTALITY AND MORBIDITY ESTIMATES

The bulk of this appendix consists of tabulated listings of reported mortality and morbidity estimates by the 271 subareas indicated in Chapter III. Tables 39 and 40 contain the actual number of deaths attributed to either heart disease, stroke, or the various cancer sites used in this study for 1960 and 1967. Tables 41 and 42 contain crude rates per thousand population for 1960 and 1967. For heart disease and stroke the rates on the latter two tables are for mortality as reported. For the cancers, morbidity estimates have been attempted.

The underlying assumption for making estimates for the cancers is that sufficient studies have been completed which indicate that there are identifiable and measurable ratios between actual incidence and mortality for the various cancer sites. Due to the fact that Illinois does not maintain a registry, multiplicative constants were developed from ratios suggested by the studies of Bailer, et al., of the National Cancer Institute. The ratios mentioned above are based largely upon previous findings of mortality-morbidity differentials in Connecticut, New York State (excluding New York City), California, and various urban populations.

Basically, the National Cancer Institute work arrived at the conclusion that in the immediate future, the incidence of cancer will continue to rise, but mortality rates will either rise at a much slower rate or remain essentially what they were in 1965. In addition, the ratios for various sites will change at different rates. Some sites, however, as is the case with leukemia, show nearly the same rate for mortality as for incidence. As a result, eight multiplicative constants were required for the conversions. The constants were used as scalars applied to all areas for which there was mortality reporting. The scalars are shown on Table 38.

TABLE 38

SCALARS USED FOR ESTIMATING CANCER MORBIDITY, 1960 AND 1967

Site Groups	1960	1967
TOTAL CANCER	1.93	2.04
Digestive cancer	1.27	1.35
Respiratory cancer	1.12	1.12
Genital cancer (M and F)	2.42	2.43
Breast cancer	2.33	2.53
Leukemia and aleukemia	1.05	1.05
Buccal cavity and pharynx	2.25	2.30
Skin cancer	2.60	2.76
All other or unspecified	2.60	2.76

TABLE 39

DEATHS REPORTED FOR HEART DISEASE, STROKE AND CANCER, 1960

Unit Area	Reported Mortality										
	Heart Disease	Stroke	Total Cancer	Cancer of Digestive Organs (1)	Respiratory Cancer (2)	Cancer of the Genital Organs (M & F) (3)	Breast Cancer (4)	Leukemia (5)	Cancer of the Buccal Cavity and Pharynx (6)	Skin Cancer (7)	Cancer Sites Unspecified (Also All Other) (8)
1	252	70	120	18	13	9	15	1	1	1	62
2	290	58	109	22	21	5	16	0	0	0	45
3	874	172	290	46	62	29	29	1	2	2	119
4	257	62	132	22	21	12	13	0	0	0	64
5	260	47	97	14	14	9	14	1	1	1	43
6	678	111	259	43	41	23	23	2	1	4	122
7	473	98	185	23	43	15	21	0	1	2	80
8	402	58	143	18	35	10	11	0	1	0	68
9	37	17	12	1	2	1	2	0	0	0	6
10	138	36	77	10	7	8	6	1	0	1	44
11	113	24	49	9	8	2	4	0	0	1	25
12	72	16	22	4	2	1	4	0	0	0	11
13	69	16	29	3	3	2	3	0	0	0	18
14	292	62	111	20	17	9	11	0	1	1	52
15	292	86	142	21	31	14	8	0	0	1	67
16	269	52	114	9	14	9	16	0	1	0	65
17	146	29	72	20	9	3	7	0	0	1	32
18	65	14	29	5	7	3	0	0	0	0	14

19	287	36	125	16	16	11	8	0	0	0	74
20	79	19	30	6	5	3	6	1	0	0	9
21	183	29	70	10	9	6	7	0	0	1	37
22	470	86	163	23	32	13	9	1	3	0	82
23	286	50	139	21	17	17	13	2	2	0	67
24	599	99	255	41	40	25	19	0	3	1	126
25	640	106	270	51	49	20	21	1	1	0	127
26	212	41	68	11	11	5	4	1	0	1	35
27	219	50	72	13	11	9	9	0	0	0	30
28	727	109	173	23	41	12	10	0	0	0	87
29	278	67	111	17	14	19	11	0	0	0	50
30	321	55	123	19	21	8	10	0	3	1	61
31	227	31	93	11	17	12	6	1	2	1	43
32	110	15	19	3	5	0	1	0	0	1	9
33	71	24	22	3	3	2	4	0	1	0	9
34	72	18	29	6	4	2	4	0	0	0	13
35	246	61	88	15	16	14	9	0	0	1	33
36	97	23	37	5	5	6	4	0	1	0	16
37	47	7	15	2	3	3	3	0	0	0	4
38	499	127	182	27	23	30	12	0	0	0	90
39	133	32	56	10	10	4	6	1	0	0	25
40	265	62	108	19	12	20	9	1	0	0	47
41	217	46	887	22	16	4	9	0	1	1	34
42	300	72	115	17	15	15	15	0	2	0	51
43	444	84	174	28	31	10	19	0	2	0	84
44	133	37	70	10	6	12	7	0	1	0	34
45	53	11	24	5	5	1	4	0	0	0	9
46	255	48	86	9	12	11	5	0	2	1	46
47	9	3	3	0	0	0	0	0	0	0	3
48	65	14	35	5	8	2	0	0	0	0	20
49	220	53	98	18	17	8	7	0	0	1	47
50	41	2	17	1	3	2	1	0	0	0	10
51	54	10	29	4	5	2	3	0	0	0	15
52	81	20	34	6	5	4	2	0	0	0	17
53	122	19	51	11	9	5	4	0	0	0	22
54	17	2	5	0	0	1	0	0	0	0	4

TABLE 39--Continued

Unit Area	Reported Mortality										
	Heart Disease	Stroke	Total Cancer	(1)	(2)	(3)	(4)	(5)	(6)	(7)	(8)
55	24	3	13	3	2	1	1	0	0	0	6
56	92	13	32	6	2	1	4	0	0	0	19
57	31	9	25	3	4	2	3	1	1	0	11
58	170	39	71	5	11	8	6	0	3	0	38
59	95	10	27	7	5	3	1	0	0	0	11
60	200	22	74	10	11	4	6	0	2	1	40
61	348	44	117	14	25	6	7	0	1	0	64
62	45	2	20	5	3	1	0	0	0	0	11
63	126	22	52	8	9	4	6	0	0	1	24
64	51	11	25	2	4	2	5	0	0	0	12
65	87	18	54	7	6	2	7	0	0	1	31
66	257	41	112	13	24	8	16	1	0	1	49
67	319	58	112	18	15	8	8	0	1	2	60
68	264	72	118	27	19	16	7	0	0	1	48
69	240	51	76	11	12	14	5	0	2	0	32
70	54	6	36	6	6	2	2	0	0	0	20
71	296	57	108	14	19	12	12	0	2	2	47
72	98	24	37	7	5	5	4	0	0	0	16
73	118	27	50	8	7	1	5	0	0	0	29
74	57	8	28	5	2	3	7	0	0	0	11
75	98	28	45	9	6	7	5	0	0	0	18
76	87	19	20	9	4	2	1	1	0	0	3
77	51	9	21	7	3	3	4	1	0	1	2
78	315	68	123	46	19	13	11	2	5	1	26
79	112	19	36	14	7	4	2	0	0	0	9
80	91	9	41	13	6	6	4	2	1	0	9
81	71	14	32	10	2	7	5	1	2	1	4

82	125	34	56	15	11	12	5	1	1	1	10
83	344	81	135	54	19	12	20	7	4	2	17
84	122	25	33	10	5	2	5	3	1	1	6
85	34	12	15	2	6	1	2	0	0	0	4
86	103	18	51	21	8	2	4	3	2	0	11
87	405	101	140	50	21	17	19	6	4	1	22
88	77	18	23	8	4	3	2	1	0	0	5
89	94	25	27	14	1	5	4	1	0	0	2
90	42	5	23	7	4	2	4	2	1	1	2
91	41	13	31	12	2	2	4	1	1	1	8
92	107	25	49	17	6	7	6	1	3	1	8
93	41	4	21	6	4	1	2	1	2	0	5
94	68	21	25	12	3	1	3	1	0	0	5
95	49	8	14	6	1	1	2	0	1	0	3
96	39	4	21	6	2	5	4	0	0	0	4
97	29	4	10	3	1	1	3	0	0	0	2
98	139	27	48	17	7	5	5	4	0	0	10
99	96	21	36	14	7	2	4	2	0	0	7
100	46	5	28	13	3	4	3	2	0	1	2
101	34	8	20	6	6	2	2	1	0	0	3
102	59	12	27	12	2	3	3	3	0	1	3
103	32	6	15	4	1	3	3	0	0	0	4
104	22	6	8	2	2	1	1	1	0	0	1
105	37	2	9	4	3	1	0	1	0	0	0
106	118	17	46	18	5	2	3	1	0	3	4
107	391	82	142	54	18	16	16	9	4	1	24
108	38	12	18	4	2	3	3	3	2	1	3
109	30	7	15	3	2	1	2	3	0	0	4
110	106	21	45	14	6	6	8	2	2	0	7
111	48	13	20	7	4	3	1	1	0	0	4
112	46	14	29	8	7	3	2	1	0	0	8
113	8	1	9	1	1	2	3	1	0	0	1
114	130	36	76	25	10	8	9	6	3	1	14
115	42	6	25	4	4	8	2	2	0	0	5
116	106	34	30	13	5	4	4	1	1	0	2
117	42	13	34	15	3	4	4	0	0	0	8

TABLE 39--Continued

Unit Area	Reported Mortality										
	Heart Disease	Stroke	Total Cancer	(1)	(2)	(3)	(4)	(5)	(6)	(7)	(8)
118	7	1	5	1	0	1	2	0	0	0	1
119	28	4	7	2	1	0	0	1	0	0	3
120	16	4	7	3	0	2	1	1	0	0	0
121	9	0	2	1	1	0	0	0	0	0	0
122	24	1	5	0	0	3	0	1	0	0	1
123	17	1	3	0	0	2	1	0	0	0	0
124	13	2	2	0	2	0	0	0	0	0	0
125	12	4	3	2	1	0	0	0	0	0	0
126	8	1	5	1	1	1	0	0	0	0	2
127	11	0	12	5	1	2	2	0	0	0	2
128	29	5	14	3	3	0	2	1	0	0	5
129	20	1	5	1	1	1	0	1	0	0	1
130	13	4	5	1	2	0	0	1	0	0	1
131	11	2	5	0	2	2	1	0	0	0	0
132	16	4	7	5	1	0	0	0	1	0	0
133	4	1	1	0	0	1	0	0	0	0	0
134	8	2	2	0	1	0	0	1	0	0	0
135	8	2	7	1	0	1	2	2	0	0	1
136	15	2	6	2	2	1	0	0	1	0	0
137	29	2	6	1	1	1	2	0	0	0	1
138	32	8	18	8	2	3	1	0	1	0	3
139	17	6	10	5	1	0	1	0	0	0	3
140	9	4	3	1	0	0	1	0	1	0	0
141	48	8	12	4	2	2	1	1	0	0	2
142	5	3	4	1	0	1	1	0	0	0	1
143	23	4	10	4	0	2	2	1	0	0	1
144	17	1	5	1	0	1	0	0	0	0	3

145	3	1	0	0	0	0	0	0	0	0	0
146	7	2	7	5	0	0	1	1	0	0	0
147	4	2	6	0	2	1	1	1	1	0	0
148	18	2	5	1	1	1	1	0	0	0	1
149	9	3	7	1	2	2	0	0	0	0	2
150	26	9	15	5	2	1	2	0	0	0	5
151	54	11	23	9	0	4	3	0	0	0	7
152	34	7	16	6	4	2	2	0	0	0	2
153	0	2	0	0	0	0	0	0	0	0	0
154	16	5	4	1	1	1	0	0	0	0	1
155	15	5	3	1	1	1	0	0	0	0	0
156	29	8	11	7	1	1	0	0	0	0	2
157	30	8	8	0	3	2	1	0	1	0	1
158	8	3	3	2	0	0	1	0	0	0	0
159	7	0	1	1	0	0	0	0	0	0	0
160	35	7	18	6	4	2	0	0	0	0	4
161	5	3	3	1	0	1	0	0	0	0	1
162	20	1	11	4	0	1	1	2	0	0	3
163	31	14	7	1	1	1	2	0	0	0	2
164	7	2	2	0	1	0	0	0	0	0	1
165	29	1	12	2	4	3	0	1	0	0	2
166	13	5	6	0	1	3	1	0	0	0	1
167	10	3	2	2	0	0	0	0	0	0	0
168	8	2	1	0	0	1	0	0	0	0	0
169	20	1	7	1	0	4	0	1	0	1	1
170	95	34	34	14	7	1	2	0	1	1	9
171	30	4	17	6	2	3	4	0	0	0	2
172	40	6	18	8	4	0	2	1	0	1	3
173	32	3	12	4	1	3	0	1	2	0	1
174	20	1	5	3	0	0	1	0	0	0	1
175	12	1	2	1	0	0	0	0	0	0	1
176	70	7	26	10	5	3	3	3	0	1	5
177	31	8	13	7	2	1	2	1	0	0	0
178	85	24	36	11	2	3	5	6	3	1	5
179	44	13	17	9	2	1	0	1	0	1	3
180	199	36	67	26	7	11	7	6	3	1	6

TABLE 39--Continued

Unit Area	Reported Mortality										
	Heart Disease	Stroke	Total Cancer	(1)	(2)	(3)	(4)	(5)	(6)	(7)	(8)
181	21	12	12	6	3	0	2	1	0	0	0
182	22	11	11	3	0	5	1	0	0	0	2
183	9	4	4	1	0	1	1	0	0	0	1
184	11	3	7	2	3	0	0	0	0	0	1
185	13	3	3	1	1	0	0	1	0	0	0
186	40	7	18	8	2	5	1	0	0	1	1
187	10	2	4	1	1	1	1	0	0	0	0
188	37	8	11	4	2	2	1	0	0	0	2
189	17	0	13	7	2	1	2	0	0	1	0
190	9	1	4	3	0	1	0	0	0	0	0
191	6	0	3	2	1	0	0	0	0	0	0
192	12	3	3	3	0	0	0	0	0	0	0
193	9	2	6	2	0	1	0	1	0	0	2
194	44	9	22	11	6	3	1	0	0	0	1
195	38	3	21	6	2	9	2	1	0	0	1
196	19	6	7	4	1	1	0	1	0	0	0
197	29	3	12	5	3	1	2	0	0	0	1
198	42	8	15	4	2	4	1	1	0	0	3
199	16	2	3	1	0	2	0	0	0	1	0
200	8	0	4	2	1	0	0	0	0	0	1
201	21	5	6	2	1	2	0	0	0	1	1
202	24	5	6	1	1	2	0	0	0	0	1
203	19	3	4	2	2	0	0	0	0	0	0
204	14	1	10	0	4	0	2	1	0	2	2
205	300	79	123	45	14	17	17	7	1	4	18
206	21	6	14	5	3	0	1	0	0	0	5
207	240	69	81	27	11	10	10	7	1	0	15

208	50	2	11	3	2	2	0	1	1	0	2
209	33	9	8	4	0	1	1	0	0	0	2
210	8	2	2	1	0	1	0	0	0	0	0
211	33	6	11	6	2	0	0	0	1	0	0
212	30	10	14	2	4	3	1	1	0	0	0
213	15	7	10	7	1	1	0	1	0	0	0
214	19	8	7	2	1	2	2	0	0	0	0
215	7	1	4	2	1	0	1	0	0	0	0
216	10	3	0	0	0	0	0	0	0	0	0
217	14	0	2	1	0	0	0	0	0	0	1
218	16	3	7	3	2	1	0	0	0	0	1
219	37	10	12	4	2	4	0	0	0	0	2
220	30	8	21	8	3	3	2	0	0	1	4
221	15	10	6	3	0	1	1	0	0	0	1
222	24	7	10	1	1	2	0	0	1	1	4
223	18	6	5	3	0	2	0	0	0	0	0
224	45	17	17	11	1	2	1	0	0	0	2
225	14	10	7	5	0	0	0	0	1	0	1
226	7	3	5	3	0	1	1	0	0	0	0
227	41	16	28	9	3	5	3	2	1	1	4
228	113	24	39	16	4	7	2	2	0	1	8
229	61	17	36	8	5	7	4	4	1	0	7
230	111	28	55	19	7	7	8	0	0	2	12
231	49	15	23	3	5	3	3	2	0	0	7
232	72	14	16	8	1	4	0	0	0	0	2
233	61	21	27	7	4	3	5	2	0	0	6
234	43	6	16	5	3	3	2	0	0	0	3
235	45	7	25	10	2	5	3	0	0	0	5
236	56	13	27	7	7	4	3	1	0	0	5
237	14	1	6	1	2	0	0	1	0	0	2
238	38	10	23	10	3	3	0	2	1	0	4
239	11	4	15	4	2	1	3	2	0	0	3
240	15	3	4	1	0	0	3	0	0	0	0
241	9	2	3	0	0	0	0	0	0	0	3
242	12	0	9	3	1	3	1	1	0	0	0
243	21	1	11	1	1	2	3	1	0	0	3

TABLE 39--Continued

Unit Area	Reported Mortality										
	Heart Disease	Stroke	Total Cancer	(1)	(2)	(3)	(4)	(5)	(6)	(7)	(8)
244	21	3	12	5	1	2	1	0	0	0	3
245	7	3	8	3	2	0	2	0	0	0	1
246	10	3	5	1	1	1	1	0	0	0	1
247	33	7	19	4	1	4	4	1	1	0	4
248	15	1	4	2	0	1	0	1	0	0	0
249	35	11	17	9	3	2	2	1	0	0	0
250	22	5	10	3	0	4	1	0	0	1	2
251	55	14	13	5	2	1	1	0	0	0	4
252	38	12	15	3	2	2	4	0	2	1	2
253	355	77	112	40	13	13	17	6	4	3	16
254	5	2	2	2	0	0	0	0	0	0	0
255	12	5	11	1	1	2	2	0	0	1	5
256	40	4	13	3	1	1	0	3	1	0	4
257	1	1	2	0	0	0	2	0	0	0	0
258	7	2	3	1	1	1	0	0	0	0	0
259	28	5	6	3	0	0	0	1	0	0	2
260	5	1	4	1	0	0	0	2	0	0	1
261	31	8	5	1	0	2	0	0	0	0	2
262	40	7	13	3	1	1	0	3	1	0	4
263	93	14	31	7	3	6	4	3	0	1	8
264	28	4	9	3	0	0	0	1	0	1	5
265	28	4	9	3	2	0	0	1	0	0	3
266	16	3	5	2	0	0	1	0	0	0	2
267	5	1	1	1	0	0	0	0	0	0	0
268	19	5	6	2	2	1	0	0	0	0	1
269	14	2	4	1	1	1	1	0	0	0	0
270	14	2	4	1	0	0	2	0	0	0	1
271	13	1	3	0	1	0	0	1	0	0	1

TABLE 40

DEATHS REPORTED FOR HEART DISEASE, STROKE AND CANCER, 1967

Unit Area	Reported Mortality										
	Heart Disease	Stroke	Total Cancer	Cancer of Digestive Organs (1)	Respiratory Cancer (2)	Cancer of the Genital Organs (M & F) (3)	Breast Cancer (4)	Leukemia (5)	Cancer of the Buccal Cavity and Pharynx (6)	Skin Cancer (7)	Cancer Sites Unspecified (Also All Other) (8)
1	280	53	113	16	26	11	11	1	1	5	42
2	353	51	142	31	17	4	15	0	0	0	71
3	951	164	285	47	56	25	34	0	3	0	120
4	278	54	115	11	30	11	10	0	0	0	53
5	229	40	81	13	21	5	14	0	0	0	28
6	714	129	245	35	53	30	18	0	1	4	104
7	387	69	135	18	19	19	11	0	0	4	64
8	420	76	129	17	24	9	15	1	1	0	62
9	39	9	18	0	4	1	6	0	0	0	7
10	186	30	76	14	12	7	9	0	0	1	33
11	148	27	65	11	12	3	6	0	0	2	31
12	79	19	37	4	11	4	5	0	0	0	13
13	81	14	42	7	3	3	8	1	0	1	19
14	261	55	106	20	21	4	7	6	2	3	49
15	345	88	144	24	21	11	15	0	0	3	70
16	293	67	120	15	25	11	15	2	2	0	50
17	203	32	69	13	7	4	12	0	0	1	32
18	62	16	20	3	2	1	2	1	0	0	11

TABLE 40--Continued

Unit Area	Reported Mortality										
	Heart Disease	Stroke	Total Cancer	(1)	(2)	(3)	(4)	(5)	(6)	(7)	(8)
19	296	53	125	22	26	6	7	0	2	0	62
20	108	22	45	7	9	1	1	0	0	0	27
21	216	32	79	7	18	9	10	0	0	1	35
22	470	77	158	17	29	11	11	0	0	1	89
23	319	58	125	13	30	11	15	0	2	0	54
24	611	103	226	41	46	14	13	1	2	2	107
25	555	103	194	29	46	14	16	3	2	0	84
26	106	26	43	4	11	5	6	0	0	0	17
27	172	50	80	5	15	13	2	0	2	2	41
28	609	79	148	21	32	18	12	0	0	0	65
29	265	52	103	12	23	15	12	0	1	2	38
30	265	68	106	16	12	10	6	0	1	1	60
31	194	29	49	9	13	5	4	0	0	0	18
32	99	6	30	4	5	3	0	0	0	0	18
33	50	7	17	1	3	1	1	0	0	2	9
34	57	12	24	7	6	3	2	0	0	0	6
35	193	37	62	5	15	11	4	0	0	0	27
36	101	26	25	3	4	2	1	0	0	0	15
37	42	12	12	1	3	3	2	0	0	0	3
38	536	129	194	24	38	31	14	0	1	0	86
39	168	37	57	8	11	10	6	0	0	1	21
40	277	63	117	23	21	11	9	0	0	1	52
41	155	26	58	12	5	4	5	0	0	1	31
42	279	68	118	9	15	16	12	0	2	1	63
43	404	87	155	22	32	13	13	1	1	0	73
44	134	40	72	10	12	8	8	1	0	1	32
45	53	11	18	1	6	1	1	0	0	0	9

46	251	28	82	10	20	4	7	0	0	1	40
47	20	6	6	0	3	0	0	0	0	0	3
48	91	12	36	5	6	1	3	0	0	1	20
49	280	47	90	18	9	12	5	1	1	1	33
50	28	6	10	2	2	0	0	0	0	0	6
51	87	9	32	4	12	0	1	0	0	0	15
52	71	22	44	7	6	6	4	0	0	1	20
53	133	16	45	5	6	4	3	0	0	0	27
54	23	5	4	1	2	0	0	0	0	0	1
55	40	5	11	1	5	2	1	0	0	0	2
56	91	11	46	4	11	4	1	0	1	0	25
57	47	9	24	5	2	3	3	0	0	1	10
58	168	31	67	13	10	3	11	1	0	0	29
59	77	15	32	9	5	2	1	0	0	0	15
60	213	41	70	3	13	7	9	1	1	1	35
61	303	41	105	16	22	14	4	0	1	0	48
62	58	11	20	5	2	2	1	0	0	0	10
63	133	19	52	12	12	4	4	0	0	1	19
64	55	21	19	3	5	0	0	0	0	0	11
65	97	16	44	6	8	8	5	0	1	0	16
66	274	38	127	19	17	7	22	1	0	1	60
67	276	56	92	15	19	8	8	0	0	0	42
68	320	63	119	12	15	25	7	0	2	0	58
69	213	54	96	11	18	12	16	0	0	0	39
70	107	14	41	4	9	3	7	0	0	0	18
71	242	42	115	17	18	9	17	0	0	2	52
72	66	16	38	8	4	6	5	0	0	0	15
73	100	19	35	6	7	1	4	0	1	1	15
74	22	8	18	1	3	2	1	0	0	0	11
75	92	16	46	4	8	5	5	0	1	0	23
76	123	23	49	13	4	6	6	3	4	0	13
77	67	12	33	7	10	7	1	0	1	0	7
78	360	87	155	48	28	29	9	10	6	2	23
79	125	19	49	22	9	8	4	1	1	0	4
80	101	19	39	16	8	5	5	1	0	0	4
81	110	25	43	10	6	11	4	2	1	1	8

TABLE 40--Continued

Unit Area	Reported Mortality										
	Heart Disease	Stroke	Total Cancer	(1)	(2)	(3)	(4)	(5)	(6)	(7)	(8)
82	159	40	52	20	8	6	5	3	0	0	10
83	418	87	142	41	34	16	16	4	3	1	27
84	205	40	79	14	21	14	7	2	1	0	20
85	58	19	25	9	5	6	2	2	0	1	0
86	115	29	56	21	9	9	7	0	0	0	10
87	449	138	143	50	25	15	13	12	2	3	23
88	115	31	53	25	9	3	3	3	1	0	9
89	101	21	32	5	13	1	2	2	3	0	6
90	56	10	18	3	3	5	2	1	0	0	4
91	100	32	48	13	8	3	4	5	4	1	10
92	163	23	45	10	9	6	9	3	1	1	6
93	68	10	33	12	8	2	2	3	0	0	6
94	96	21	41	14	9	7	3	1	0	0	7
95	72	19	23	6	4	6	1	0	1	1	4
96	54	15	34	12	5	3	4	0	1	1	8
97	50	7	21	8	3	1	4	1	0	0	4
98	143	13	37	11	9	4	3	1	0	1	8
99	89	16	50	13	12	8	5	2	0	2	8
100	76	11	34	11	5	2	5	1	1	1	8
101	75	18	29	12	6	5	3	0	0	1	2
102	112	21	38	11	11	3	3	3	0	1	6
103	63	10	20	7	9	1	2	0	0	1	0
104	51	11	30	8	4	3	5	4	0	0	6
105	35	4	18	7	6	0	3	1	0	0	1
106	224	30	84	25	17	13	5	8	0	3	13
107	404	105	151	45	24	24	22	3	4	4	25
108	65	15	29	11	5	4	5	2	0	1	1

109	36	6	21	5	2	3	3	1	0	0	7
110	185	26	65	28	5	3	12	3	1	0	13
111	56	9	29	10	6	3	3	0	0	1	6
112	51	14	31	7	2	6	7	1	0	0	8
113	13	5	6	1	1	0	0	2	0	0	2
114	14	472	115	37	17	14	24	10	0	2	11
115	63	14	31	14	6	2	4	1	0	0	4
116	143	26	54	12	11	8	7	1	1	1	13
117	47	10	27	9	0	4	3	2	1	0	8
118	21	2	9	1	2	1	1	1	0	0	3
119	31	5	9	2	0	1	2	0	1	0	3
120	16	3	7	0	2	1	1	1	0	0	2
121	10	2	7	1	2	1	2	1	0	0	0
122	37	4	9	1	3	1	3	1	0	0	0
123	17	6	13	4	2	0	3	1	1	0	2
124	13	1	5	2	2	0	1	0	0	0	0
125	22	4	1	1	0	0	0	0	0	0	0
126	18	3	10	1	1	1	1	1	0	0	5
127	23	3	8	1	0	4	1	0	0	0	2
128	35	10	7	0	2	4	0	0	0	0	1
129	31	10	14	2	4	1	1	2	1	0	3
130	27	4	7	1	1	0	4	0	0	0	1
131	24	6	6	1	2	1	0	0	0	0	2
132	28	12	12	2	5	0	2	1	0	0	2
133	12	2	6	4	1	1	0	0	0	0	0
134	18	5	6	2	1	0	0	1	0	0	2
135	18	6	2	1	0	0	0	0	0	0	1
136	5	2	3	1	0	1	1	0	0	0	0
137	34	4	5	4	0	1	0	0	0	0	0
138	44	6	15	5	4	2	1	0	0	0	3
139	40	8	10	3	1	2	2	0	1	0	1
140	11	4	5	0	1	1	1	1	0	0	1
141	52	13	15	3	4	3	1	1	1	0	2
142	14	2	7	3	0	3	1	0	0	0	0
143	33	8	19	6	3	2	1	1	0	0	6
144	33	2	18	9	4	2	0	1	0	0	2

TABLE 40--Continued

Unit Area	Reported Mortality										
	Heart Disease	Stroke	Total Cancer	(1)	(2)	(3)	(4)	(5)	(6)	(7)	(8)
145	11	2	4	1	0	2	0	0	0	0	1
146	25	8	12	1	3	2	3	1	0	0	2
147	22	12	4	1	1	0	2	0	0	0	0
148	12	2	8	1	1	2	0	1	0	0	3
149	12	2	6	2	2	1	1	0	0	0	0
150	49	8	16	5	3	2	1	0	0	0	5
151	42	7	14	10	0	0	3	0	0	0	1
152	44	18	15	7	2	0	0	2	0	0	4
153	5	1	4	1	0	2	0	1	0	0	0
154	13	2	17	10	3	2	1	0	0	0	1
155	23	7	5	1	0	1	1	0	1	0	1
156	41	9	17	5	3	2	3	0	0	0	4
157	43	14	6	2	0	0	2	1	0	0	1
158	7	2	5	1	2	1	0	1	0	0	0
159	5	3	6	1	1	0	1	0	1	0	2
160	43	11	9	4	2	2	1	0	0	0	0
161	7	1	4	1	2	0	0	1	0	0	0
162	36	7	22	5	3	1	3	0	1	0	9
163	55	12	19	6	5	1	3	1	0	0	3
164	28	1	9	3	2	3	0	0	0	0	1
165	34	1	16	5	2	4	1	1	0	0	3
166	5	0	6	3	2	0	1	0	0	0	0
167	15	1	2	2	0	0	0	0	0	0	0
168	8	2	1	0	0	0	0	0	0	0	1
169	18	3	5	2	1	1	0	0	0	1	0
170	63	16	20	2	2	4	1	0	10	1	3
171	5	1	4	2	1	0	0	1	0	0	0

172	46	11	16	8	4	1	2	0	0	1	1
173	25	2	7	3	2	0	0	1	0	0	1
174	24	2	4	1	0	2	1	0	0	0	0
175	1	1	0	0	0	0	0	0	0	0	0
176	40	15	12	4	6	2	0	0	0	0	0
177	27	7	7	3	0	3	0	1	0	0	0
178	84	34	36	15	4	4	6	0	1	0	6
179	50	12	19	5	4	2	3	1	0	0	4
180	26	382	105	26	24	15	10	6	2	0	22
181	27	11	19	2	5	3	3	0	0	0	6
182	34	3	8	1	1	2	1	0	0	0	3
183	19	2	4	0	1	0	3	0	0	0	0
184	15	7	9	2	1	1	0	0	1	0	4
185	11	4	8	3	2	2	0	0	0	0	1
186	42	10	20	8	2	2	1	0	0	0	5
187	14	3	4	2	0	0	1	0	0	0	1
188	44	16	18	7	5	2	0	0	0	0	4
189	37	6	15	3	1	0	4	0	2	0	4
190	13	3	4	2	1	1	0	0	0	0	0
191	12	0	4	3	1	0	0	0	0	0	0
192	18	5	4	1	2	0	0	0	1	0	0
193	16	0	4	0	1	1	0	1	0	0	1
194	36	10	11	3	4	1	1	0	0	0	2
195	40	11	21	10	6	2	0	0	0	0	3
196	34	8	7	3	3	4	3	0	1	0	3
197	36	7	18	8	4	1	2	1	1	0	1
198	28	12	24	5	4	4	0	0	0	0	1
199	13	1	4	1	1	0	1	0	0	0	1
200	13	4	3	1	2	0	0	0	0	0	0
201	32	2	6	1	1	0	1	0	0	0	1
202	20	3	11	4	1	1	1	1	0	0	3
203	26	3	7	2	3	0	0	1	0	0	1
204	7	2	5	0	0	0	1	1	0	1	3
205	335	90	151	45	34	22	19	8	2	0	21
206	31	11	12	4	3	1	2	1	0	0	1
207	273	63	75	20	18	7	8	2	2	0	10

TABLE 40--Continued

Unit Area	Reported Mortality										
	Heart Disease	Stroke	Total Cancer	(1)	(2)	(3)	(4)	(5)	(6)	(7)	(8)
208	45	3	17	4	4	3	1	1	1	0	3
209	42	17	19	5	2	2	5	0	1	0	4
210	10	1	2	1	0	0	0	0	0	0	1
211	59	17	18	6	5	0	2	2	0	0	3
212	35	3	4	1	0	1	2	0	0	0	0
213	26	7	6	2	1	2	0	0	0	0	1
214	27	7	7	2	2	2	0	0	1	0	0
215	22	8	9	1	2	3	0	0	0	0	3
216	4	1	0	0	0	0	0	0	0	0	0
217	11	1	2	1	1	0	0	0	0	0	0
218	19	6	3	1	0	1	1	0	0	0	0
219	24	4	7	3	3	0	0	0	0	0	1
220	41	14	12	5	2	1	2	0	1	0	1
221	24	13	6	2	1	2	1	0	0	0	0
222	32	9	20	4	6	1	1	1	2	1	4
223	20	3	8	1	2	0	1	0	0	1	3
224	63	24	23	13	0	0	3	1	0	0	6
225	5	26	8	1	1	2	0	0	2	1	1
226	5	26	7	1	2	0	1	0	0	0	3
227	16	13	20	4	6	1	1	1	2	1	4
228	5	27	20	3	4	5	3	0	1	1	3
229	102	17	53	12	11	8	6	4	1	0	11
230	141	29	59	14	13	5	6	3	3	0	15
231	54	16	20	4	3	3	5	0	0	0	5
232	40	11	25	10	5	1	2	0	0	0	7
233	79	12	32	8	7	3	6	1	0	0	7
234	59	18	21	6	2	3	2	1	1	0	6

235	54	15	36	11	9	2	1	2	0	0	11
236	98	13	34	14	6	4	4	1	0	0	5
237	26	2	11	2	5	1	1	2	0	0	0
238	49	13	26	9	5	4	1	2	0	0	5
239	27	2	12	4	2	2	1	2	0	0	1
240	13	4	6	0	3	1	1	0	0	0	1
241	15	2	8	0	3	1	0	1	0	0	3
242	14	2	5	2	1	1	1	0	0	0	0
243	26	4	9	2	0	2	2	1	1	0	1
244	42	8	19	8	2	3	2	1	0	0	3
245	17	12	9	1	4	2	0	1	0	0	1
246	12	3	3	0	0	0	0	1	0	0	2
247	29	7	10	2	3	2	0	1	0	0	2
248	25	3	15	5	4	2	0	1	0	0	3
249	35	9	14	4	3	1	3	2	0	0	1
250	34	7	9	2	3	0	0	1	0	0	3
251	45	8	21	6	3	3	4	0	0	1	5
252	60	16	13	6	1	1	2	2	0	1	1
253	428	109	156	48	30	19	19	7	5	0	28
254	19	4	7	5	0	0	1	0	0	0	1
255	14	0	7	2	1	0	1	0	0	0	3
256	41	10	9	6	2	0	0	0	0	0	1
257	3	2	4	1	1	1	0	0	0	0	1
258	12	1	10	3	3	1	0	1	0	0	2
259	20	2	8	4	0	0	1	0	2	0	1
260	5	1	2	1	0	0	0	1	0	0	0
261	31	9	12	3	5	2	0	0	1	0	1
262	20	4	12	4	2	4	0	0	2	0	0
263	67	15	16	11	1	2	0	0	0	0	2
264	18	7	19	4	6	2	2	1	0	1	4
265	27	7	8	0	2	1	1	2	0	0	2
266	1	10	5	2	0	0	1	0	0	0	2
267	1	10	5	2	0	0	1	0	0	0	2
268	8	2	11	6	2	0	1	0	0	0	2
269	4	1	4	2	1	0	0	0	0	0	1
270	7	2	4	2	0	0	2	0	0	0	0
271	5	3	7	1	2	1	2	0	0	0	1

TABLE 41

CRUDE RATES PER 1,000 FOR HEART DISEASE, STROKE AND CANCER, 1960

Unit Area	Reported Mortality		Estimated Cancer Morbidity								
	Heart Disease	Stroke	Total Cancer	Cancer of Digestive Organs (1)	Respiratory Cancer (2)	Cancer of the Genital Organs (M & F) (3)	Breast Cancer (4)	Leukemia (5)	Cancer of the Buccal Cavity and Pharynx (6)	Skin Cancer (7)	Cancer Sites Unspecified (Also All Other) (8)
1	4.430	1.230	4.071	0.402	0.256	0.369	0.638	0.018	0.040	2.834	0.046
2	4.539	0.908	3.293	0.437	0.368	0.182	0.606	0.0	0.0	1.831	0.0
3	6.845	1.347	4.384	0.458	0.544	0.529	0.550	0.008	0.035	2.423	0.041
4	5.155	1.244	5.111	0.560	0.472	0.561	0.631	0.0	0.0	3.338	0.0
5	5.926	0.071	4.267	0.405	0.357	0.478	0.772	0.024	0.051	2.548	0.059
6	5.709	0.935	4.209	0.460	0.387	0.451	0.469	0.018	0.019	2.671	0.088
7	5.324	1.103	4.019	0.329	0.542	0.393	0.572	0.0	0.025	2.341	0.059
8	5.324	0.768	3.655	0.303	0.519	0.309	0.353	0.0	0.030	2.341	0.0
9	2.944	1.353	1.843	0.101	0.178	0.185	0.385	0.0	0.0	1.241	0.0
10	3.370	0.879	3.629	0.310	0.191	0.455	0.355	0.026	0.0	2.793	0.063
11	4.110	0.873	3.440	0.416	0.326	0.169	0.352	0.0	0.0	2.364	0.095
12	3.745	0.832	2.208	0.264	0.116	0.121	0.503	0.0	0.0	1.487	0.0
13	3.862	0.896	3.133	0.213	0.188	0.261	0.406	0.0	0.0	2.620	0.0
14	5.905	1.254	4.332	0.514	0.385	0.424	0.538	0.0	0.046	2.734	0.053
15	4.429	1.305	4.157	0.405	0.527	0.495	0.294	0.0	0.0	2.642	0.039
16	4.614	0.892	3.774	0.196	0.269	0.360	0.664	0.0	0.039	2.899	0.0
17	3.507	0.697	3.338	0.610	0.242	0.168	0.407	0.0	0.0	1.999	0.062
18	5.508	1.186	4.742	0.538	0.664	0.592	0.0	0.0	0.0	3.084	0.0

19	4.714	0.591	3.963	0.334	0.294	0.421	0.318	0.0	0.0	3.160	0.0
20	3.687	0.887	2.702	0.356	0.261	0.326	0.678	0.049	0.0	1.092	0.0
21	4.604	0.730	3.399	0.320	0.254	0.352	0.426	0.0	0.0	2.420	0.065
22	4.958	0.907	3.318	0.308	0.378	0.320	0.230	0.011	0.071	2.249	0.0
23	3.994	0.698	3.746	0.372	0.266	0.553	0.439	0.029	0.063	2.433	0.0
24	4.289	0.709	3.524	0.373	0.321	0.417	0.329	0.0	0.048	2.346	0.019
25	5.115	0.847	4.164	0.518	0.439	0.372	0.406	0.008	0.018	2.639	0.0
26	4.648	0.899	2.877	0.306	0.270	0.255	0.212	0.023	0.0	1.995	0.057
27	3.275	0.748	2.078	0.247	0.184	0.314	0.326	0.0	0.0	1.166	0.0
28	5.742	0.861	2.637	0.231	0.363	0.221	0.191	0.0	0.0	1.787	0.0
29	2.225	0.536	0.715	0.173	0.126	0.354	0.213	0.0	0.0	1.041	0.0
30	5.267	0.903	3.895	0.396	0.386	0.306	0.397	0.0	0.111	2.603	0.043
31	4.685	0.640	3.705	0.288	0.393	0.577	0.300	0.022	0.093	2.308	0.054
32	25.363	3.459	8.455	0.878	1.291	0.0	0.558	0.0	0.0	5.395	0.599
33	6.860	2.319	4.102	0.368	0.325	0.450	0.935	0.0	0.217	2.261	0.0
34	4.562	1.140	3.546	0.483	0.284	0.295	0.613	0.0	0.0	2.142	0.0
35	4.701	1.166	3.246	0.364	0.342	0.623	0.416	0.0	0.0	1.640	0.050
36	3.979	0.943	2.929	0.260	0.230	0.573	0.397	0.0	0.092	1.706	0.0
37	3.858	0.575	2.377	0.209	0.276	0.574	0.596	0.0	0.0	0.854	0.0
38	6.235	1.587	4.389	0.428	0.322	0.873	0.363	0.0	0.0	2.924	0.0
39	3.202	0.770	2.602	0.306	0.270	0.224	0.350	0.025	0.0	1.565	0.0
40	6.065	1.419	4.771	0.552	0.308	1.607	0.499	0.024	0.0	2.7972	0.0
41	4.761	1.009	3.684	0.613	0.393	0.204	0.478	0.0	0.049	1.940	0.057
42	3.691	0.886	2.731	0.266	0.207	0.430	0.447	0.0	0.055	1.631	0.0
43	6.075	1.149	4.595	0.487	0.475	0.319	0.629	0.0	0.062	2.988	0.0
44	3.170	0.882	3.220	0.303	0.160	0.666	0.404	0.0	0.054	2.107	0.0
45	4.170	0.865	3.644	0.500	0.441	0.183	0.762	0.0	0.0	1.841	0.0
46	5.109	0.962	3.325	0.229	0.269	0.513	0.242	0.0	0.090	2.396	0.052
47	2.599	0.866	1.672	0.0	0.0	0.0	0.0	0.0	0.0	2.252	0.0
48	3.359	0.723	3.491	0.328	0.463	0.241	0.0	0.0	0.0	2.687	0.0
49	3.745	0.902	3.219	0.389	0.324	0.317	0.288	0.0	0.0	2.080	0.044
50	4.874	0.238	3.900	0.151	0.399	0.554	0.288	0.0	0.0	3.091	0.0
51	2.873	0.532	2.978	0.270	0.298	0.248	0.386	0.0	0.0	2.075	0.0
52	3.489	0.862	2.827	0.328	0.241	0.401	0.208	0.0	0.0	1.904	0.0
53	3.447	0.537	2.781	0.395	0.285	0.329	0.273	0.0	0.0	1.616	0.0
54	1.485	0.175	0.843	0.0	0.0	0.204	0.0	0.0	0.0	0.908	0.0

TABLE 41--Continued

Unit Area	Reported Mortality		Estimated Cancer Morbidity								
	Heart Disease	Stroke	Total Cancer	(1)	(2)	(3)	(4)	(5)	(6)	(7)	(8)
55	2.686	0.336	2.808	0.426	0.251	0.261	0.271	0.0	0.0	1.746	0.0
56	2.274	0.321	1.527	0.188	0.055	0.058	0.239	0.0	0.0	1.221	0.0
57	2.929	0.850	4.559	0.360	0.423	0.440	0.686	0.099	0.213	2.702	0.0
58	4.471	1.026	3.604	0.167	0.324	0.490	0.383	0.0	0.178	2.599	0.0
59	5.619	0.591	3.082	0.526	0.331	0.413	0.143	0.0	0.0	1.692	0.0
60	4.812	0.529	3.436	0.306	0.296	0.224	0.349	0.0	0.108	2.502	0.063
61	5.161	0.653	3.349	0.264	0.415	0.207	0.251	0.0	0.033	2.468	0.0
62	3.166	0.141	2.715	0.447	0.236	0.164	0.0	0.0	0.0	2.012	0.0
63	4.461	0.779	3.553	0.360	0.357	0.330	0.514	0.0	0.0	2.209	0.092
64	2.713	0.585	2.567	0.135	0.238	0.248	0.644	0.0	0.0	1.660	0.0
65	3.233	0.669	3.873	0.330	0.250	0.173	0.630	0.0	0.0	2.995	0.097
66	5.005	0.798	4.210	0.322	0.523	0.363	0.754	0.020	0.0	2.481	0.051
67	5.452	0.991	3.694	0.391	0.287	0.319	0.331	0.0	0.038	0.089	2.666
68	2.705	0.738	2.334	0.351	0.218	0.382	0.174	0.0	0.0	0.027	1.279
69	3.799	0.807	2.322	0.221	0.213	0.516	0.192	0.0	0.071	0.0	1.317
70	1.398	0.155	1.798	0.197	0.174	0.121	0.125	0.0	0.0	0.0	1.346
71	4.976	0.958	3.504	0.299	0.358	0.470	0.488	0.0	0.076	0.087	2.054
72	3.949	0.967	2.878	0.358	0.226	0.469	0.390	0.0	0.0	0.0	1.676
73	3.961	0.906	3.239	0.341	0.263	0.078	0.406	0.0	0.0	0.0	2.531
74	2.598	0.365	2.463	0.289	0.102	0.319	0.772	0.0	0.0	0.0	1.303
75	3.511	1.003	3.112	0.410	0.241	0.584	0.434	0.0	0.0	0.0	1.677
76	3.121	0.682	1.385	0.410	0.161	0.167	0.087	0.038	0.0	0.0	0.280
77	2.460	0.434	1.955	0.429	0.162	0.337	0.467	0.051	0.0	0.125	0.251
78	5.809	1.254	4.378	1.077	0.392	0.559	0.491	0.039	0.207	0.048	1.247
79	5.709	0.968	3.542	0.906	0.400	0.475	0.247	0.0	0.0	0.0	1.193
80	4.454	0.441	3.873	0.808	0.329	0.684	0.474	0.103	0.110	0.0	1.145
81	2.840	0.560	2.470	0.508	0.090	0.652	0.484	0.042	0.180	0.104	0.416

82	3.641	0.990	3.148	0.555	0.359	0.814	0.352	0.031	0.066	0.076	0.757
83	4.976	1.172	3.769	0.992	0.308	0.404	0.700	0.106	0.130	0.075	0.639
84	3.497	0.717	1.826	0.364	0.161	0.134	0.347	0.090	0.064	0.075	0.447
85	1.814	0.640	1.544	0.135	0.358	0.124	0.258	0.0	0.0	0.0	0.555
86	4.316	0.754	4.124	1.117	0.375	0.195	0.406	0.132	0.189	0.0	1.198
87	5.108	1.274	3.408	0.801	0.297	0.500	0.580	0.079	0.114	0.033	0.721
88	3.185	0.744	1.836	0.420	0.185	0.289	0.200	0.043	0.0	0.0	0.538
89	6.504	1.730	3.606	1.230	0.077	0.806	0.670	0.073	0.0	0.0	0.360
90	2.292	0.273	2.423	0.485	0.245	0.254	0.528	0.115	0.123	0.142	0.284
91	2.261	0.717	3.300	0.841	0.124	0.257	0.534	0.058	0.124	0.143	1.147
92	3.681	0.860	3.253	0.743	0.231	0.561	0.499	0.036	0.232	0.089	0.715
93	3.066	0.299	3.031	0.570	0.335	0.174	0.362	0.079	0.337	0.0	0.972
94	4.449	1.374	3.157	0.997	0.220	0.152	0.475	0.069	0.0	0.0	0.851
95	3.553	0.580	1.959	0.552q	0.081	0.169	0.351	0.0	0.163	0.0	0.566
96	2.155	0.221	2.239	0.421	0.124	0.644	0.535	0.0	0.0	0.0	0.575
97	2.469	0.341	1.643	0.324	0.095	0.198	0.618	0.0	0.0	0.0	0.443
98	5.086	0.988	3.390	0.790	0.287	0.426	0.443	0.154	0.0	0.0	0.951
99	4.307	0.942	3.117	0.798	0.352	0.209	0.434	0.094	0.0	0.0	0.816
100	2.240	0.244	2.632	0.804	0.164	0.454	0.354	0.102	0.0	0.127	0.253
101	1.798	0.423	2.042	0.403	0.355	0.246	0.256	0.056	0.0	0.0	0.413
102	2.893	0.588	2.555	0.747	0.110	0.343	0.356	0.154	0.0	0.127	0.382
103	2.272	0.426	2.055	0.361	0.080	0.496	0.515	0.0	0.0	0.0	0.738
104	1.891	0.516	1.327	0.218	0.193	0.200	0.208	0.090	0.0	0.0	0.223
105	3.004	0.162	0.410	0.412	0.273	0.189	0.0	0.085	0.0	0.0	0.0
106	4.295	0.619	3.232	0.832	0.204	0.170	0.264	0.038	0.0	0.284	1.325
107	6.400	1.342	4.486	1.123	0.330	0.610	0.634	0.155	0.147	0.043	1.021
108	3.303	1.043	3.020	0.442	0.195	0.608	0.631	0.183	0.196	0.0	0.678
109	1.000	0.233	0.965	0.127	0.075	0.078	0.161	0.105	0.0	0.0	0.347
110	3.246	0.643	2.659	0.544	0.206	0.428	0.593	0.064	0.138	0.0	0.557
111	3.997	1.083	3.215	0.740	0.373	0.582	0.202	0.087	0.0	0.0	0.866
112	3.623	1.103	4.409	0.800	0.618	0.551	0.381	0.083	0.0	0.0	1.638
113	0.735	0.092	1.597	0.117	0.103	0.428	0.667	0.097	0.0	0.0	0.239
114	2.190	0.606	2.471	0.535	0.189	0.314	0.367	0.106	0.114	0.044	0.613
115	2.321	0.332	2.667	0.281	0.248	1.030	0.268	0.116	0.0	0.0	0.719
116	3.750	1.203	2.048	0.584	0.198	0.330	0.342	0.037	0.080	0.0	0.184
117	3.142	0.972	4.909	0.425	0.251	0.697	0.724	0.0	0.0	0.0	1.556

TABLE 41--Continued

Unit Area	Reported Mortality		Estimated Cancer Morbidity								
	Heart Disease	Stroke	Total Cancer	(1)	(2)	(3)	(4)	(5)	(6)	(7)	(8)
118	1.857	0.265	2.560	0.337	0.0	0.618	1.284	0.0	0.0	0.0	0.690
119	5.153	0.736	2.486	0.467	0.206	0.0	0.0	0.193	0.0	0.0	1.435
120	2.762	0.691	2.333	0.658	0.0	0.805	0.418	0.181	0.0	0.0	0.0
121	1.227	0.0	0.526	0.173	0.153	0.0	0.0	0.0	0.0	0.0	0.0
122	2.795	0.116	1.124	0.0	0.0	0.814	0.0	0.122	0.0	0.0	0.303
123	2.012	0.118	0.685	0.0	0.0	0.552	0.286	0.0	0.0	0.0	0.0
124	2.262	0.348	0.672	0.0	0.390	0.0	0.0	0.0	0.0	0.0	0.0
125	3.901	1.300	1.882	0.826	0.364	0.0	0.0	0.0	0.0	0.0	0.0
126	1.211	0.151	1.460	0.192	0.169	0.353	0.0	0.0	0.0	0.0	0.787
127	2.379	0.0	5.009	1.373	0.242	1.008	1.047	0.0	0.0	0.0	1.125
128	2.769	0.477	2.580	0.364	0.321	0.0	0.462	0.100	0.0	0.0	0.241
129	3.516	0.176	1.697	0.223	0.197	0.410	0.0	0.185	0.0	0.0	0.457
130	2.095	0.645	1.555	0.205	0.361	0.0	0.0	0.169	0.0	0.0	0.419
131	4.064	0.739	3.565	0.0	0.827	1.721	0.894	0.0	0.0	0.0	0.0
132	2.053	0.513	1.733	0.815	0.144	0.0	0.0	0.0	0.289	0.0	0.0
133	0.482	0.121	0.233	0.0	0.0	0.281	0.0	0.0	0.0	0.0	0.0
134	1.070	0.267	0.516	0.0	0.150	0.0	0.0	0.140	0.0	0.0	0.0
135	2.854	0.714	4.820	0.453	0.0	0.831	1.727	0.749	0.0	0.0	0.928
136	5.069	0.676	3.913	0.858	0.757	0.787	0.0	0.0	0.760	0.0	0.0
137	8.537	0.589	3.409	0.374	0.330	0.686	1.425	0.0	0.0	0.0	0.765
138	3.221	0.805	3.496	1.023	0.225	0.704	0.244	0.0	0.226	0.0	0.785
139	1.452	0.513	1.649	0.543	0.096	0.0	0.207	0.0	0.0	0.0	0.666
140	2.791	1.240	1.795	0.394	0.0	0.0	0.750	0.0	0.698	0.0	0.0
141	7.267	1.211	3.506	0.769	0.339	0.706	0.366	0.159	0.0	0.0	0.787
142	1.248	0.749	1.928	0.317	0.0	0.582	0.604	0.0	0.0	0.0	0.649
143	2.879	0.501	2.416	0.636	0.0	0.583	0.606	0.131	0.0	0.0	0.325
144	4.565	0.269	2.591	0.341	0.0	0.626	0.0	0.0	0.0	0.0	2.095

145	1.157	0.386	0.0	0.0	0.0	0.0	0.0	0.0	0.0	0.0	0.0
146	1.854	0.530	3.579	1.682	0.0	0.0	0.641	0.278	0.0	0.0	0.0
147	1.062	0.531	3.075	0.0	0.595	0.619	0.643	0.279	0.597	0.0	0.0
148	4.283	0.476	2.296	0.302	0.266	0.554	0.576	0.0	0.0	0.0	0.619
149	1.992	0.664	2.991	0.281	0.496	1.032	0.0	0.0	0.0	0.0	1.151
150	3.072	1.063	3.420	0.750	0.265	0.275	0.572	0.0	0.0	0.0	1.536
151	5.538	1.128	4.553	1.172	0.0	0.956	0.745	0.0	0.0	0.0	1.867
152	4.527	0.932	4.111	1.015	0.596	0.620	0.644	0.0	0.0	0.0	0.692
153	0.0	0.427	0.0	0.0	0.0	0.0	0.0	0.0	0.0	0.0	0.457
154	2.813	0.879	1.357	0.223	0.197	0.410	0.0	0.0	0.0	0.0	0.457
155	3.710	1.237	1.432	0.314	0.277	0.576	0.0	0.0	0.0	0.0	0.0
156	2.785	0.768	2.039	0.854	0.108	0.224	0.0	0.0	0.0	0.0	0.499
157	4.808	1.282	2.475	0.0	0.539	0.747	0.388	0.0	0.361	0.0	0.417
158	2.633	0.987	1.906	0.836	0.0	0.0	0.797	0.0	0.0	0.0	0.0
159	1.452	0.0	0.400	0.263	0.0	0.0	0.0	0.0	0.0	0.0	0.0
160	3.374	0.675	3.349	0.735	0.432	0.449	0.0	0.0	0.0	0.0	1.003
161	1.727	1.036	2.000	0.439	0.0	0.805	0.0	0.0	0.0	0.0	0.898
162	3.129	0.156	3.321	0.795	0.0	0.365	0.379	0.329	0.0	0.0	1.220
163	2.860	1.292	1.247	0.117	0.103	0.215	0.447	0.0	0.0	0.0	0.480
164	0.976	0.279	0.538	0.0	0.156	0.0	0.0	0.0	0.0	0.0	0.363
165	3.538	0.122	2.826	0.310	0.547	0.853	0.0	0.128	0.0	0.0	0.634
166	2.229	0.857	1.985	0.0	0.192	1.198	0.415	0.0	0.0	0.0	0.446
167	3.167	0.950	1.222	0.804	0.0	0.0	0.0	0.0	0.0	0.0	0.0
168	3.425	0.856	0.826	0.0	0.0	0.997	0.0	0.0	0.0	0.0	0.0
169	2.139	0.107	1.445	0.136	0.0	0.997	0.0	0.112	0.0	0.278	0.278
170	1.637	0.586	1.131	0.306	0.135	0.040	0.083	0.0	0.039	0.045	0.403
171	1.512	0.202	1.653	0.384	0.113	0.352	0.488	0.0	0.0	0.0	0.262
172	1.616	0.242	1.403	0.410	0.181	0.0	0.196	0.042	0.0	0.105	0.315
173	1.476	0.138	1.068	0.234	0.052	0.322	0.0	0.048	0.208	0.0	0.120
174	5.997	0.300	2.894	1.142	0.0	0.0	0.726	0.0	0.0	0.0	0.780
175	2.867	0.239	0.922	0.303	0.0	0.0	0.0	0.0	0.0	0.0	0.621
176	1.465	0.046	1.050	0.266	0.117	0.146	0.152	0.066	0.0	0.054	0.272
177	1.066	0.275	0.863	0.306	0.077	0.080	0.166	0.036	0.0	0.0	0.0
178	3.329	0.940	2.721	0.547	0.088	0.274	0.474	0.247	0.264	0.102	0.509
179	2.145	0.634	1.599	0.557	0.109	0.114	0.0	0.051	0.0	0.127	0.380
180	3.571	0.646	2.321	0.593	0.141	0.460	0.304	0.113	0.121	0.047	0.280

TABLE 41--Continued

Unit Area	Reported Mortality		Estimated Cancer Morbidity								
	Heart Disease	Stroke	Total Cancer	(1)	(2)	(3)	(4)	(5)	(6)	(7)	(8)
181	1.782	1.018	1.965	0.647	0.285	0.0	0.411	0.089	0.0	0.0	0.0
182	5.946	2.973	5.738	1.030	0.0	3.149	0.654	0.0	0.0	0.0	1.405
183	2.392	1.063	2.052	0.338	0.0	0.619	0.643	0.0	0.0	0.0	0.691
184	2.445	0.667	3.003	0.565	0.747	0.0	0.0	0.0	0.0	0.0	0.578
185	3.721	0.859	1.657	0.363	0.321	0.0	0.0	0.301	0.0	0.0	0.0
186	3.743	0.655	3.251	0.951	0.210	1.090	0.226	0.0	0.0	0.243	0.243
187	2.892	0.578	2.233	0.367	0.324	0.674	0.700	0.0	0.0	0.0	0.0
188	4.322	0.935	2.480	0.593	0.262	0.544	0.283	0.0	0.0	0.0	0.607
189	1.615	0.0	2.384	0.845	0.213	0.221	0.460	0.0	0.0	0.247	0.0
190	1.796	0.200	1.541	0.760	0.0	0.465	0.0	0.0	0.0	0.0	0.0
191	2.339	0.0	2.257	0.990	0.437	0.0	0.0	0.0	0.0	0.0	0.0
192	3.719	0.930	1.794	1.181	0.0	0.0	0.0	0.0	0.0	0.0	0.0
193	2.339	0.520	3.009	0.660	0.0	0.606	0.0	0.273	0.0	0.0	1.351
194	4.993	1.021	4.818	1.585	0.763	0.793	0.275	0.0	0.0	0.0	0.295
195	4.679	0.369	4.990	0.938	0.276	2.582	0.596	0.129	0.0	0.0	0.320
196	3.524	1.113	2.506	0.942	0.208	0.432	0.0	0.195	0.0	0.0	0.0
197	5.559	0.575	4.439	1.217	0.644	0.447	0.928	0.0	0.0	0.0	0.498
198	3.554	0.677	1.450	0.430	0.190	0.789	0.205	0.089	0.0	0.0	0.660
199	2.394	0.299	0.867	0.190	0.0	0.697	0.0	0.0	0.0	0.389	0.0
200	2.149	0.0	2.074	0.682	0.301	0.0	0.0	0.0	0.0	0.0	0.698
201	2.543	0.606	1.402	0.308	0.136	0.564	0.0	0.0	0.0	0.315	0.315
202	4.931	1.027	2.379	0.261	0.230	0.479	0.994	0.0	0.0	0.0	0.534
203	2.867	0.453	1.165	0.383	0.338	0.0	0.0	0.0	0.0	0.0	0.0
204	0.306	0.022	0.422	0.0	0.098	0.0	0.106	0.023	0.0	0.114	0.114
205	4.708	1.240	3.726	0.897	0.246	0.622	0.646	0.115	0.035	0.163	0.735
206	1.205	0.344	1.551	0.364	0.193	0.0	0.139	0.0	0.0	0.0	0.746
207	4.854	1.395	3.162	0.693	0.249	0.471	0.489	0.149	0.046	0.0	0.789

208	6.670	0.267	2.832	0.508	0.299	0.622	0.0	0.140	0.300	0.0	0.694
209	4.316	1.177	2.019	0.664	0.0	0.305	0.317	0.0	0.0	0.0	0.680
210	3.049	0.762	1.471	0.484	0.0	0.888	0.0	0.0	0.0	0.0	0.0
211	3.560	0.647	2.290	0.822	0.242	0.0	0.0	0.0	0.243	0.0	0.0
212	11.858	3.953	10.680	1.004	1.771	2.763	0.957	0.415	0.0	0.0	3.083
213	2.731	1.275	3.514	1.619	0.204	0.424	0.0	0.191	0.0	0.0	0.0
214	2.234	0.941	1.588	0.299	0.132	0.548	0.569	0.0	0.0	0.0	0.0
215	1.496	0.214	1.650	0.543	0.239	0.0	0.517	0.0	0.0	0.0	0.0
216	2.922	0.877	0.0	0.0	0.0	0.0	0.0	0.0	0.0	0.0	0.0
217	2.290	0.0	0.631	0.208	0.0	0.0	0.0	0.0	0.0	0.0	0.425
218	3.196	0.599	2.698	0.761	0.447	0.465	0.0	0.0	0.0	0.0	0.519
219	2.195	0.593	1.374	0.301	0.133	0.553	0.0	0.0	0.0	0.0	0.308
220	3.608	0.962	4.643	1.222	0.404	0.841	0.582	0.0	0.0	0.313	1.251
221	3.531	2.354	2.726	0.897	0.0	0.548	0.570	0.0	0.0	0.0	0.612
222	7.194	2.098	5.207	0.381	0.336	1.397	0.0	0.0	0.674	0.779	3.118
223	5.045	1.682	2.705	1.068	0.0	1.306	0.0	0.0	0.0	0.0	0.0
224	5.058	1.911	3.688	1.570	0.126	0.524	0.272	0.0	0.0	0.0	0.584
225	3.177	2.270	3.066	1.441	0.0	0.0	0.0	0.0	0.511	0.0	0.590
226	1.921	0.823	2.648	1.046	0.0	0.639	0.664	0.0	0.0	0.0	0.0
227	2.978	1.162	3.785	0.830	0.244	0.846	0.527	0.153	0.163	0.189	0.755
228	3.321	0.705	2.212	0.597	0.132	0.479	0.142	0.062	0.0	0.076	0.611
229	2.884	0.804	3.284	0.480	0.265	0.771	0.458	0.199	0.106	0.0	0.860
230	3.001	0.757	2.870	0.652	0.212	0.441	0.523	0.0	0.0	0.141	0.843
231	3.068	0.939	2.779	0.239	0.351	0.438	0.455	0.131	0.0	0.0	0.404
232	5.599	1.089	2.401	0.790	0.087	0.725	0.0	0.0	0.0	0.0	0.404
233	2.704	0.931	2.310	0.394	0.199	0.310	0.536	0.093	0.0	0.0	0.691
234	3.325	0.464	2.388	0.491	0.260	0.540	0.374	0.0	0.0	0.0	0.603
235	2.207	0.343	2.366	0.623	0.110	0.571	0.356	0.0	0.0	0.0	0.638
236	2.303	0.535	2.143	0.366	0.322	0.383	0.299	0.043	0.0	0.0	0.535
237	2.077	0.148	1.718	0.188	0.332	0.0	0.0	0.156	0.0	0.0	0.771
238	4.157	1.094	4.856	1.389	0.368	0.765	0.0	0.230	0.246	0.0	1.138
239	1.869	0.680	4.919	0.863	0.381	0.396	1.234	0.357	0.0	0.0	1.325
240	4.209	0.842	2.166	0.356	0.0	0.0	2.037	0.0	0.0	0.0	0.0
241	2.133	0.474	1.372	0.0	0.0	0.0	0.0	0.0	0.0	0.0	1.849
242	3.351	0.0	4.851	1.064	0.313	1.952	0.676	0.293	0.0	0.0	0.0
243	3.064	0.146	3.097	0.185	0.163	0.680	1.059	0.153	0.0	0.0	1.138

TABLE 41--Continued

Unit Area	Reported Mortality		Estimated Cancer Morbidity								
	Heart Disease	Stroke	Total Cancer	(1)	(2)	(3)	(4)	(5)	(6)	(7)	(8)
244	3.502	0.500	3.862	1.059	0.187	0.777	0.404	0.0	0.0	0.0	1.301
245	2.279	0.977	5.028	1.241	0.729	0.0	1.576	0.0	0.0	0.0	0.847
246	3.250	0.975	3.136	0.413	0.364	0.757	0.786	0.0	0.0	0.0	0.845
247	2.008	0.426	2.231	0.309	0.068	0.567	0.589	0.064	0.137	0.0	0.633
248	1.005	0.067	0.517	0.170	0.0	0.156	0.0	0.070	0.0	0.0	0.0
249	0.681	0.214	0.639	0.223	0.065	0.091	0.094	0.020	0.0	0.0	0.0
250	0.753	0.171	0.661	0.130	0.0	0.319	0.083	0.0	0.0	0.089	0.178
251	0.825	0.210	0.376	0.095	0.034	0.035	0.036	0.0	0.0	0.0	0.156
252	0.288	0.091	0.220	0.029	0.017	0.035	0.073	0.0	0.034	0.020	0.039
253	5.316	1.153	3.237	0.761	0.218	0.454	0.616	0.094	0.135	0.117	0.623
254	0.849	0.340	0.656	0.431	0.0	0.0	0.0	0.0	0.0	0.0	0.0
255	3.465	1.444	6.131	0.367	0.323	1.346	1.398	0.0	0.0	0.751	3.754
256	5.291	0.529	3.319	0.504	0.148	0.308	0.0	0.417	0.298	0.0	1.376
257	0.280	0.280	1.080	0.0	0.0	0.0	1.354	0.0	0.0	0.0	0.0
258	1.088	0.311	0.900	0.197	0.174	0.362	0.0	0.0	0.0	0.0	0.0
259	6.651	1.188	2.751	0.905	0.0	0.0	0.575	0.0	0.0	0.0	1.235
260	2.264	0.453	3.496	0.575	0.0	0.0	0.0	0.951	0.0	0.0	1.178
261	3.430	0.885	1.068	0.141	0.0	0.516	0.0	0.0	0.0	0.0	0.575
262	2.942	0.515	1.845	0.280	0.082	0.171	0.0	0.232	0.165	0.0	0.765
263	3.402	0.512	2.189	0.325	0.123	0.511	0.354	0.115	0.0	0.095	0.761
264	2.716	0.388	1.685	0.370	0.0	0.0	0.0	0.102	0.0	0.252	1.261
265	4.333	0.619	2.688	0.590	0.347	0.0	0.0	0.162	0.0	0.0	1.207
266	2.400	0.450	1.447	0.381	0.0	0.0	0.363	0.0	0.0	0.0	0.780
267	4.102	0.820	1.583	1.042	0.0	0.0	0.0	0.0	0.0	0.0	0.0
268	4.145	1.091	2.526	0.554	0.489	0.508	0.0	0.0	0.0	0.0	0.567
269	2.539	0.363	1.400	0.230	0.203	0.423	0.439	0.0	0.0	0.0	0.0
270	7.576	1.082	4.177	0.687	0.0	0.0	2.619	0.0	0.0	0.0	1.407
271	3.296	0.254	1.468	0.0	0.284	0.0	0.0	0.266	0.0	0.0	0.659

TABLE 42

CRUDE RATES PER 1,000 FOR HEART DISEASE, STROKE AND CANCER, 1967

Unit Area	Reported Mortality		Estimated Cancer Morbidity								
	Heart Disease	Stroke	Total Cancer	Cancer of Digestive Organs (1)	Respiratory Cancer (2)	Cancer of the Genital Organs (M & F) (3)	Breast Cancer (4)	Leukemia (5)	Cancer of the Buccal Cavity and Pharynx (6)	Skin Cancer (7)	Cancer Sites Unspecified (Also All Other) (8)
1	4.982	0.943	4.120	0.384	0.518	0.476	0.495	0.019	0.041	0.246	2.063
2	5.456	0.788	4.477	0.647	0.294	0.150	0.587	0.0	0.0	0.171	3.029
3	7.530	1.298	4.603	0.502	0.497	0.481	0.681	0.0	0.055	0.0	2.622
4	5.928	1.151	5.002	0.317	0.716	0.570	0.539	0.0	0.0	0.0	3.119
5	5.572	0.973	4.020	0.427	0.572	0.296	0.862	0.0	0.0	0.0	1.880
6	6.220	1.124	4.354	0.412	0.517	0.635	0.397	0.0	0.020	0.096	2.500
7	4.685	0.835	3.334	0.294	0.258	0.559	0.337	0.0	0.0	0.134	2.138
8	5.364	0.971	3.361	0.293	0.343	0.279	0.485	0.013	0.029	0.0	2.185
9	2.889	0.667	2.720	0.0	0.332	0.180	1.124	0.0	0.0	0.0	1.431
10	4.326	0.698	3.606	0.440	0.313	0.396	0.530	0.0	0.0	0.064	2.118
11	5.502	1.004	4.929	0.552	0.500	0.271	0.564	0.0	0.0	0.205	3.181
12	4.247	1.022	4.058	0.290	0.662	0.523	0.680	0.0	0.0	0.0	1.929
13	4.682	0.809	4.953	0.546	0.194	0.421	1.170	0.061	0.0	0.160	3.031
14	5.613	1.183	4.650	0.581	0.506	0.209	0.381	0.0	0.099	0.178	2.908
15	5.468	1.395	4.655	0.513	0.373	0.424	0.601	0.0	0.0	0.131	3.062
16	5.251	1.201	4.387	0.363	0.502	0.479	0.680	0.038	0.082	0.0	2.473
17	4.915	0.775	3.408	0.425	0.190	0.235	0.735	0.0	0.0	0.067	2.138
18	5.439	1.404	3.579	0.355	0.196	0.213	0.444	0.092	0.0	0.0	2.663

TABLE 42--Continued

Unit Area	Reported Mortality		Estimated Cancer Morbidity								
	Heart Disease	Stroke	Total Cancer	(1)	(2)	(3)	(4)	(5)	(6)	(7)	(8)
19	5.148	0.922	4.435	0.517	0.506	0.254	0.308	0.0	0.080	0.0	2.976
20	5.347	1.089	4.545	0.468	0.499	0.120	0.125	0.0	0.0	0.0	3.689
21	5.775	0.856	4.309	0.253	0.539	0.520	0.676	0.0	0.0	0.074	2.583
22	5.027	0.824	3.447	0.245	0.347	0.286	0.298	0.0	0.0	0.030	2.627
23	4.726	0.859	3.778	0.260	0.498	0.396	0.562	0.0	0.068	0.0	2.208
24	4.696	0.792	3.544	0.425	0.396	0.261	0.253	0.008	0.035	0.042	2.270
25	4.703	0.873	3.354	0.332	0.437	0.288	0.343	0.027	0.039	0.0	1.965
26	2.500	0.613	2.069	0.127	0.291	0.287	0.358	0.0	0.0	0.0	1.107
27	2.743	0.797	2.603	0.108	0.268	0.504	0.081	0.0	0.073	0.088	1.805
28	5.250	0.681	2.603	0.244	0.309	0.377	0.262	0.0	0.0	0.0	1.547
29	2.169	0.426	1.719	0.133	0.211	0.298	0.248	0.0	0.019	0.045	0.858
30	4.625	1.187	3.774	0.377	0.235	0.424	0.265	0.0	0.040	0.048	2.890
31	4.273	0.639	2.202	0.268	0.321	0.268	0.223	0.0	0.0	0.0	1.094
32	20.625	1.250	12.750	1.125	1.167	1.519	0.0	0.0	0.0	0.0	10.350
33	4.310	0.603	2.990	0.116	0.290	0.209	0.218	0.0	0.0	0.476	2.141
34	4.488	0.945	3.855	0.744	0.529	0.574	0.398	0.0	0.0	0.0	1.304
35	3.923	0.752	2.571	0.137	0.341	0.543	0.206	0.0	0.0	0.0	1.515
36	3.840	0.989	1.939	0.154	0.170	0.185	0.096	0.0	0.0	0.0	1.574
37	4.000	1.143	2.331	0.129	0.320	0.694	0.482	0.0	0.0	0.0	0.789
38	6.419	1.545	4.740	0.388	0.510	0.902	0.424	0.0	0.028	0.0	2.843
39	4.386	0.966	3.036	0.282	0.322	0.634	0.396	0.0	0.0	0.072	1.513
40	6.472	1.472	5.577	0.725	0.550	0.625	0.532	0.0	0.0	0.064	3.353
41	3.780	0.634	2.886	0.395	0.137	0.237	0.309	0.0	0.0	0.067	2.087
42	3.568	0.870	3.078	0.155	0.215	0.497	0.388	0.0	0.059	0.035	2.224
43	5.580	1.202	4.367	0.410	0.495	0.436	0.454	0.015	0.032	0.0	2.783
44	2.965	0.885	3.250	0.299	0.297	0.430	0.448	0.023	0.0	0.061	1.954
45	4.309	0.894	2.985	0.110	0.546	0.198	0.206	0.0	0.0	0.0	2.020

46	5.273	0.588	3.514	0.284	0.471	0.204	0.372	0.0	0.0	0.058	2.319
47	6.061	1.818	3.709	0.0	1.018	0.0	0.0	0.0	0.0	0.0	2.509
48	4.619	0.609	3.728	0.343	0.341	0.123	0.385	0.0	0.0	0.140	2.802
49	4.746	0.797	3.112	0.412	0.361	0.494	0.214	0.018	0.039	0.047	1.544
50	3.415	0.732	2.488	0.329	0.273	0.0	0.0	0.0	0.0	0.0	2.020
51	4.508	0.466	3.382	0.280	0.696	0.0	0.131	0.0	0.0	0.0	2.145
52	2.983	0.924	3.771	0.397	0.282	0.613	0.425	0.0	0.0	0.116	2.319
53	3.437	0.413	2.372	0.174	0.174	0.251	0.196	0.0	0.0	0.0	1.926
54	1.983	0.431	0.703	0.116	0.193	0.0	0.0	0.0	0.0	0.0	0.238
55	3.846	0.481	2.158	0.130	0.538	0.467	0.243	0.0	0.0	0.0	0.531
56	2.136	0.258	2.203	0.127	0.289	0.228	0.059	0.0	0.054	0.0	1.620
57	4.434	0.849	4.619	0.637	0.211	0.688	0.716	0.0	0.0	0.260	2.604
58	4.603	0.849	3.745	0.481	0.307	0.200	0.762	0.029	0.0	0.0	2.193
59	4.813	0.938	4.080	0.759	0.350	0.304	0.158	0.0	0.0	0.0	2.587
60	5.532	1.065	3.709	0.105	0.378	0.442	0.591	0.027	0.060	0.072	2.509
61	4.794	0.649	3.389	0.342	0.390	0.538	0.160	0.0	0.036	0.0	2.096
62	4.056	0.769	2.853	0.472	0.157	0.340	0.177	0.0	0.0	0.0	1.930
63	4.963	0.709	3.958	0.604	0.501	0.363	0.378	0.0	0.0	0.103	1.957
64	2.466	0.942	1.738	0.182	0.251	0.0	0.0	0.0	0.0	0.0	1.361
65	3.593	0.593	3.324	0.300	0.332	0.720	0.469	0.0	0.085	0.0	1.636
66	5.615	0.779	5.309	0.526	0.390	0.349	1.141	0.022	0.0	0.057	3.393
67	4.902	0.995	3.334	0.360	0.378	0.345	0.360	0.0	0.0	0.0	2.059
68	3.493	0.688	2.650	0.177	0.183	0.663	0.193	0.0	0.050	0.0	1.748
69	3.486	0.884	3.205	0.243	0.330	0.477	0.663	0.0	0.0	0.0	1.762
70	2.388	0.313	1.867	0.121	0.225	0.163	0.395	0.0	0.0	0.0	1.109
71	4.223	0.733	4.094	0.401	0.352	0.382	0.751	0.0	0.0	0.096	2.505
72	2.727	0.661	3.203	0.446	0.185	0.602	0.523	0.0	0.0	0.0	1.711
73	3.226	0.613	2.303	0.261	0.253	0.078	0.326	0.0	0.074	0.089	1.335
74	0.932	0.339	1.556	0.057	0.142	0.206	0.107	0.0	0.0	0.0	1.286
75	3.382	0.588	3.450	0.199	0.329	0.447	0.465	0.0	0.085	0.0	2.334
76	2.817	0.527	2.289	0.402	0.103	0.334	0.348	0.072	0.211	0.0	0.822
77	2.623	0.470	2.636	0.370	0.439	0.666	0.099	0.0	0.090	0.0	0.756
78	6.446	1.558	5.662	1.160	0.562	1.262	0.408	0.188	0.247	0.099	1,137
79	4.955	0.753	3.963	1.177	0.400	0.771	0.401	0.042	0.091	0.0	0.438
80	4.371	0.822	3.443	0.935	0.388	0.526	0.547	0.045	0.0	0.0	0.478
81	3.475	0.790	2.771	0.426	0.212	0.844	0.320	0.066	0.073	0.087	0.697

TABLE 42--Continued

Unit Area	Reported Mortality		Estimated Cancer Morbidity								
	Heart Disease	Stroke	Total Cancer	(1)	(2)	(3)	(4)	(5)	(6)	(7)	(8)
82	3.593	0.904	2.397	0.610	0.202	0.329	0.286	0.071	0.0	0.0	0.624
83	5.871	1.222	4.068	0.777	0.535	0.546	0.569	0.059	0.097	0.039	1.047
84	3.716	0.725	2.922	0.343	0.426	0.617	0.321	0.038	0.042	0.0	1.001
85	2.443	0.800	2.148	0.512	0.236	0.614	0.213	0.088	0.0	0.116	0.0
86	3.639	0.918	3.615	0.897	0.319	0.692	0.560	0.0	0.0	0.0	0.873
87	5.397	1.659	3.506	0.811	0.337	0.438	0.395	0.151	0.055	0.100	0.763
88	3.744	1.009	3.520	1.099	0.328	0.237	0.247	0.103	0.075	0.0	0.809
89	6.179	1.285	3.994	0.413	0.891	0.149	0.310	0.128	0.422	0.0	1.013
90	2.308	0.412	1.514	0.167	0.139	0.501	0.209	0.043	0.0	0.0	0.455
91	4.114	1.316	4.028	0.722	0.369	0.300	0.416	0.216	0.378	0.114	1.135
92	4.428	0.625	2.494	0.367	0.274	0.396	0.619	0.086	0.062	0.075	0.450
93	3.868	0.569	3.829	0.921	0.510	0.276	0.288	0.179	0.0	0.0	0.942
94	5.145	1.125	4.483	1.013	0.540	0.912	0.407	0.056	0.0	0.0	1.035
95	4.615	1.218	3.007	0.519	0.287	0.934	0.162	0.0	0.147	0.177	0.708
96	2.356	0.655	3.027	0.707	0.244	0.318	0.442	0.0	0.100	0.120	0.963
97	3.471	0.486	2.974	0.750	0.233	0.169	0.703	0.073	0.0	0.0	0.767
98	4.766	0.433	1.233	0.366	0.300	0.133	0.100	0.033	0.0	0.033	0.266
99	3.254	0.585	3.729	0.642	0.491	0.711	0.462	0.077	0.0	0.202	0.807
100	3.018	0.437	2.754	0.590	0.222	0.193	0.502	0.042	0.091	0.110	0.877
101	2.327	0.558	1.835	0.503	0.208	0.377	0.235	0.0	0.0	0.086	0.171
102	4.112	0.771	2.846	0.545	0.452	0.268	0.279	0.116	0.0	0.101	0.608
103	3.378	0.536	2.188	0.507	0.540	0.130	0.271	0.0	0.0	0.148	0.0
104	3.272	0.706	3.926	0.693	0.287	0.468	0.812	0.269	0.0	0.0	1.062
105	2.378	0.272	2.495	0.642	0.457	0.0	0.516	0.071	0.0	0.0	0.188
106	6.419	0.860	4.910	0.967	0.546	0.905	0.362	0.241	0.0	0.237	1.028
107	6.420	1.669	4.895	0.965	0.427	0.927	0.885	0.050	0.146	0.175	1.097
108	3.963	0.915	3.607	0.905	0.341	0.593	0.771	0.128	0.0	0.168	0.168

109	0.944	0.157	1.123	0.177	0.059	0.191	0.199	0.028	0.0	0.0	0.506
110	3.911	0.550	2.803	0.799	0.118	0.154	0.642	0.067	0.049	0.0	0.758
111	3.669	0.590	3.876	0.884	0.440	0.478	0.498	0.0	0.0	0.181	1.085
112	3.552	0.975	4.404	0.658	0.156	1.015	1.233	0.073	0.0	0.0	1.538
113	0.838	0.322	0.789	0.087	0.072	0.0	0.0	0.135	0.0	0.0	0.356
114	0.193	6.500	3.231	0.688	0.262	0.468	0.836	0.145	0.0	0.076	0.418
115	3.078	0.684	3.090	0.924	0.328	0.237	0.495	0.051	0.0	0.0	0.539
116	4.604	0.837	3.546	0.522	0.397	0.626	0.570	0.034	0.074	0.089	1.155
117	3.200	0.681	3.750	0.827	0.0	0.662	0.517	0.143	0.157	0.0	1.503
118	4.385	0.418	3.834	0.282	0.468	0.507	0.528	0.219	0.0	0.0	1.729
119	3.531	0.569	2.091	0.308	0.0	0.277	0.576	0.0	0.262	0.0	0.943
120	2.442	0.458	2.180	0.0	0.342	0.371	0.386	0.160	0.0	0.0	0.843
121	1.117	0.223	1.595	0.151	0.250	0.271	0.565	0.117	0.0	0.0	0.0
122	3.809	0.412	1.890	0.139	0.346	0.250	0.781	0.108	0.0	0.0	0.0
123	1.562	0.551	2.437	0.496	0.206	0.0	0.697	0.096	0.211	0.0	0.507
124	1.780	0.137	1.397	0.370	0.307	0.0	0.346	0.0	0.0	0.0	0.0
125	5.650	1.027	0.524	0.347	0.0	0.0	0.0	0.0	0.0	0.0	0.0
126	1.464	0.244	1.659	1.110	0.091	0.198	0.206	0.085	0.0	0.0	1.122
127	3.953	0.516	2.805	0.232	0.0	1.671	0.435	0.0	0.0	0.0	0.949
128	2.762	0.789	1.127	0.0	0.177	0.767	0.0	0.0	0.0	0.0	0.218
129	4.229	1.364	3.896	0.368	0.611	0.331	0.345	0.286	0.314	0.0	1.129
130	3.176	0.471	1.680	0.159	0.132	0.0	1.191	0.0	0.0	0.0	0.325
131	6.595	1.649	3.364	0.371	0.616	0.668	0.0	0.0	0.0	0.0	1.517
132	3.176	1.361	2.777	0.306	0.635	0.0	0.574	0.119	0.0	0.0	0.626
133	1.004	0.167	0.024	0.452	0.094	0.203	0.0	0.0	0.0	0.0	0.0
134	1.895	0.526	1.288	0.284	0.118	0.0	0.0	0.111	0.0	0.0	0.581
135	5.262	1.754	1.193	0.395	0.0	0.0	0.0	0.0	0.0	0.0	0.807
136	1.538	0.615	1.882	0.415	0.0	0.747	0.778	0.0	0.0	0.0	0.0
137	7.482	0.880	2.245	1.188	0.0	0.535	0.0	0.0	0.0	0.0	0.0
138	3.628	0.495	2.523	0.557	0.369	0.401	0.209	0.0	0.0	0.0	0.683
139	2.375	0.475	1.211	0.240	0.067	0.289	0.300	0.0	0.137	0.0	0.164
140	2.682	0.975	2.487	0.0	0.273	0.593	0.617	0.256	0.0	0.0	0.673
141	5.322	1.331	3.132	0.415	0.459	0.746	0.259	0.107	0.235	0.0	0.565
142	2.608	0.373	2.660	0.754	0.0	1.358	0.471	0.0	0.0	0.0	0.0
143	2.746	0.666	3.225	0.674	0.280	0.404	0.211	0.087	0.0	0.0	1.378
144	5.990	0.363	6.665	2.205	0.813	0.882	0.0	0.191	0.0	0.0	1.002

TABLE 42--Continued

Unit Area	Reported Mortality		Estimated Cancer Morbidity								
	Heart Disease	Stroke	Total Cancer	(1)	(2)	(3)	(4)	(5)	(6)	(7)	(8)
145	2.424	0.441	1.798	0.297	0.0	1.071	0.0	0.0	0.0	0.0	0.608
146	5.040	1.613	4.935	0.272	0.677	0.980	1.530	0.212	0.0	0.0	1.113
147	4.344	2.369	1.611	0.267	0.221	0.0	0.999	0.0	0.0	0.0	0.0
148	2.255	0.376	3.067	0.254	0.210	0.913	0.0	0.197	0.0	0.0	1.556
149	1.796	0.299	1.832	0.404	0.335	0.364	0.379	0.0	0.0	0.0	0.0
150	4.373	0.714	2.913	0.602	0.300	0.434	0.226	0.0	0.0	0.0	1.232
151	3.808	0.635	2.590	1.224	0.0	0.0	0.688	0.0	0.0	0.0	0.250
152	4.424	1.810	3.077	0.950	0.225	0.0	0.0	0.211	0.0	0.0	1.110
153	0.828	0.166	1.351	0.223	0.0	0.805	0.0	0.174	0.0	0.0	0.0
154	1.727	0.266	4.606	1.793	0.446	0.646	0.336	0.0	0.0	0.0	0.367
155	4.415	1.344	1.958	0.259	0.0	0.466	0.486	0.0	0.441	0.0	0.530
156	3.110	0.683	2.630	0.512	0.255	0.369	0.576	0.0	0.0	0.0	0.837
157	3.954	1.318	1.152	0.254	0.0	0.0	0.476	0.099	0.0	0.0	0.260
158	2.037	0.582	2.969	0.393	0.652	0.707	0.0	0.306	0.0	0.0	0.0
159	0.595	0.357	1.457	0.161	0.133	0.0	0.301	0.0	0.274	0.0	0.657
160	3.396	0.869	1.450	0.426	0.177	0.384	0.200	0.0	0.0	0.0	0.0
161	1.910	0.273	2.226	0.368	0.611	0.0	0.0	0.286	0.0	0.0	0.0
162	3.745	0.728	4.668	0.702	0.349	0.253	0.789	0.0	0.239	0.0	2.584
163	4.157	0.907	2.930	0.612	0.423	0.184	0.574	0.079	0.0	0.0	0.626
164	2.494	0.089	1.635	0.361	0.200	0.649	0.0	0.0	0.0	0.0	0.246
165	3.218	0.095	3.089	0.639	0.212	0.920	0.239	0.099	0.0	0.0	0.784
166	0.696	0.0	1.705	0.564	0.312	0.0	0.352	0.0	0.0	0.0	0.0
167	2.158	0.144	0.587	0.388	0.0	0.0	0.0	0.0	0.0	0.0	0.0
168	0.590	0.147	0.150	0.0	0.0	0.0	0.0	0.0	0.0	0.0	0.203
169	1.350	0.225	0.765	0.203	0.084	0.182	0.0	0.0	0.0	0.207	0.0
170	0.779	0.198	0.505	0.033	0.028	0.060	0.031	0.0	0.284	0.034	0.102
171	0.237	0.047	0.386	0.128	0.053	0.0	0.0	0.050	0.0	0.0	0.0

172	1.491	0.357	1.058	0.350	0.145	0.079	0.164	0.0	0.0	0.089	0.089
173	0.819	0.066	0.468	0.133	0.073	0.0	0.0	0.0	0.34	0.0	0.090
174	5.442	0.454	1.850	0.306	0.0	1.102	0.574	0.0	0.0	0.0	0.0
175	0.132	0.132	0.0	0.0	0.0	0.0	0.0	0.0	0.0	0.0	0.0
176	0.652	0.245	0.399	0.088	0.110	0.079	0.0	0.0	0.0	0.0	0.0
177	1.292	0.335	0.683	0.194	0.0	0.349	0.0	0.050	0.0	0.0	0.0
178	2.343	0.948	2.048	0.565	0.125	0.271	0.423	0.0	0.064	0.0	0.462
179	1.735	0.416	1.345	0.234	0.155	0.169	0.263	0.036	0.0	0.0	0.383
180	0.332	4.882	2.737	0.449	0.343	0.466	0.323	0.081	0.059	0.0	0.776
181	1.631	0.665	2.342	0.163	0.338	0.440	0.459	0.0	0.0	0.0	1.000
182	6.697	0.591	3.214	0.266	0.221	0.957	0.498	0.0	0.0	0.0	1.631
183	3.543	0.373	1.522	0.0	0.209	0.0	1.415	0.0	0.0	0.0	0.0
184	2.375	1.108	2.906	0.427	0.177	0.385	0.0	0.0	0.364	0.0	1.748
185	2.242	0.815	3.326	0.825	0.456	0.990	0.0	0.0	0.0	0.0	0.562
186	2.798	0.666	2.718	0.720	0.149	0.324	0.169	0.0	0.0	0.0	0.919
187	3.188	0.683	1.858	0.615	0.0	0.0	0.576	0.0	0.0	0.0	0.629
188	4.220	1.534	3.522	0.906	0.537	0.466	0.0	0.0	0.0	0.0	1.059
189	2.535	0.411	2.096	0.277	0.077	0.0	0.693	0.0	0.315	0.0	0.756
190	1.682	0.388	1.056	0.349	0.145	0.314	0.0	0.0	0.0	0.0	0.0
191	3.146	0.0	2.139	1.062	0.294	0.0	0.0	0.0	0.0	0.0	0.0
192	3.383	0.940	1.534	0.254	0.421	0.0	0.0	0.0	0.432	0.0	0.0
193	2.299	0.0	1.172	0.0	0.161	0.349	0.0	0.151	0.0	0.0	0.397
194	3.197	0.888	1.993	0.360	0.398	0.216	0.225	0.0	0.0	0.0	0.490
195	3.666	1.008	3.927	1.237	0.616	0.445	0.0	0.0	0.0	0.0	0.759
196	4.163	0.979	4.246	0.496	0.411	1.190	0.929	0.0	0.282	0.0	1.014
197	5.347	1.040	5.454	1.604	0.665	0.361	0.752	0.156	0.342	0.0	0.410
198	1.649	0.707	1.682	0.398	0.264	0.572	0.0	0.0	0.0	0.0	0.163
199	0.597	0.046	0.375	0.062	0.051	0.0	0.116	0.0	0.0	0.0	0.127
200	3.279	1.009	1.544	0.340	0.565	0.0	0.0	0.0	0.0	0.0	0.0
201	2.487	0.155	0.951	0.105	0.087	0.0	0.197	0.0	0.0	0.0	0.215
202	2.747	0.412	3.082	0.742	0.154	0.334	0.347	0.144	0.0	0.0	1.137
203	2.251	0.260	1.236	0.234	0.291	0.0	0.0	0.091	0.0	0.0	0.239
204	0.176	0.050	0.257	0.0	0.0	0.0	0.064	0.026	0.0	0.070	0.209
205	4.482	1.204	4.121	0.813	0.509	0.715	0.643	0.112	0.062	0.0	0.775
206	1.218	0.432	0.962	0.212	0.132	0.096	0.199	0.041	0.0	0.0	0.108
207	5.257	1.213	2.946	0.520	0.388	0.328	0.390	0.040	0.089	0.0	0.531

TABLE 42--Continued

Unit Area	Reported Mortality		Estimated Cancer Morbidity								
	Heart Disease	Stroke	Total Cancer	(1)	(2)	(3)	(4)	(5)	(6)	(7)	(8)
208	4.845	0.323	3.734	0.581	0.482	0.785	0.272	0.113	0.248	0.0	0.891
209	4.985	2.018	4.601	0.801	0.266	0.577	0.501	0.0	0.273	0.0	1.310
210	2.465	0.247	1.006	0.333	0.0	0.0	0.0	0.0	0.0	0.0	0.680
211	4.715	1.359	2.935	0.647	0.448	0.0	0.404	0.168	0.0	0.0	0.662
212	12.385	1.062	2.887	0.478	0.0	0.860	1.791	0.0	0.0	0.0	0.0
213	3.898	1.049	1.835	0.405	0.168	0.729	0.0	0.0	0.0	0.0	0.414
214	2.368	0.614	1.252	0.237	0.196	0.426	0.0	0.0	0.202	0.0	0.0
215	2.812	1.023	2.347	0.173	0.286	0.932	0.0	0.0	0.0	0.0	1.058
216	0.322	0.080	0.0	0.0	0.0	0.0	0.0	0.0	0.0	0.0	0.0
217	1.583	0.144	0.587	0.194	0.161	0.0	0.0	0.0	0.0	0.0	0.0
218	3.145	0.993	1.013	0.223	0.0	0.402	0.419	0.0	0.0	0.0	0.0
219	1.239	0.207	0.737	0.209	0.173	0.0	0.0	0.0	0.0	0.0	0.142
220	2.883	0.985	1.722	0.475	0.158	0.171	0.356	0.0	0.162	0.0	0.194
221	4.983	2.699	2.542	0.561	0.233	1.009	0.525	0.0	0.0	0.0	0.0
222	4.988	1.403	6.041	0.842	1.047	0.379	0.394	0.164	0.717	0.430	1.721
223	5.079	0.762	3.626	0.343	0.569	0.0	0.642	0.0	0.0	0.701	2.103
224	5.226	1.991	3.892	1.456	0.0	0.0	0.630	0.087	0.0	0.0	1.374
225	1.036	5.390	2.960	0.280	0.232	1.007	0.0	0.0	0.954	0.572	0.572
226	1.256	6.529	3.586	0.339	0.563	0.0	0.635	0.0	0.0	0.0	2.079
227	1.104	0.897	2.674	0.373	0.464	0.168	0.175	0.072	0.317	0.190	0.762
228	0.124	0.672	1.016	0.101	0.112	0.313	0.189	0.0	0.057	0.069	0.206
229	4.241	0.707	4.496	0.674	0.512	0.808	0.631	0.175	0.096	0.0	1.262
230	2.752	0.566	2.349	0.369	0.284	0.237	0.296	0.061	0.135	0.0	0.808
231	2.582	0.765	1.951	0.258	0.161	0.349	0.606	0.0	0.0	0.0	0.660
232	2.876	0.791	3.667	0.971	0.403	0.175	0.364	0.0	0.0	0.0	1.389
233	2.853	0.433	2.358	0.390	0.283	0.263	0.548	0.038	0.0	0.0	0.698
234	3.222	0.983	2.340	0.442	0.122	0.398	0.276	0.057	0.126	0.0	0.904

235	1.912	0.531	2.601	0.526	0.357	0.172	0.090	0.074	0.0	0.0	1.075
236	3.078	0.408	2.179	0.594	0.211	0.305	0.318	0.033	0.0	0.0	0.433
237	2.785	0.214	2.404	0.289	0.600	0.260	0.271	0.225	0.0	0.0	0.0
238	3.870	1.027	4.190	0.960	0.442	0.768	0.200	0.166	0.0	0.0	1.090
239	3.751	0.278	3.401	0.750	0.311	0.675	0.351	0.292	0.0	0.0	0.383
240	2.634	0.811	2.480	0.0	0.681	0.492	0.513	0.0	0.0	0.0	0.559
241	2.860	0.381	3.112	0.0	0.641	0.463	0.0	0.200	0.0	0.0	1.579
242	1.795	0.256	1.308	0.346	0.144	0.312	0.324	0.0	0.0	0.0	0.0
243	3.346	0.515	2.363	0.347	0.0	0.625	0.651	0.135	0.296	0.0	0.355
244	5.870	1.118	5.417	1.509	0.313	1.019	0.707	0.147	0.0	0.0	1.157
245	3.998	2.822	4.318	0.317	1.054	0.143	0.0	0.247	0.0	0.0	0.649
246	2.643	0.661	1.348	0.0	0.0	0.0	0.0	0.231	0.0	0.0	1.216
247	2.435	0.588	1.713	0.227	0.282	0.408	0.0	0.088	0.0	0.0	0.463
248	1.218	0.146	1.491	0.329	0.218	0.237	0.0	0.051	0.0	0.0	0.403
249	2.413	0.621	1.969	0.372	0.232	0.168	0.523	0.145	0.0	0.0	0.190
250	2.124	0.437	1.147	0.169	0.210	0.0	0.0	0.066	0.0	0.0	0.517
251	1.295	0.230	1.233	0.233	0.097	0.210	0.291	0.0	0.0	0.079	0.397
252	1.477	0.394	0.653	0.199	0.028	0.060	0.125	0.052	0.0	0.068	0.068
253	5.803	1.478	4.315	0.879	0.456	0.626	0.652	0.100	0.156	0.0	1.048
254	2.848	0.600	2.140	1.012	0.0	0.0	0.379	0.0	0.0	0.0	0.414
255	3.274	0.0	3.340	0.631	0.262	0.0	0.592	0.0	0.0	0.0	1.936
256	4.785	1.167	2.143	0.945	0.261	0.0	0.0	0.0	0.0	0.0	0.322
257	0.336	0.224	0.913	0.151	0.125	0.272	0.0	0.0	0.0	0.0	0.309
258	1.492	0.124	2.537	0.504	0.418	0.302	0.0	0.131	0.0	0.0	0.686
259	4.541	0.454	3.706	1.226	0.0	0.0	0.574	0.0	1.045	0.0	0.627
260	0.655	0.131	0.535	0.177	0.0	0.0	0.0	0.138	0.0	0.0	0.0
261	2.291	0.665	1.809	0.299	0.414	0.359	0.0	0.0	0.170	0.0	0.204
262	1.311	0.262	1.605	0.354	0.147	0.637	0.0	0.0	0.302	0.0	0.0
263	2.015	0.451	0.982	0.447	0.034	0.146	0.0	0.0	0.0	0.0	0.166
264	1.331	0.518	20.867	0.399	0.497	0.359	0.374	0.078	0.0	0.204	0.817
265	2.711	0.703	1.639	0.0	0.225	0.244	0.254	0.211	0.0	0.0	0.554
266	0.050	0.500	0.510	0.135	0.0	0.0	0.127	0.0	0.0	0.0	0.276
267	0.784	7.843	8.000	2.118	0.0	0.0	1.984	0.0	0.0	0.0	4.329
268	0.380	0.0	4.266	1.540	0.426	0.0	0.481	0.0	0.0	0.0	1.049
269	0.162	0.0	1.320	0.437	0.181	0.0	0.0	0.0	0.0	0.0	0.447
270	0.402	0.0	1.641	0.543	0.0	0.0	1.017	0.0	0.0	0.0	0.0
271	0.627	0.0	2.984	0.282	0.468	0.508	1.057	0.0	0.0	0.0	0.577

APPENDIX C

A MODEL FOR FORECASTING RACIAL CHANGE IN THE CHICAGO AREA

A MODEL FOR FORECASTING RACIAL CHANGE IN THE CHICAGO AREA

The search for a method which would accurately replicate and subsequently aid in forecasting racial change in the Chicago area was based on the simple assumption that American residential neighborhoods are largely segregated, and that black ghetto areas have spread outward from core areas in patterns which can be described as a function of time and distance. Many studies specific to the above subject as well as general ones of the urban social ecology have indicated that it is possible to trace such patterns, and that ghetto expansion is axial or "sectorial" in nature often following major transportation lines. Data for per cent black were for the years 1950, 1960, and 1967 available for 159 (Fig. 68) of the 271 subareas of this study, and they were tested with the linear regression model shown as equation (2). The equation proved to be too linear for a good fit thus suggesting that barriers to expansion, for limited periods of time at least, are sufficient to suggest that the function might be exponential in some manner. Additional results which would appear to be fairly reliable were obtained then by using suggestions put forth by Morrill.[1]

Applications of the trend surface method in the construction of racial response surfaces

The trend surface analysis method which was utilized to smooth the disease distributions discussed in Chapter III has some polynomial expansion characteristics applicable to the problem proposed here. We have assumed that Per Cent Black (Z) is a function of Distance from Loop (Y) and Time (X) making three-space relationship that can be expressed in terms of an estimated trend surface. In addition, the surface can be successively smoothed through the polynomial expansions. The most basic form of the equation is a plane expressed by

$$Z_{trend} = A + BX + CY, \qquad (25)$$

but this is essentially the linear function already mentioned. The second degree is a

---

[1]Richard Morrill, "The Shape of Diffusion in Space and Time," Economic Geography, XLVI, No. 2, Supplement (Proceedings of the International Geographical Union Commission on Quantitative Methods, June, 1970), 259-68.

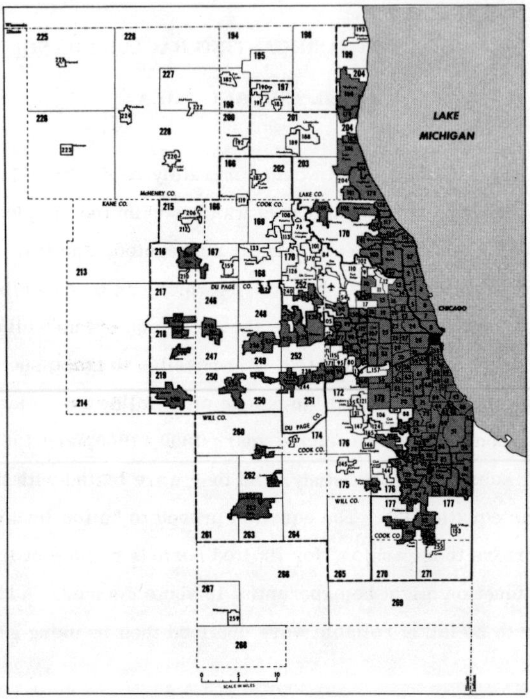

Fig. 68.--Communities for which racial forecasts could be made

paraboloid expressed by

$$Z = A + BX + CY + DX^2 + EXY + FY^2, \tag{26}$$

and the third degree by

$$Z = A + BX + CY + DX^2 + EXY + FY^2 + GX^3 + HX^2Y + IXY^2 + JY^3, \tag{27}$$

and so on to six degrees with computer programs currently available. In fact, the number of terms generated by a sixth degree expansion may be more than necessary for describing a surface.

It is possible to develop a racial response surface which can extrapolate to a future time by extending the appropriate axis. In other words, data for Per Cent Black are known for three times, t_1, t_2, and t_3. The axis is extended to time t_4, and the resultant surface has been forced to estimate to the end of the axis. The basic problem with use of this method to extrapolate occurs at the higher degree levels of the polynomial expansion wherein the method is simply doing its job so well that the data points which do not exist are recognized as such. The true utility of this method thus appears to be within the third and fourth degree polynomial expansions. The latter is at least true for the Chicago tests.

The Chicago area response surfaces

Initially data for all 159 points were put to the trend surface analysis. The result was a fairly weak fit, the coefficient of determination being only .167. The points were then separated into five sectors intended to represent paths of varied ghetto growth (or lack thereof) and different social status areas within the context of factorial ecology. Five functional relationships were thus obtained and utilized in the forecasting process. The surfaces are shown on Figure 68, and the equations are given on Table 43 along with the surfaces selected. The actual Per Cent Black for each of the 159 units in 1980 was then obtained by substituting for X and Y in each of the five equations.

Each of the five sectors has a "ghetto expansion wave" which is different, and this is most apparent in Figure 69. In these illustrations, the "X" values actually existed for 1950, 1960, and 1967 while all values beyond those in time were extrapolated. It should be pointed out that all industrial satellites were removed as data collection points due mostly to the age of the cities and the duration for which black populations have existed.

The best fit turned out to be for the Northern Sector. And this becomes particularly intriguing because the North Shore area has not traditionally been a "Black Belt" or ghetto area in the ecological context. However, Per Cent Black still appears to be a function of distance from the Loop and time.

The Northwest Sector did not display a very strong fit. In addition, the number of black persons in the area has not increased substantially over the years, and many communities have never had black populations. The inner city part of the sector is characterized by large concentrations of blue collar workers with strong residual ethnic tendencies. The suburban parts of the sector are comprised of communities with upper middle class residents who are usually white collar workers. Incomes are generally not so high in these areas as in the Northern Sector, but there are fewer blacks.

The Western Sector had a fairly good fit. The inner city part of this sector is characterized by a ghetto area fairly new by Chicago standards, and this growth shows up very nicely on the graph. Immediately adjacent to the West Side ghetto area are neighborhoods and communities which have, for periods of time, managed to resist the movement of black people into their areas. The latter areas show up as the large blank area on the graph. Beyond the areas of strong resistance are areas with a statistically significant number of black people. The model here suggests that the farther areas will eventually

TABLE 43

EQUATIONS FOR RACIAL RESPONSE SURFACES

A. Northern Sector (Third Degree Surface) — $R^2 = .556$

$$Z = 20.46665 + (-0.82252)X + 2.58163Y + (-0.00715)X^2 + 0.07265XY + (-0.31950)Y^2 + 0.00022X^3 + (-0.00137)X^2Y + 0.00273XY^2 + 0.00354Y^3$$

B. Northwestern Sector (Third Degree Surface) — $R^2 = .185$

$$Z = -375.35669 + 20.19775X + (-4.64304)Y + (-0.35534)X^2 + 0.08786XY + 0.28926Y^2 + 0.00207X^3 + (-0.00068)X^2Y + (-0.00096)XY^2 + (-0.00947)Y^3$$

C. Western Sector (Fourth Degree Surface) — $R^2 = .322$

$$Z = -281.32881 + 5.82529X + 22.23707Y + 0.11232X^2 + (-0.57879)XY + (-0.87451)Y^2 + (-0.00325)X^3 + 0.00254X^2Y + 0.01524XY^2 + 0.02123Y^2 + 0.00002X^4 + 0.00001X^3Y + (-0.00011)X^2Y^2 + 0.00002XY^3 + (-0.00036)Y^4$$

D. Southwestern Sector (Fourth Degree Surface) — $R^2 = .110$

$$Z = -28.65113 + 1.40947X + (-3.91186)Y + (-0.01642)X^2 + 0.13094XY + 0.19862Y^2 + (-0.00030)X^3 + 0.00131X^2Y + (-0.01306)XY^2 + 0.00507Y^3 + 0.00000X^4 + (-0.00002)X^3Y + 0.00008X^2Y^2 + 0.00008XY^3 + (-0.00011)Y^4$$

E. Southern Sector (Third Degree Surface) — $R^2 = .428$

$$Z = -13.60893 + (-0.91704)X + 0.09119Y + 0.11046X^2 + (-0.43966)XY + 0.75549Y^2 + (-0.00097)X^3 + 0.00311X^2Y + (-0.00024)XY^2 + (-0.01283)Y^3$$

link up with movement to areas adjacent to the ghetto as resistance in the middle areas eventually relaxes.

The Southwestern Sector displayed a very weak fit, and the graph does not tell much of a story either. Simply stated, there are few blacks in the area. The black people in these areas have been there for a long time, and they are nearly evenly spread throughout (at least by community). There are no large ghetto areas at this level of aggregation. Two small pockets do show up. One is suggested to be comprised of communities of the inner city adjacent to large ghetto areas, and the other is near Joliet.

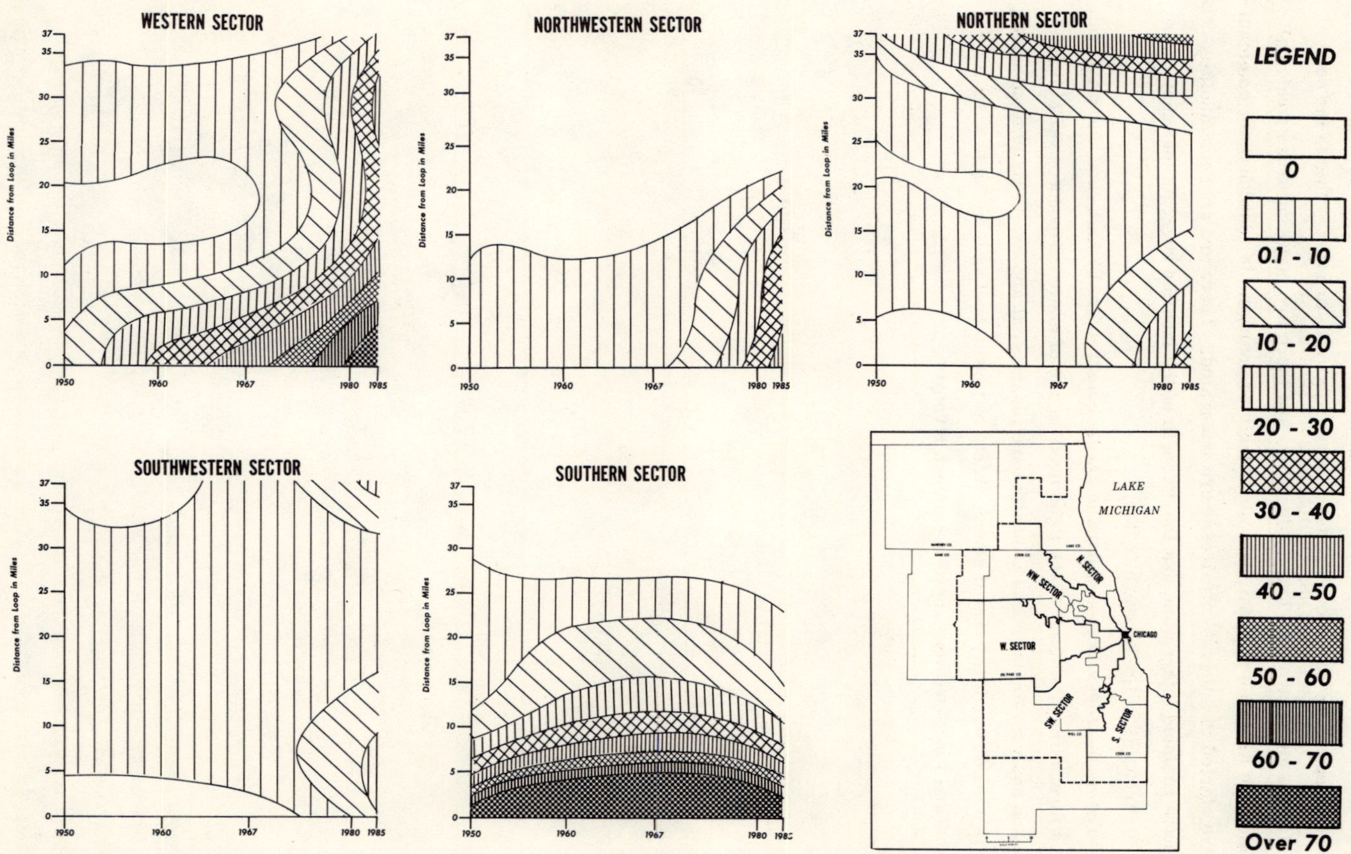

Fig. 69.--Racial response surfaces for five sectors of the metropolis

The Southern Sector also displayed a good fit. As indicated by the graph, Per Cent Black appears to be a slow but steady outward growth function. This is the sector containing the ghetto areas of longest duration, and there are many suburban municipalities which are all black and have been since their beginnings. In addition many communities have started to integrate or already are integrated. There are also communities which have resisted integration, but the strength of the function suggests that resistance is not so strong as in the Western Sector.

The methodology proposed here is hardly construed to be foolproof, but for purposes of forecasting Per Cent Black to be used as one of many independent variables in a regression analysis for purposes of health care planning, it appears to be quite adequate. There is a good possibility that if census tracts had been used as modifiable units the mathematical functions would have been much stronger.

APPENDIX D

DEMOGRAPHIC AND SOCIO-ECONOMIC FORECASTS

FOR 1967 AND 1980

TABLE 44

DEMOGRAPHIC AND SOCIO-ECONOMIC FORECASTS FOR 1967 AND 1980
(RMP Subareas Are Numbered in the Left-Hand Column.
1980 Forecasts Are Shown Directly Below Those for 1967)

Subarea	Population	Population Density/ Sq. Mile	Income (Dollars)	Per Cent Nonwhite	Age Groups (%)			
					<15	15-44	45-65	>65
1	56200	305.4	8672	1.30	17.97	36.73	30.26	15.04
	53000	288.0	11200	16.00	18.13	35.02	30.90	15.95
2	64700	182.8	10530	0.20	21.37	35.44	32.55	10.63
	75000	211.9	13200	16.50	21.24	33.81	33.98	10.97
3	126300	315.8	9177	4.80	39.56	6.85	34.96	18.63
	127000	317.5	11000	20.50	43.54	4.16	33.59	18.72
4	46900	183.9	9150	1.00	20.40	34.43	31.12	14.05
	37000	145.1	11100	20.00	20.83	32.51	31.94	14.71
5	41100	204.5	8420	0.40	24.90	35.44	26.62	13.03
	34000	169.2	10300	22.00	25.92	33.70	26.85	13.53
6	114800	363.3	9802	3.10	20.46	36.20	29.73	13.61
	113000	357.6	13700	22.50	21.42	33.99	30.31	14.27
7	82600	260.6	8102	7.50	25.06	39.40	24.03	11.51
	76000	239.7	11400	24.30	26.48	37.47	24.13	11.91
8	78300	313.2	12205	37.60	26.87	37.74	24.86	10.53
	70000	280.0	18200	37.60	29.32	34.87	24.96	10.85
9	13500	117.4	10610	0.0	30.85	32.76	26.36	10.03
	12000	104.3	13100	0.0	32.34	31.22	26.12	10.33
10	43000	101.7	10850	0.20	26.87	34.34	29.42	9.37
	47000	111.1	14300	26.00	27.14	32.01	31.12	9.73
11	26900	109.3	10040	0.0	23.77	34.95	29.24	12.04
	27300	111.0	13600	27.00	24.26	32.68	30.30	12.77
12	18600	62.8	13040	1.10	23.65	29.94	36.47	9.95
	16500	55.7	16200	27.00	23.58	27.60	38.51	10.30
13	17300	68.7	10770	7.60	20.97	33.96	33.84	11.24
	15000	59.5	12900	27.80	20.58	30.95	36.65	11.82
14	46500	242.2	8020	1.40	23.34	32.69	28.41	15.56
	46000	239.6	10400	28.20	24.11	30.34	28.88	16.67
15	63100	158.9	9640	0.20	23.15	34.06	28.78	14.01
	61000	153.7	13500	26.50	23.89	31.98	29.21	14.92
16	55800	174.4	8830	0.50	23.54	35.71	27.93	12.82
	56000	175.0	11300	28.50	24.43	33.68	28.49	13.40

TABLE 44--Continued

Subarea	Population	Population Density/ Sq. Mile	Income (Dollars)	Per Cent Nonwhite	Age Groups (%)			
					<15	15-44	45-65	>65
17	41300	123.7	9720	0.10	24.45	36.48	29.47	9.60
	42000	125.7	13200	27.00	24.49	34.42	30.98	10.10
18	11400	114.0	9150	0.10	22.57	34.69	29.75	12.99
	25000	250.0	11700	27.50	22.61	32.10	31.44	13.85
19	57500	145.2	9070	0.60	22.75	36.25	27.98	13.01
	53000	133.8	11500	28.00	23.23	33.92	28.87	13.98
20	20200	169.7	8500	0.30	24.06	36.48	26.99	12.47
	26750	224.8	10900	29.00	24.87	34.76	27.28	13.09
21	37400	187.9	8260	0.20	26.27	30.73	31.03	11.97
	34100	171.4	10600	29.20	27.16	22.96	37.31	12.57
22	93500	267.1	7780	0.90	26.89	38.34	23.77	11.00
	98000	280.0	10100	29.50	28.22	36.38	23.98	11.42
23	67500	190.7	8020	2.90	27.50	38.78	23.38	10.35
	65300	184.5	9900	29.50	28.87	36.72	23.65	10.76
24	130100	281.6	7210	2.40	31.75	39.13	19.94	9.18
	128000	277.1	8900	31.00	33.87	36.67	19.96	9.49
25	118000	163.9	9230	0.60	22.56	35.02	28.69	13.74
	123000	170.8	11700	50.00	23.23	33.26	29.09	14.42
26	42400	331.3	5670	68.70	33.51	40.99	17.45	8.05
	57000	445.3	6500	60.00	36.48	39.16	16.37	7.99
27	62700	326.6	5260	87.50	41.95	42.14	11.62	4.29
	61000	317.7	5900	87.50	46.78	38.81	10.34	4.07
28	116000	205.3	4860	60.10	43.40	34.78	16.12	5.70
	111000	196.5	6500	68.00	48.13	30.84	15.47	5.56
29	122200	377.2	5670	94.60	47.78	38.96	10.22	3.04
	121500	375.0	7300	94.60	53.55	35.04	8.66	2.75
30	57300	140.4	7370	6.60	26.71	38.51	23.98	10.79
	54000	132.4	9100	62.00	28.27	36.04	24.37	11.32
31	45400	183.8	5830	1.30	32.87	39.11	18.89	9.14
	40000	161.9	6600	67.00	35.24	36.68	18.74	9.34
32	4800	32.0	0	5.80	1.32	34.33	43.17	21.18
	4000	26.7	0	0.0	1.31	30.73	45.49	22.47
33	11600	70.7	4050	63.10	45.51	32.15	14.15	8.19
	16000	86.6	5600	95.00	51.52	27.01	13.30	8.17
34	12700	127.0	5990	63.20	37.68	36.79	16.94	8.59
	12000	120.0	7300	87.00	39.83	34.23	17.04	8.90
35	49200	303.7	7222	89.60	43.06	35.45	15.36	6.13
	55000	339.5	8900	82.50	47.71	31.46	14.73	6.10

TABLE 44--Continued

Subarea	Population	Population Density/ Sq. Mile	Income (Dollars)	Per Cent Nonwhite	Age Groups (%)			
					<15	15-44	45-65	>65
36	26300	453.4	4050	98.30	49.80	31.56	14.01	4.64
	24600	424.1	5400	78.00	56.86	25.40	13.30	4.45
37	10500	145.8	5180	72.00	44.32	34.96	16.44	4.29
	10000	138.9	6100	97.30	48.62	30.99	16.19	4.19
38	10800	61.4	5100	70.00	30.45	33.84	25.79	9.91
	83500	474.4	6500	99.10	33.34	29.87	26.38	10.42
39	38300	364.8	7340	83.50	34.90	42.64	16.77	5.69
	41000	390.4	9100	60.00	39.10	39.91	15.56	5.42
40	42800	285.3	5990	55.00	24.53	36.02	29.13	10.32
	45000	300.0	7500	99.00	26.27	32.21	30.58	10.94
41	41000	253.1	9050	32.80	22.10	45.35	20.87	11.68
	44000	271.6	12000	50.00	23.34	44.91	19.97	11.78
42	78200	363.7	5508	98.30	32.88	43.77	17.19	6.16
	82000	381.4	7100	98.30	36.99	41.13	15.90	5.98
43	72400	249.7	8662	43.60	18.12	30.46	34.62	16.80
	78000	269.0	10000	43.60	18.21	28.08	35.83	17.87
44	45200	153.7	8420	88.00	23.48	43.92	23.76	8.84
	51000	173.5	10400	88.00	23.95	44.30	22.81	8.94
45	12300	97.6	8750	25.60	27.17	32.97	28.08	11.79
	11000	87.3	9100	25.60	28.16	31.12	28.39	12.34
46	47600	144.7	7700	5.40	28.95	35.66	25.46	9.93
	45000	136.8	9100	27.00	30.21	32.78	26.59	10.43
47	3300	53.2	7700	4.10	29.12	37.78	22.54	10.56
	2000	32.3	10100	25.00	30.06	35.20	23.58	11.15
48	19700	112.6	9880	6.20	31.73	37.32	23.49	7.45
	18000	102.9	11100	25.00	33.70	34.64	24.02	7.65
49	59000	122.2	8500	24.90	27.38	33.63	27.82	11.16
	63000	130.4	10100	24.90	28.14	30.96	29.23	11.67
50	8200	33.5	8020	0.10	27.72	36.23	26.57	9.49
	15000	61.2	9800	23.00	28.28	33.68	28.12	9.92
51	19300	32.2	8990	0.30	36.09	37.11	20.06	6.73
	18750	31.3	9800	16.00	37.72	33.26	21.86	7.17
52	23800	64.0	8830	0.10	9.20	47.70	32.45	10.64
	23000	61.8	11100	22.50	7.91	45.67	35.06	11.37
53	38700	106.6	8590	2.80	31.77	36.55	22.51	9.18
	40900	112.7	10200	17.00	33.59	33.82	23.13	9.46
54	11600	32.2	3810	86.50	60.61	30.19	6.56	2.63
	13500	37.5	4400	86.50	64.23	26.89	6.30	2.57

TABLE 44--Continued

Subarea	Popu-lation	Population Density/ Sq. Mile	Income (Dollars)	Per Cent Nonwhite	Age Groups (%)			
					<15	15-44	45-65	>65
55	10400	20.6	8830	0.40	31.73	40.90	19.62	7.75
	18750	37.1	12200	13.00	33.36	38.84	19.87	7.94
56	42600	100.9	9560	5.50	39.59	38.64	16.94	4.83
	43500	101.2	10000	6.00	43.05	35.22	16.85	4.88
57	10600	48.4	8990	1.80	27.60	39.97	21.19	11.24
	44000	104.3	11600	16.00	28.99	37.46	21.47	12.07
58	11800	53.9	7860	1.30	26.83	39.56	22.58	11.03
	36500	126.3	10900	18.00	27.95	37.09	23.22	11.74
59	16000	97.0	8180	0.20	29.71	38.24	22.10	9.96
	34000	117.6	10100	17.20	31.18	35.84	22.54	10.44
60	38500	182.5	7370	0.40	31.51	38.09	20.57	9.83
	15000	90.9	10100	16.40	33.06	35.81	20.90	10.23
61	63200	126.9	7940	0.40	31.36	39.32	20.13	9.19
	36000	170.6	9100	15.80	32.83	37.09	20.51	9.57
62	14300	122.2	9720	0.30	26.75	39.58	26.05	7.62
	10500	21.1	10100	17.20	27.01	36.76	28.14	8.09
63	26800	121.8	8910	0.10	23.97	32.59	29.78	13.65
	26500	226.5	12200	17.40	25.58	27.03	32.11	15.29
64	22300	87.8	8750	0.10	33.37	43.60	18.17	4.86
	26000	118.2	11000	18.00	34.86	41.69	18.51	4.94
65	27000	95.7	9640	0.20	29.03	39.32	23.91	7.74
	23000	90.6	10900	15.00	30.29	37.20	24.50	8.01
66	48800	138.2	9150	0.20	20.52	34.02	32.28	13.18
	25000	88.7	12000	16.30	20.76	31.37	33.85	14.03
67	56300	178.2	7610	31.40	28.69	36.47	23.60	11.24
	50000	141.6	11600	17.00	30.20	34.23	23.85	11.72
68	52000	164.6	6080	31.40	38.98	38.55	16.00	6.48
	91600	298.4	9500	82.60	43.01	35.96	14.79	6.24
69	61100	171.1	7130	96.90	29.89	42.01	21.24	6.85
	95000	309.4	7100	82.60	31.57	41.22	20.53	6.68
70	44800	89.8	10370	0.10	40.44	39.03	16.50	4.03
	65000	182.1	8600	96.90	41.84	36.48	17.51	4.16
71	48500	97.2	9560	15.30	21.98	31.15	31.81	15.05
	57300	153.6	13000	34.70	22.13	28.76	33.04	16.07
72	24200	75.4	13690	0.10	28.63	27.71	31.33	12.33
	61500	164.9	11600	34.70	29.90	25.75	31.67	12.69
73	22500	70.1	9960	23.00	27.76	32.99	27.98	11.27
	31000	106.9	15400	37.20	28.71	30.92	28.55	11.82

TABLE 44--Continued

Subarea	Population	Population Density/ Sq. Mile	Income (Dollars)	Per Cent Nonwhite	Age Groups (%)			
					<15	15-44	45-65	>65
74	23600	107.8	10210	0.10	36.07	35.31	22.56	6.05
	34000	117.2	11600	37.20	37.73	31.32	24.54	6.41
75	22000	85.0	9880	14.00	31.98	32.27	24.76	10.99
	27200	100.5	13100	33.20	33.38	29.97	25.30	11.35
76	27000	36.9	12300	0.0	42.60	37.69	14.97	4.75
	43670	84.4	12100	33.20	46.40	35.36	13.75	4.49
77	5900	5.0	10300	0.10	37.40	40.19	17.80	4.61
	26000	41.3	14300	0.0	39.76	37.80	17.81	4.63
78	26553	42.9	9660	0.10	20.84	34.41	31.45	13.30
	55850	76.3	16500	32.50	21.28	32.21	32.40	14.11
79	25225	44.8	8920	3.40	29.11	36.36	23.56	10.97
	56400	77.0	13200	46.00	30.48	34.39	23.71	11.41
80	23108	58.6	10500	0.10	30.02	36.95	29.56	3.47
	33000	58.6	12300	14.50	30.90	34.36	31.35	3.40
81	31658	26.8	9030	0.10	35.73	41.01	17.40	5.86
	24024	61.0	13900	11.00	38.32	38.85	16.90	5.93
82	44253	41.4	8920	19.50	37.36	38.99	16.62	7.03
	38790	32.8	12900	19.50	40.59	36.43	16.00	6.97
83	57500	53.8	8920	0.10	24.02	37.47	27.34	11.17
	71203	53.8	10300	23.10	24.81	35.28	28.24	11.67
84	55161	42.6	11250	0.10	36.34	39.54	18.51	5.60
	71915	85.2	12200	52.00	38.42	37.90	18.12	5.56
85	23738	35.2	10100	0.10	45.82	40.08	10.68	3.42
	78200	60.4	15600	0.10	49.65	37.13	9.94	3.28
86	31599	140.4	10700	0.20	26.21	37.31	28.09	8.38
	29120	43.1	14100	12.00	26.37	35.48	29.38	8.78
87	40000	82.1	11500	13.00	22.11	39.12	25.52	13.25
	83200	177.8	14300	27.50	23.03	37.53	25.62	13.81
88	30717	54.6	10900	0.10	32.15	46.08	16.13	5.64
	83200	82.1	15400	13.20	32.18	45.93	16.15	5.75
89	16346	48.5	9000	0.20	23.94	37.13	25.21	13.71
	40500	71.9	13100	0.10	24.69	35.71	25.40	14.20
90	24259	53.9	10200	0.20	34.82	42.66	18.24	4.28
	16995	50.4	12000	41.00	35.59	40.89	19.15	4.37
91	24307	22.7	14300	0.20	38.84	36.88	19.90	4.38
	31000	68.9	14200	25.00	40.79	34.98	19.89	4.34
92	36812	72.8	8700	8.00	32.81	40.48	19.92	6.79
	40000	37.4	12000	8.00	34.54	38.74	19.85	6.87

TABLE 44--Continued

Subarea	Population	Population Density/ Sq. Mile	Income (Dollars)	Per Cent Nonwhite	Age Groups (%)			
					<15	15-44	45-65	>65
93	17581	26.0	12000	0.40	34.13	33.84	25.19	6.85
	45200	89.3	12400	16.40	35.82	31.74	25.52	6.92
94	18659	82.9	13350	6.00	34.24	34.05	24.49	9.22
	24300	36.0	18100	5.00	33.97	32.43	24.34	9.25
95	15602	55.5	13120	0.10	29.15	35.46	26.75	8.64
	26800	119.1	20500	30.00	30.08	33.58	27.52	8.83
96	16000	31.6	9900	0.10	39.63	39.81	16.57	3.99
	22917	31.4	18700	6.00	41.64	37.68	16.67	4.01
97	14403	28.5	15960	0.40	32.46	35.98	26.68	4.88
	28113	38.5	13800	5.20	33.77	34.69	26.66	4.88
98	31000	138.0	9450	32.00	30.74	35.86	23.20	10.21
	16000	31.6	18100	14.50	32.82	33.87	22.87	10.45
99	27355	34.7	9350	0.50	32.54	43.73	17.97	5.76
	32139	142.8	13000	37.00	33.77	42.41	18.01	5.80
100	25185	49.8	12400	0.80	42.99	39.78	13.54	3.68
	31800	40.4	11800	37.50	46.79	37.32	12.35	3.54
101	32234	31.8	12080	0.20	43.62	37.84	14.68	3.86
	28000	55.3	17200	0.80	46.96	35.40	13.85	3.79
102	27238	30.3	10500	0.10	34.92	42.26	17.57	5.24
	48600	48.0	15000	0.80	35.12	41.68	17.82	5.38
103	18651	66.4	10200	0.20	39.61	40.67	14.94	4.79
	32700	36.3	13600	0.20	42.51	38.39	14.29	4.81
104	15588	9.9	14700	0.20	44.60	38.76	13.58	3.06
	23900	85.1	14400	0.20	47.77	36.09	13.14	3.00
105	14716	37.4	10300	0.10	40.72	39.48	16.39	3.42
	25200	16.0	19000	5.00	42.22	37.26	17.01	3.51
106	5000	41.0	100000	0.0	41.26	38.57	16.00	4.17
	16680	42.3	14800	0.10	44.04	35.78	15.97	4.20
107	46500	63.6	11000	0.40	23.69	32.36	28.38	15.57
	62925	79.9	14500	0.10	24.75	30.95	28.10	16.20
108	16400	17.1	10900	0.20	41.45	39.38	13.98	5.19
	63525	80.6	15000	47.50	44.29	37.54	13.15	5.01
109	27630	28.9	11100	0.40	48.66	40.97	8.73	1.65
	38151	56.5	13400	1.20	52.00	37.11	9.21	1.68
110	47304	56.0	13650	0.10	33.77	34.65	24.29	7.29
	58200	86.2	15500	1.20	35.64	33.35	23.71	7.30
111	15263	19.4	9980	0.10	32.70	35.98	24.90	6.43
	61000	72.3	17900	0.10	33.59	33.75	26.05	6.62

TABLE 44--Continued

Subarea	Population	Population Density/ Sq. Mile	Income (Dollars)	Per Cent Nonwhite	Age Groups (%) <15	15-44	45-65	>65
112	14360	28.4	17320	0.20	23.15	35.66	28.92	12.27
	19200	24.4	13000	12.00	23.87	34.18	29.26	12.69
113	15508	46.0	9240	0.10	41.45	39.38	13.98	5.19
	14928	29.5	23000	40.00	44.29	37.54	13.15	5.01
114	22617	71.7	11340	0.30	36.75	38.56	20.03	4.66
	26129	77.5	12200	0.10	38.96	36.56	19.83	4.65
115	20465	36.3	11550	0.0	35.85	38.44	21.53	4.18
	79100	78.1	14000	11.00	36.67	35.94	23.08	4.30
116	31063	36.8	16800	0.50	36.00	33.68	21.63	8.69
	21276	37.8	16000	0.0	38.69	32.24	20.55	8.53
117	14689	23.7	25520	1.50	29.39	30.78	29.40	10.43
	31063	36.8	19800	9.50	30.59	29.14	29.65	10.62
118	4789	5.7	8400	0.10	41.78	42.43	12.34	3.44
	14689	23.7	30000	8.00	43.93	41.06	11.63	3.38
119	6250	7.5	11340	0.20	31.01	33.58	24.83	10.59
	8780	19.5	20000	9.00	32.43	31.71	25.16	10.70
120	6551	23.2	10180	0.10	42.76	39.07	16.46	3.70
	12731	28.3	14900	0.20	45.53	36.50	14.27	3.69
121	5952	19.9	9240	0.10	43.25	44.85	9.86	2.03
	6811	24.2	12600	27.50	45.74	42.93	9.35	1.98
122	9714	28.8	10180	1.60	33.09	38.81	23.41	4.68
	12900	28.7	12000	0.10	33.54	36.33	25.33	4.80
123	10882	21.5	9450	0.30	43.56	40.04	13.19	3.21
	10098	30.0	13200	35.00	46.42	37.20	13.19	3.20
124	7303	32.5	9150	0.10	47.01	41.31	9.70	1.98
	13800	27.3	12000	15.00	50.68	38.72	8.71	1.90
125	3894	17.3	7250	65.00	27.70	55.65	12.02	4.63
	9700	43.1	12000	0.10	26.27	58.69	10.77	4.26
126	12294	16.8	10400	0.10	38.58	42.82	13.96	4.64
	4750	21.1	10100	65.00	40.75	41.65	13.14	4.46
127	5818	4.7	10000	0.50	34.60	32.78	26.59	6.03
	20700	28.3	14100	0.10	36.60	31.62	25.80	5.98
128	8450	6.8	25700	3.50	36.51	27.10	29.41	6.98
	12673	17.3	35000	7.00	39.42	23.86	29.66	7.06
129	7331	10.9	9150	0.10	31.45	38.53	24.33	5.70
	16500	22.6	30000	7.00	31.63	36.59	25.87	5.92
130	8500	21.6	10300	0.10	44.33	36.34	15.44	3.88
	9650	14.3	11500	26.00	48.48	33.05	14.70	3.76

TABLE 44--Continued

Subarea	Population	Population Density/ Sq. Mile	Income (Dollars)	Per Cent Nonwhite	Age Groups (%)			
					<15	15-44	45-65	>65
131	3639	9.2	9450	0.80	37.37	31.24	23.58	7.80
	12000	30.5	12500	4.00	39.66	28.03	24.46	7.86
132	8815	39.2	10290	0.20	40.26	41.83	14.52	3.39
	7300	18.5	11600	0.80	41.90	40.16	14.58	3.35
133	9165	15.2	11020	0.0	38.32	41.14	15.86	4.68
	11954	40.7	12900	29.50	40.55	39.66	15.26	4.52
134	9501	56.6	9350	0.0	41.26	38.51	16.00	4.17
	12434	15.8	15500	0.0	44.04	35.78	15.97	4.20
135	3421	20.4	9500	0.0	42.84	42.63	12.52	2.01
	12800	76.2	12600	14.20	45.79	41.02	11.80	1.39
136	3251	14.4	29500	1.00	29.16	28.08	33.93	8.83
	4900	29.2	13300	0.0	30.38	25.94	34.71	8.96
137	3251	9.0	9250	0.10	31.60	38.39	20.66	9.35
	4544	14.4	35000	9.00	33.35	37.45	19.83	9.38
138	6880	13.4	9450	0.10	31.20	40.18	21.46	7.16
	12128	43.0	12000	0.10	31.66	38.66	22.32	7.36
139	16842	23.0	9250	36.00	38.59	46.47	11.89	3.05
	17400	61.7	12000	0.10	39.21	45.74	11.84	3.20
140	4101	9.1	9660	0.0	42.62	38.03	13.91	5.44
	26300	36.0	12600	36.00	46.40	35.27	13.10	5.24
141	6200	13.8	8930	0.10	39.48	38.20	15.76	6.57
	9770	29.5	14300	0.0	41.68	36.46	15.23	6.63
142	5369	9.5	16800	0.40	36.81	34.55	24.29	4.35
	15800	47.7	10900	10.00	38.20	31.59	25.75	4.46
143	12018	71.5	10400	0.80	27.49	39.37	26.59	6.56
	18650	85.4	25000	7.00	27.69	37.00	28.62	6.69
144	5509	52.0	9450	0.0	42.94	42.68	7.31	7.07
	12495	74.4	14100	38.00	45.16	41.27	6.39	7.19
145	4538	6.7	8720	0.20	45.13	41.24	9.39	4.23
	8900	84.0	12000	4.80	48.45	38.93	8.45	4.17
146	4960	12.6	13230	0.0	37.37	31.24	23.58	7.80
	13575	20.1	11000	4.00	39.66	28.03	24.46	7.86
147	5065	6.9	9560	0.10	37.37	31.24	23.58	7.80
	8250	20.9	17500	0.0	39.66	28.03	24.46	7.86
148	5321	23.6	6820	92.00	40.41	36.75	16.26	6.58
	10150	13.9	13600	0.10	44.06	33.48	15.84	6.62
149	6681	29.7	8190	0.10	45.23	41.22	9.51	4.04
	6500	28.9	9000	92.00	49.42	37.89	8.79	3.90

TABLE 44--Continued

Subarea	Population	Population Density/ Sq. Mile	Income (Dollars)	Per Cent Nonwhite	Age Groups (%) <15	15-44	45-65	>65
150	11205	22.1	9980	0.10	32.72	40.33	21.26	5.69
	10900	48.4	10500	12.00	34.00	38.51	21.69	5.80
151	11028	49.0	13340	0.10	23.73	30.43	35.01	10.83
	14350	28.4	12000	26.30	24.06	28.22	36.57	11.15
152	9945	44.2	5980	99.00	44.28	34.31	16.83	4.58
	11466	51.0	18100	39.00	46.06	32.66	16.76	4.52
153	6041	13.4	9240	0.20	43.57	38.27	14.49	3.66
	15700	69.8	8000	99.00	47.18	35.74	13.62	3.46
154	7529	14.9	9030	0.10	39.55	41.92	14.32	4.20
	7850	17.4	12700	0.20	42.64	40.15	13.09	4.12
155	5210	6.6	8300	0.20	35.41	43.30	15.44	5.86
	9610	19.0	11000	26.00	36.99	42.25	14.94	5.82
156	13184	29.3	10820	0.10	42.59	39.90	12.42	5.09
	16700	38.5	11000	0.20	45.72	37.79	11.56	4.93
157	10621	47.2	9140	0.0	32.41	38.59	21.61	7.39
	16100	35.8	15800	16.30	34.26	36.18	21.91	7.64
158	3436	30.7	8920	0.20	39.13	42.86	14.28	3.73
	16200	72.0	12800	0.0	39.92	41.82	14.46	3.80
159	8401	12.4	8400	0.10	38.32	41.14	15.86	4.68
	9572	31.9	11000	32.00	40.55	39.66	15.26	4.52
160	12662	56.3	8400	15.00	30.74	42.44	19.88	6.94
	13871	20.5	10700	0.10	31.92	40.55	20.41	7.12
161	3665	9.3	9240	0.10	43.34	40.09	11.62	4.96
	18000	80.0	11500	15.00	47.20	38.10	10.05	4.65
162	9614	19.0	9450	0.20	45.58	37.64	11.91	4.87
	46000	116.8	13000	6.50	49.22	34.74	11.30	4.73
163	13230	33.6	15440	0.10	32.93	34.63	27.04	5.40
	22000	43.5	12000	4.00	33.93	33.39	27.30	5.38
164	11228	16.6	9030	0.20	50.83	41.75	5.72	1.71
	18900	48.0	22000	27.00	55.01	38.60	4.79	1.59
165	10567	26.8	9240	0.10	44.04	41.10	12.04	2.82
	15000	22.2	11800	5.00	47.45	38.56	11.34	2.65
166	7180	1.3	11000	0.10	30.03	35.82	27.32	6.83
	17000	43.1	12200	9.00	30.37	33.54	29.24	6.85
167	6952	2.5	9100	0.20	37.26	36.81	19.59	6.33
	13431	2.4	16000	0.10	39.27	34.58	19.66	6.28
168	10572	3.8	9000	0.20	38.32	41.14	15.86	4.68
	135680	4.8	12400	0.20	40.55	39.66	15.26	4.52

TABLE 44--Continued

Subarea	Population	Population Density/ Sq. Mile	Income (Dollars)	Per Cent Nonwhite	Age Groups (%)			
					<15	15-44	45-65	>65
169	13329	5.0	11500	0.0	35.21	35.62	20.34	8.82
	32008	11.4	12400	0.20	36.99	33.33	20.67	9.02
170	10872	12.8	12000	0.40	38.58	42.82	13.96	4.64
	22557	8.5	15000	0.0	40.75	41.65	13.14	4.46
171	21114	34.1	13200	0.0	16.86	26.40	36.23	20.50
	109000	54.6	17400	0.40	14.90	22.30	40.32	22.48
172	30852	17.7	11700	0.40	38.85	36.88	19.65	4.63
	58288	39.2	18400	27.50	41.39	34.51	19.62	4.49
173	30507	27.1	9800	0.0	29.56	53.16	14.40	2.88
	45500	26.1	17100	10.00	28.99	54.87	13.46	2.69
174	4410	2.7	9600	0.0	30.61	34.48	22.85	12.05
	48000	42.6	14600	14.00	31.30	32.13	23.83	12.75
175	7560	2.0	9400	0.10	34.70	38.73	16.82	9.75
	15400	9.4	12200	3.70	36.28	37.13	16.57	10.03
176	21323	6.1	11000	3.20	37.37	31.24	23.58	7.80
	23900	6.4	13000	3.70	39.66	28.03	24.46	7.86
177	20900	3.0	9100	0.10	43.57	38.27	14.49	3.66
	84305	8.3	15200	3.20	47.18	35.74	13.62	3.46
178	25847	4.1	17220	2.00	34.82	36.30	21.81	7.08
	29000	4.2	13200	0.10	37.35	34.37	21.23	7.04
179	28815	36.6	7560	31.00	40.89	42.33	12.32	4.46
	48400	66.2	21000	5.00	44.94	39.46	11.33	4.27
180	28254	33.9	8500	9.20	34.71	38.57	19.55	7.17
	38947	49.4	11000	31.00	37.71	36.11	19.00	7.19
181	16553	49.1	14280	0.10	44.43	38.99	12.70	3.87
	105763	45.8	12300	12.10	47.86	37.01	11.48	3.65
182	5077	7.5	8190	0.20	29.08	35.02	24.55	11.35
	22364	66.4	21000	5.00	29.57	33.32	25.39	11.72
183	5363	10.6	9870	0.0	38.76	38.54	16.51	6.20
	5825	12.6	11000	0.20	40.73	36.96	16.22	6.09
184	6317	22.5	7880	3.00	31.60	39.78	20.97	7.65
	8613	17.0	13000	0.0	33.81	37.31	21.11	7.77
185	4907	8.7	13650	0.10	36.58	36.95	20.90	5.57
	8538	30.4	10900	3.00	38.30	35.87	20.41	5.42
186	15009	8.3	15750	2.50	29.21	36.07	25.79	8.93
	6660	11.8	20000	0.10	31.52	33.62	25.78	9.08
187	4391	7.8	10500	0.20	39.27	41.98	13.47	5.28
	20300	11.3	22900	2.50	39.33	41.97	13.41	5.30

TABLE 44--Continued

Subarea	Population	Population Density/ Sq. Mile	Income (Dollars)	Per Cent Nonwhite	Age Groups (%) <15	15-44	45-65	>65
188	10427	9.8	10500	0.10	33.74	40.90	17.82	7.55
	6650	11.8	15000	0.20	35.24	39.99	17.31	7.45
189	14598	21.6	10290	0.20	48.94	38.95	8.92	3.19
	15500	14.5	14100	0.10	52.61	36.41	7.97	3.00
190	7730	46.0	9140	0.20	39.14	37.21	17.55	6.10
	15900	23.6	14500	0.20	40.68	35.94	17.21	6.17
191	3814	8.5	8820	0.60	35.01	36.55	19.28	9.17
	8700	51.8	12600	0.20	35.44	35.14	19.63	9.79
192	5320	8.6	9450	0.10	40.43	39.42	14.05	6.11
	4775	10.6	11200	0.60	43.05	38.28	12.87	5.79
193	6960	11.2	9660	0.20	41.38	42.50	12.30	3.83
	6800	11.0	12600	0.10	43.63	40.94	11.73	3.70
194	11260	2.2	7100	0.0	32.85	31.24	22.93	12.97
	14500	23.4	13000	0.20	35.11	26.68	24.28	13.93
195	10910	3.2	8300	0.10	42.69	32.66	16.83	7.82
	13500	2.6	9500	0.0	47.69	27.79	16.64	7.88
196	8168	3.7	7800	0.0	33.21	30.03	24.89	11.88
	13200	3.9	11100	0.10	35.47	25.27	26.65	12.61
197	6733	3.7	7900	0.0	39.10	33.69	19.56	7.66
	12000	5.5	10900	0.0	43.09	29.17	19.96	7.78
198	16980	2.4	9600	0.10	41.45	36.16	16.48	5.91
	10150	5.6	11000	0.0	46.05	31.82	16.27	5.86
199	21780	9.7	9400	0.40	42.38	38.59	14.70	4.32
	30000	4.2	13100	0.10	47.09	34.51	14.21	4.19
200	3965	1.5	7700	0.10	40.18	32.87	20.91	6.04
	27300	12.1	12900	0.40	44.38	28.13	21.48	6.01
201	12865	1.5	10500	0.10	40.76	33.91	19.08	6.24
	14850	1.9	14000	0.0	45.17	29.30	19.30	6.22
202	7281	3.2	9600	0.10	36.31	34.60	22.06	7.02
	30000	3.5	13800	0.10	39.48	30.32	23.07	7.13
203	11550	5.9	10500	0.10	40.08	36.23	18.14	5.56
	10500	4.7	14000	0.10	44.28	31.98	18.23	5.51
204	39682	10.2	9500	0.10	3.97	2.15	93.44	0.43
	40250	10.3	14000	0.10	2.02	0.72	97.01	0.25
205	44749	10.9	8800	6.50	31.69	38.46	19.63	10.21
	53500	13.8	13400	0.10	33.66	37.34	18.80	10.21
206	25445	23.8	8400	0.10	54.52	39.90	3.97	1.60
	89000	41.6	13100	11.10	59.86	35.89	2.92	1.32

TABLE 44--Continued

Subarea	Population	Population Density/ Sq. Mile	Income (Dollars)	Per Cent Nonwhite	Age Groups (%)			
					<15	15-44	45-65	>65
207	21934	20.7	8900	4.50	25.08	34.65	26.44	13.83
	30500	28.5	10800	0.10	26.50	32.97	26.36	14.17
208	9288	16.5	9660	3.00	33.39	34.82	20.51	11.28
	64000	37.9	12100	9.30	35.41	33.30	20.03	11.25
209	8425	18.7	11130	3.00	31.56	35.74	21.98	10.72
	13000	23.1	13100	23.50	34.06	33.54	21.59	10.80
210	4056	10.3	8700	1.00	36.66	40.19	17.77	5.37
	11350	25.2	17500	25.00	39.09	39.00	16.70	5.21
211	12512	17.1	9870	0.40	34.81	35.49	20.46	9.25
	14056	20.3	12000	0.00	37.49	33.34	20.02	9.15
212	2826	10.1	9800	0.10	30.83	36.57	20.44	12.16
	16900	23.1	13900	25.00	32.25	35.80	19.80	12.14
213	6670	0.5	6100	0.0	36.51	35.86	18.96	8.67
	8600	12.8	13500	0.10	38.32	34.04	18.83	8.81
214	11404	0.5	7100	0.0	36.43	35.72	18.75	9.09
	13000	0.9	8000	0.0	38.24	33.88	18.59	9.29
215	7823	2.5	8100	1.40	35.86	36.56	19.17	8.41
	20800	0.9	9500	0.0	37.48	34.91	19.07	8.54
216	12425	4.7	9000	1.40	33.40	36.89	22.60	7.11
	15500	4.9	10000	1.40	34.35	35.35	23.15	7.15
217	6948	2.0	9500	3.00	37.83	40.99	16.76	4.42
	22500	8.5	11600	1.40	39.61	40.03	16.11	4.26
218	6041	1.6	9300	0.80	37.24	35.82	18.98	7.95
	8750	2.5	12200	3.00	39.22	33.94	18.82	8.02
219	19369	9.3	8600	0.10	38.35	40.77	15.68	5.20
	9675	2.6	12400	0.80	40.29	39.73	14.92	5.05
220	14219	10.5	10290	0.20	37.74	35.11	18.82	8.33
	28000	13.4	11600	0.10	40.86	33.33	17.73	8.08
221	4816	43.0	8190	0.0	28.62	34.49	22.63	14.26
	17000	12.6	14000	0.20	29.48	33.71	22.49	14.32
222	6416	11.4	9140	0.10	36.31	35.46	18.20	10.03
	5525	49.3	10500	0.0	38.97	33.74	17.32	9.97
223	3938	6.4	8820	0.30	34.10	37.78	17.40	10.72
	7350	13.1	12200	0.10	36.17	37.13	16.38	10.33
224	12056	21.4	9240	0.20	32.31	34.46	21.12	12.10
	15250	28.5	10500	0.30	34.22	32.71	20.94	12.13
225	4824	0.3	7300	0.0	35.36	36.46	19.33	8.85
	17100	30.4	12000	0.20	37.01	35.21	18.87	8.91

TABLE 44--Continued

Subarea	Population	Population Density/ Sq. Mile	Income (Dollars)	Per Cent Nonwhite	Age Groups (%)			
					<15	15-44	45-65	>65
226	3982	0.3	7500	0.0	32.94	35.58	21.85	9.63
	7450	0.5	10000	0.0	34.02	34.27	21.90	9.81
227	14496	2.6	8000	0.0	37.20	36.05	17.23	9.52
	15950	4.4	9500	0.0	39.31	34.61	16.47	9.61
228	40161	1.3	8000	0.0	36.98	36.82	18.29	7.90
	17900	3.2	11000	0.0	38.98	35.54	17.63	7.85
229	24049	23.7	11100	0.10	35.90	37.26	20.48	6.35
	66200	2.2	10200	0.0	38.11	35.74	19.86	6.29
230	31230	31.0	12280	0.20	34.97	35.66	22.52	6.86
	35300	34.8	15200	25.00	37.39	33.63	22.11	6.86
231	20913	31.0	12180	0.30	36.93	35.64	20.98	6.44
	85000	151.0	16000	26.00	39.23	34.41	20.08	6.28
232	13909	49.5	14180	0.70	33.36	33.64	24.89	8.11
	31500	46.7	14100	25.00	35.39	32.04	24.54	8.03
233	27687	44.7	10600	0.10	40.92	37.86	16.05	5.17
	36150	57.5	19500	26.00	44.00	35.94	15.00	5.06
234	18309	14.8	11760	0.20	36.47	40.02	16.81	6.69
	34000	54.9	14500	25.00	39.64	37.59	16.27	6.50
235	28240	33.4	10710	0.10	39.64	39.83	15.53	4.99
	28500	23.0	16200	25.00	42.54	38.37	14.22	4.86
236	31834	35.4	11500	1.50	37.71	40.80	15.86	5.63
	46700	55.3	14600	25.00	41.17	38.30	15.06	5.46
237	9336	23.7	9450	0.10	45.68	45.22	7.04	2.06
	47700	53.0	15600	25.00	45.59	45.30	7.04	2.07
238	12660	32.1	9350	0.20	37.57	40.90	15.85	5.68
	15400	39.1	11800	25.00	39.79	39.78	14.95	5.48
239	7198	32.0	12600	0.20	36.71	36.63	21.46	5.19
	21000	53.3	11200	15.50	38.35	34.59	21.81	5.26
240	4935	12.5	10080	0.0	39.53	37.85	17.08	5.54
	8850	39.3	16400	25.00	42.48	36.42	15.83	5.27
241	5245	13.3	10600	0.0	36.47	40.02	16.81	6.69
	8100	20.6	13300	0.0	39.64	37.59	16.27	6.50
242	7800	19.8	10500	0.0	43.39	40.47	12.13	4.00
	10000	25.4	14900	25.00	46.89	38.61	10.77	3.72
243	7770	13.8	8610	0.30	38.69	38.05	16.22	7.04
	8800	22.3	14200	0.0	41.36	36.84	14.99	6.81
244	7155	25.5	9240	0.40	33.59	38.29	19.81	8.31
	8440	15.0	11500	25.00	35.13	36.65	19.60	8.62

TABLE 44--Continued

Subarea	Population	Population Density/ Sq. Mile	Income (Dollars)	Per Cent Nonwhite	Age Groups (%)			
					<15	15-44	45-65	>65
245	4252	15.1	9980	0.20	34.90	37.22	21.14	6.74
	13655	48.6	12100	25.00	36.06	35.83	21.17	6.94
246	4540	1.4	9100	0.10	33.79	40.51	19.29	6.41
	7000	24.9	13100	10.00	34.81	39.54	19.21	6.44
247	11910	3.4	9000	0.10	38.05	36.24	18.59	7.13
	13750	4.2	12000	25.00	40.27	34.17	18.35	7.20
248	20523	5.8	10400	0.0	44.03	39.63	12.83	3.50
	25500	7.3	12000	0.10	47.38	37.58	11.72	3.32
249	14503	5.5	10000	0.0	36.08	39.61	18.15	6.15
	40600	11.4	14100	0.0	37.66	38.33	17.85	6.15
250	16010	2.5	10500	0.0	37.11	41.87	17.06	3.96
	21750	8.2	14000	0.0	38.74	40.87	16.53	3.86
251	34754	13.7	10100	0.0	35.34	38.23	20.22	6.20
	39800	6.2	12600	0.0	36.71	37.26	20.02	6.01
252	40630	10.0	10500	0.40	38.25	38.35	18.01	5.38
	52500	20.7	14400	0.0	40.40	36.65	17.63	5.32
253	63752	13.6	8610	9.20	30.67	37.89	21.20	10.24
	67150	16.6	14800	9.00	32.73	36.30	20.64	10.34
254	6672	10.8	8400	0.20	41.11	41.37	13.27	4.25
	84533	38.5	11400	14.10	43.61	38.59	13.47	4.32
255	4276	9.5	10400	0.0	32.47	37.68	21.75	8.10
	9100	14.7	11400	10.00	34.14	36.27	21.50	8.10
256	8568	21.7	9140	2.30	32.61	38.65	20.37	8.37
	5600	12.4	16500	0.0	34.73	36.92	19.91	8.44
257	8935	19.9	8920	1.00	52.44	44.95	2.11	0.49
	11800	29.9	12000	5.50	55.75	42.26	1.57	0.41
258	8042	23.9	8400	0.50	37.40	42.43	14.35	5.82
	10500	23.3	12500	3.00	39.33	40.80	14.00	5.87
259	4404	8.7	7770	0.10	33.97	39.93	23.13	2.98
	10500	31.2	11000	0.50	34.56	38.49	24.09	2.87
260	7633	1.0	9000	0.0	36.79	37.57	18.61	7.04
	5200	10.3	9800	0.10	39.58	35.16	18.31	6.95
261	13531	1.9	9000	0.0	40.71	38.53	14.78	5.98
	13900	1.8	11800	5.50	44.40	35.96	13.88	5.77
262	15256	6.2	9000	0.0	27.07	56.48	13.59	2.86
	25700	3.6	12500	0.0	26.40	58.63	12.36	2.61
263	33255	19.1	9200	0.0	35.34	37.76	19.54	7.36
	21200	8.6	12000	6.00	37.77	35.48	19.44	7.31

TABLE 44--Continued

Subarea	Population	Population Density/ Sq. Mile	Income (Dollars)	Per Cent Nonwhite	Age Groups (%)			
					<15	15-44	45-65	>65
264	13520	1.9	9500	0.20	39.88	37.91	16.67	5.54
	42100	24.1	12600	11.00	43.39	35.30	15.98	5.33
265	9960	1.2	8400	0.10	37.21	36.36	18.20	8.23
	28900	4.0	13000	0.20	40.18	33.73	17.87	8.22
266	20000	1.1	7300	0.0	38.04	37.03	17.24	7.69
	21100	2.6	11400	0.10	41.19	34.45	16.74	7.62
267	1275	0.3	7300	0.0	27.89	22.84	12.21	37.06
	14000	0.7	9400	0.0	27.30	18.05	10.95	43.70
268	5260	1.0	6800	1.00	38.45	34.59	17.92	9.04
	6525	2.4	9400	0.0	41.62	31.45	17.44	9.49
269	6180	0.5	7000	0.20	30.55	33.96	21.88	13.61
	6600	1.2	8900	1.00	31.67	31.00	22.26	15.08
270	4973	1.3	8900	0.0	40.26	32.65	18.02	9.08
	9300	0.7	9800	0.20	43.82	29.04	17.45	9.68
271	4786	1.0	8900	0.0	46.04	39.06	11.52	3.38
	10400	2.8	12000	0.0	50.66	35.81	10.20	3.33

APPENDIX E

DISEASE FORECASTS FOR 1980

TABLE 45

DISEASE FORECASTS FOR 1980

Community	Heart Disease		Stroke		Cancer	
	Rate[a]	Deaths	Rate[a]	Deaths	Cases	Rate[b]
1	6.02	319.30	1.23	65.10	191.57	1.54
2	5.99	449.01	1.12	83.71	229.65	1.31
3	10.69	1357.06	6.69	849.81	939.16	3.16
4	6.87	254.11	1.46	53.99	162.42	1.87
5	7.37	250.57	1.56	52.92	129.26	1.62
6	7.06	797.93	1.42	160.14	371.79	1.40
7	6.51	494.77	1.39	105.64	251.54	1.41
8	5.68	397.41	1.28	89.95	145.27	0.89
9	4.16	49.87	0.93	11.13	27.30	0.97
10	5.17	242.78	0.87	41.07	146.83	1.33
11	5.92	161.51	1.05	28.77	82.68	1.29
12	5.81	95.84	1.00	16.57	41.43	1.07
13	5.63	84.39	1.05	15.73	46.68	1.33
14	7.38	339.51	1.58	72.75	172.80	1.60
15	6.16	375.95	1.24	75.70	210.31	1.47
16	6.30	352.99	1.17	65.34	189.40	1.44
17	5.41	227.35	0.88	36.86	125.47	1.28
18	6.37	159.34	1.22	30.58	94.40	1.61
19	6.58	348.89	1.12	59.46	188.37	1.52
20	5.37	143.55	0.94	25.05	71.56	1.14
21	6.37	217.32	1.09	37.22	108.43	1.36
22	6.40	627.26	1.25	122.46	302.80	1.32
23	5.67	370.28	1.00	65.64	225.29	1.47
24	5.68	726.97	1.05	134.69	420.28	1.40
25	6.90	849.05	1.27	156.03	444.33	1.54
26	5.25	299.38	1.13	64.15	182.45	1.37
27	4.18	255.18	0.86	52.78	158.21	1.11
28	5.87	651.76	1.40	155.87	288.48	1.11
29	3.31	402.69	0.61	74.28	259.35	0.91
30	6.46	348.69	1.33	71.91	193.75	1.53
31	6.40	256.19	1.15	45.98	150.99	1.61
32	5.10	60.42	8.20	32.79	27.49	2.93
33	7.00	42.01	2.37	14.22	21.73	1.55
34	5.62	67.42	1.30	15.61	40.96	1.46
35	5.11	281.03	1.27	69.63	131.69	1.02
36	4.51	110.86	1.04	25.55	68.74	1.19
37	4.67	46.74	0.96	9.59	27.26	1.16
38	7.56	81.69	2.41	26.04	46.11	1.82
39	3.99	163.43	0.83	34.15	96.26	1.00
40	6.08	273.57	1.62	72.80	178.18	1.69
41	5.41	238.04	1.22	53.87	137.72	1.34

TABLE 45--Continued

Community	Heart Disease		Stroke		Cancer	
	Rate[a]	Deaths	Rate[a]	Deaths	Cases	Rate[b]
42	4.38	358.90	0.97	79.30	225.93	1.18
43	6.85	534.44	1.52	118.80	320.33	1.75
44	4.25	216.58	0.83	42.39	155.34	1.30
45	5.95	65.47	1.10	12.05	41.89	1.63
46	6.22	279.83	1.31	59.02	150.19	1.43
47	4.96	9.91	0.85	1.70	4.49	0.96
48	5.16	92.89	0.88	15.83	61.89	1.47
49	4.77	300.62	0.97	61.03	198.90	1.35
50	5.85	87.69	0.89	13.30	50.01	1.42
51	4.57	85.62	0.72	13.45	58.68	1.34
52	5.69	130.83	0.91	20.90	64.32	1.19
53	4.97	203.26	0.82	33.59	116.54	1.22
54	2.76	37.29	0.39	5.29	21.85	0.69
55	3.74	70.14	0.56	10.56	41.64	0.95
56	5.69	250.54	3.73	164.18	265.62	2.58
57	4.14	48.88	0.60	7.10	42.16	1.53
58	6.76	229.88	1.45	49.38	118.00	1.48
59	6.69	100.39	1.10	16.51	43.95	1.25
60	6.74	242.59	1.30	46.78	118.88	1.41
61	6.22	65.33	1.34	14.12	33.14	1.35
62	6.33	167.84	0.72	19.09	93.22	1.50
63	5.57	144.95	1.12	29.11	77.46	1.27
64	4.20	96.53	0.66	15.31	58.17	1.08
65	4.99	124.70	0.86	21.50	89.93	1.54
66	6.97	348.52	1.40	69.93	188.78	1.61
67	6.14	319.11	1.39	72.49	167.41	1.37
68	3.94	373.98	0.81	77.07	237.33	1.07
69	4.31	280.04	0.90	58.39	172.51	1.13
70	3.17	153.86	0.35	17.22	113.21	1.00
71	6.91	424.74	1.31	80.89	202.02	1.40
72	5.07	114.03	0.86	19.43	68.51	1.30
73	5.32	180.88	1.10	37.46	99.91	1.25
74	4.53	99.56	0.59	12.92	57.30	1.11
75	4.30	116.23	0.98	26.46	76.09	1.20
76	3.68	21.69	0.80	4.72	8.86	0.64
77	5.05	134.11	0.81	21.44	71.58	1.15
78	7.88	444.61	1.73	97.48	188.87	1.43
79	6.30	208.01	1.15	37.97	83.73	1.08
80	5.71	137.15	0.89	21.43	80.25	1.43
81	3.55	137.73	0.72	27.84	66.58	0.73
82	4.46	256.62	0.97	55.72	159.02	1.18
83	6.92	497.39	1.38	99.20	255.17	1.52
84	4.28	334.68	0.78	60.67	130.38	0.71
85	2.68	78.16	0.41	11.85	34.86	0.51
86	6.71	268.24	1.03	41.04	146.46	1.56
87	5.78	481.06	1.56	130.08	227.99	1.17
88	4.44	179.85	0.66	26.83	64.26	0.68
89	6.13	104.17	1.51	25.69	47.32	1.19

TABLE 45--Continued

Community	Heart Disease		Stroke		Cancer	
	Rate[a]	Deaths	Rate[a]	Deaths	Cases	Rate[b]
90	4.19	129.76	0.57	17.81	74.49	1.03
91	3.02	120.89	0.58	23.29	104.43	1.11
92	4.95	223.56	0.90	40.92	89.35	0.84
93	3.48	84.65	0.55	13.31	56.30	0.99
94	5.61	150.40	1.14	30.45	84.35	1.34
95	4.68	75.89	0.76	12.31	23.96	0.63
96	3.23	90.89	0.54	15.29	37.87	0.58
97	3.63	58.14	0.52	8.25	36.37	0.97
98	6.53	209.81	1.41	45.19	89.19	1.18
99	4.44	141.11	1.04	33.09	65.61	0.88
100	4.04	113.04	0.51	14.30	80.25	1.22
101	2.57	124.89	0.47	22.98	77.21	0.68
102	3.68	120.47	0.63	20.45	68.68	0.90
103	3.69	88.24	0.50	11.91	52.99	0.95
104	1.59	40.02	0.46	11.61	10.03	0.17
105	5.07	84.52	0.56	9.32	23.29	0.60
106	4.89	227.30	1.11	51.49	127.50	1.17
107	6.65	422.53	1.76	112.07	241.06	1.62
108	3.19	88.22	0.65	17.91	45.88	0.71
109	2.70	157.21	0.34	19.80	103.13	0.76
110	3.89	236.99	0.73	44.66	149.72	1.05
111	3.50	67.22	0.78	14.95	31.14	0.69
112	5.18	77.33	0.92	13.68	64.28	1.84
113	4.05	105.72	0.29	7.64	22.83	0.37
114	3.28	259.23	0.69	54.85	210.24	1.13
115	3.50	74.48	0.43	9.16	47.35	0.95
116	4.41	136.94	1.12	34.77	80.30	1.10
117	4.09	60.13	0.73	10.79	65.33	1.90
118	1.98	12.54	0.36	2.28	2.92	0.20
119	6.96	88.63	1.17	14.94	27.35	0.92
120	3.71	25.29	0.63	4.27	13.94	0.87
121	2.88	37.11	0.35	4.55	12.86	0.43
122	3.93	39.64	0.56	5.71	17.34	0.73
123	3.39	46.80	0.47	6.47	13.06	0.40
124	3.85	37.33	0.47	4.61	13.00	0.57
125	3.49	16.56	0.87	4.13	5.29	0.48
126	3.81	78.89	0.40	8.23	27.89	0.58
127	1.67	14.11	0.37	3.13	20.68	1.05
128	4.40	72.66	0.72	11.84	48.43	1.25
129	3.96	38.24	0.60	5.79	1.24	0.05
130	3.92	47.03	0.54	6.46	26.34	0.94
131	4.69	34.23	0.76	5.58	15.80	0.92
132	3.86	35.37	0.57	5.24	22.86	1.07
133	3.52	43.72	0.24	3.03	3.77	0.13
134	3.42	43.81	0.32	4.11	15.88	0.53
135	3.06	14.99	0.52	2.53	15.38	1.34
136	4.47	14.52	1.05	3.42	10.47	1.38
137	6.86	47.20	1.86	12.81	3.53	0.22

TABLE 45--Continued

Community	Heart Disease		Stroke		Cancer	
	Rate[a]	Deaths	Rate[a]	Deaths	Cases	Rate[b]
138	5.22	90.79	0.93	16.22	61.91	1.52
139	1.93	50.84	0.42	11.05	30.89	0.50
140	2.53	15.66	0.52	3.20	5.93	0.41
141	7.46	117.80	1.88	29.70	48.81	1.32
142	1.72	14.90	0.32	2.75	11.45	0.57
143	5.28	65.93	0.70	8.80	23.24	0.79
144	5.37	47.82	0.74	6.55	18.36	0.88
145	0.86	11.73	0.28	3.87	25.79	0.81
146	3.14	25.91	0.40	3.30	26.52	1.37
147	1.88	19.09	0.32	3.22	12.13	0.51
148	4.66	30.28	0.78	5.09	12.67	0.83
149	3.74	40.75	0.54	5.94	31.64	1.24
150	3.76	54.02	0.82	11.77	40.35	1.20
151	7.54	86.51	1.33	15.27	49.66	1.85
152	5.68	89.11	1.04	16.38	27.09	0.74
153	2.48	19.44	0.14	1.11	1.49	0.08
154	3.53	33.90	0.73	6.98	14.37	0.64
155	3.48	23.30	0.86	5.79	5.47	0.35
156	4.72	75.94	0.84	13.55	45.92	1.22
157	5.86	94.99	1.05	17.01	31.80	0.84
158	3.25	11.60	0.51	1.84	5.71	1.68
159	3.89	54.02	0.38	5.21	2.11	0.06
160	4.54	81.79	0.80	14.38	60.58	1.44
161	1.72	79.21	0.38	17.60	24.44	0.23
162	2.67	58.71	0.44	9.71	37.46	0.73
163	4.02	76.05	0.75	14.19	39.72	0.90
164	1.92	28.77	0.28	4.26	9.54	0.27
165	4.71	79.99	0.65	11.01	46.65	1.17
166	0.23	3.06	0.52	6.99	24.44	0.23
167	2.76	29.17	0.61	6.50	3.26	0.13
168	1.51	48.18	0.64	20.37	24.44	0.23
169	2.29	51.58	0.40	9.02	24.08	0.46
170	2.88	313.75	0.60	64.96	160.13	0.63
171	2.97	72.24	0.28	6.70	52.88	0.93
172	2.73	124.26	0.44	20.11	35.47	0.33
173	3.10	148.76	0.36	17.07	44.49	0.40
174	1.51	23.27	0.65	10.05	35.47	0.33
175	1.09	25.95	0.49	11.67	116.37	0.59
176	2.63	221.65	0.45	37.72	116.37	0.59
177	2.12	61.43	0.30	8.64	18.22	0.27
178	5.83	282.01	0.90	43.35	198.33	1.75
179	2.67	104.01	0.51	19.98	3.68	0.04
180	4.08	431.49	0.94	99.38	221.53	0.89
181	3.27	73.18	0.38	8.52	53.85	1.03
182	3.05	17.79	1.32	7.68	8.47	0.62
183	3.52	30.33	0.66	5.66	19.81	0.98
184	3.40	29.03	0.58	4.92	20.64	1.03
185	2.98	19.85	0.78	5.17	8.37	0.54

TABLE 45--Continued

Community	Heart Disease		Stroke		Cancer	
	Rate[a]	Deaths	Rate[a]	Deaths	Cases	Rate[b]
186	3.58	72.66	1.02	20.70	49.54	1.04
187	3.66	24.36	0.49	3.25	6.59	0.42
188	4.66	72.25	1.20	18.55	32.43	0.89
189	3.00	47.76	0.38	6.00	35.96	0.97
190	3.40	29.61	0.36	3.16	14.42	0.71
191	1.86	8.90	0.38	1.81	2.52	0.23
192	3.70	25.14	0.89	6.08	10.72	0.67
193	3.01	43.71	0.54	7.83	34.53	1.02
194	1.35	18.22	1.16	15.72	2.28	0.07
195	4.87	64.34	0.89	11.73	55.58	1.80
196	3.83	45.95	0.81	9.68	23.31	0.83
197	4.49	45.61	1.03	10.43	30.56	1.29
198	2.32	69.71	0.92	27.71	32.11	0.46
199	3.06	83.44	0.42	11.49	26.99	0.42
200	0.97	4.73	0.30	1.47	4.23	0.37
201	2.56	76.86	0.76	22.67	28.13	0.40
202	4.42	46.43	0.83	8.72	18.30	0.74
203	3.49	70.61	0.64	12.91	27.42	0.58
204	2.24	119.91	0.23	12.50	62.94	0.50
205	5.68	505.81	1.34	119.09	300.94	1.44
206	2.28	69.40	0.28	8.64	38.46	0.54
207	5.14	329.12	1.46	93.71	196.04	1.31
208	5.28	68.64	0.82	10.69	27.94	0.92
209	5.13	58.19	1.05	11.97	23.47	0.88
210	3.12	12.67	0.57	2.32	1.58	0.17
211	4.75	80.24	1.05	17.78	43.33	1.09
212	8.66	31.19	2.61	9.39	22.80	2.70
213	0.05	0.65	0.92	11.99	17.42	0.36
214	1.97	41.05	0.62	12.83	17.42	0.36
215	3.45	53.43	0.30	4.64	41.98	1.16
216	1.97	44.43	0.55	12.43	9.23	0.25
217	1.54	13.48	0.38	3.35	4.50	0.22
218	3.19	30.88	0.69	6.71	18.43	0.81
219	4.61	129.00	0.68	18.93	63.90	0.97
220	3.53	60.05	0.75	12.69	59.28	1.49
221	5.57	30.75	0.89	4.93	14.92	1.15
222	3.48	25.56	1.88	13.80	20.45	1.19
223	4.28	22.45	1.23	6.47	10.17	0.83
224	6.29	107.51	1.69	28.89	63.07	1.57
225	0.01	0.05	0.81	6.06	4.58	0.33
226	1.53	9.10	0.50	3.00	4.58	0.33
227	6.53	116.94	1.04	18.60	80.52	1.92
228	2.40	159.01	0.96	63.87	59.15	0.38
229	5.92	208.89	0.64	22.59	153.77	1.86
230	5.19	441.26	0.80	67.81	252.01	1.27
231	3.29	103.49	0.62	19.42	58.21	0.79
232	6.80	109.80	1.20	19.36	43.24	1.14
233	4.12	140.13	0.83	28.07	55.55	0.70

TABLE 45--Continued

Community	Heart Disease		Stroke		Cancer	
	Rate[a]	Deaths	Rate[a]	Deaths	Cases	Rate[b]
234	3.24	92.42	0.65	18.66	39.69	0.59
235	4.05	189.03	0.54	25.40	98.52	0.90
236	3.39	161.74	0.55	26.17	92.13	0.82
237	3.19	49.17	0.33	5.14	17.98	0.50
238	5.10	107.00	0.99	20.80	79.97	1.63
239	3.26	28.84	0.42	3.76	36.43	1.76
240	3.83	31.03	0.86	7.00	8.72	0.46
241	3.19	31.93	0.52	5.16	13.85	0.59
242	3.75	33.03	0.53	4.64	27.85	1.35
243	3.54	29.90	0.63	5.35	18.71	0.95
244	5.63	76.88	0.78	10.59	49.35	1.54
245	2.93	20.48	0.49	3.43	22.75	1.39
246	0.36	4.89	0.74	10.16	22.75	1.39
247	3.29	83.77	0.51	13.10	49.30	0.83
248	1.82	73.78	0.27	10.94	26.10	0.27
249	3.49	75.91	0.28	6.18	8.90	0.17
250	0.98	39.19	0.25	9.85	25.91	0.28
251	2.62	137.76	0.27	14.23	73.18	0.60
252	1.37	91.73	0.19	12.53	21.30	0.14
253	6.39	539.89	1.38	116.65	239.88	1.21
254	1.87	17.01	0.18	1.65	3.82	0.18
255	11.67	65.33	5.78	32.36	35.89	2.74
256	5.93	69.98	1.25	14.71	31.23	1.13
257	1.31	13.73	0.17	1.79	6.11	0.25
258	2.58	27.07	0.33	3.43	12.67	0.52
259	4.62	24.03	1.33	6.91	8.80	0.72
260	0.02	0.24	0.48	6.63	129.30	3.97
261	4.02	103.42	0.84	21.57	30.58	0.51
262	4.69	99.49	0.66	13.91	47.45	0.96
263	5.39	227.11	0.84	35.44	107.27	1.09
264	0.76	21.88	0.50	14.36	63.86	0.94
265	1.64	34.62	0.74	15.71	6.92	0.14
266	0.59	8.27	0.48	6.74	37.88	1.16
267	2.77	4.23	0.57	0.87	0.61	0.17
268	0.46	3.01	0.86	5.70	20.99	1.36
269	0,12	1.13	0.37	3.41	1.67	0.08
270	0.43	4.42	0.75	7.77	33.21	1.36
271	0.13	0.84	0.35	2.21	1.67	0.11

[a]Mortality per 1,000 persons.

[b]Morbidity per 1,000 persons.

SELECTED BIBLIOGRAPHY

SELECTED BIBLIOGRAPHY

Health Care Facilities Planning

Abbe, Leslie Morgan, and Anna Mae Baney. The Nation's Health Facilities: Ten Years of the Hill-Burton Hospital and Medical Facilities Program, 1946-1956. Washingington, D.C.: U.S. Department of Health, Education, and Welfare, Public Health Service, 1958.

Ament, Richard P. "Medicare Boosts Bed Usage by Elderly." The Modern Hospital, Vol. CVIII (1967).

Beal, Frank. The Urban Planner in Health Planning. Washington, D.C.: U.S. Department of Health, Education, and Welfare and the American Society of Planning Officials, 1968.

Bloom, Lawrence S., Peter Bonavich, and Daniel Sudran. "Medicaid in Cook County." Inquiry, V (1968), 1-12.

Borhani, Nemat, and John S. Meyer. Medical Basis for Comprehensive Community Stroke Programs. Washington, D.C.: National Heart Institute and National Institute of Neurological Diseases and Blindness, 1968.

Cavanaugh, James H. "Areawide Planning for Hospitals and Related Health Facilities: A National Survey." Ann Arbor: University Microfilms, Inc., 1964.

________. "Past, Present, and Future Goals and Philosophy in Comprehensive Health Planning." Paper presented at the American Hospital Association Invitational Conference on Comprehensive Health Planning, 1968.

Commission on Hospital Care. Hospital Care in the United States. New York: The Commonwealth Fund, 1947.

Letourneau, Charles U. "Medicare, Its Effect upon Hospitals and Health Facilities." Hospital Management (August 1966), pp. 31-33.

Lerner, Monroe, and Odin W. Anderson. Health Progress in the United States, 1900-1960. Chicago: University of Chicago Press, 1963.

May, J. Joel. Health Planning: Its Past and Potential. Health Administration Perspectives No. A5. Chicago: Center for Health Administration, 1967.

Rorem, Rufus. "Areawide Planning Is Here to Stay, Auspices and Areas." The Modern Hospital (August, 1964).

Sox, Ellis D. "New Resources for Urban Health Programs." American Journal of Public Health, LVIII (1968), 1030-35.

Stone, Charles I. "Areawide Planning for Health Facilities." Hospitals, XLI (1967), 51-53.

Stump, Dennis E., Jr. "The Major Aspects of Medical Assistance under Title XIX." Public Health Reports, LXXXI (1966), 867-69.

Treloar, Alan E., and Don Chill. Patient Care Facilities: Construction Needs and Hill-Burton Accomplishments. Hospital Monograph Series No. 10. Chicago: American Hospital Association, 1961.

U.S. Department of Health, Education, and Welfare. "A Brief Explanation of 'Medicare' Health Insurance for the Aged." OASI-1965-2. Washington, D.C., 1965.

________. "Areawide Planning for Hospitals and Related Health Facilities." Public Health Service Publication No. 885. Washington, D.C.: U.S. Government Printing Office, 1961.

________. "Procedures for Areawide Health Facility Planning." Washington, D.C.: Public Health Service Division of Hospital and Medical Facilities, 1963.

Wilbur, Dwight L. "Quality and Availability of Care under Regional Medical Programs." The Journal of the American Medical Association, CCIII (1968), 143-47.

Winston, Ellen. "The New Medical Assistance Program." Public Health Reports, LXXXI (1966), 863-66.

Heart Disease and Stroke

Berkson, D. M., and J. Stamler. "Epidemiological Findings on Cerebrovascular Disease and Their Implications." Journal of Arteriosclerosis Research, V (1965), 189-202.

________. "Bethesda Conference Report." The American Journal of Cardiology, XXIII (1969), 603-18.

Cooper, James K., Knight Steel, and James P. Christodoulou. "Mobile Coronary Care - A Controversial Innovation." New England Journal of Medicine, CCLXXXI (1969), 906-7.

Enterline, P. E. "Death Rates for Coronary Heart Disease in Metropolitan and Other Areas." Public Health Reports, LXXV (1960), 525-34.

Epstein, Frederick H. "The Epidemiology of Coronary Heart Disease." Journal of Chronic Diseases, XVIII (1965), 735-74.

Gelperin, Abraham. "Rehabilitation." Chicago Medicine, LXXII (1969), 859-62.

Hechter, H. H., and N. O. Borhani. "Mortality and Geographic Distribution of Arteriosclerotic Heart Disease." Public Health Reports, LXXX (1965), 11-24.

Kuller, Lewis. "Nationwide Cerebrovascular Disease Morbidity Study." Stroke, I (1970), 86-99.

Kowal, John S., Lawrence M. White, and Stanley A. Forward. "Cardiac Resuscitation Program." Hospitals, XLIV (1970), 77-80.

Moriyama, Iwao. "Factors in Diagnosis and Classification of Deaths from CVR Diseases." Public Health Reports, LXXV (1960), 189-95.

Most, Albert S., and Donald R. Peterson. "Myocardial Infarction Surveillance in a Metropolitan Community." The Journal of the American Medical Association, CCVIII (1969), 2433-38.

Phibbs, Brendan. The Human Heart. St. Louis: C. U. Mosby Company, 1967.

Rose, Geoffrey. "The Distribution of Mortality from Hypertension Within the United States." Journal of Chronic Diseases, XV (1962), 1017-24.

Shapiro, Sam, Eve Weinblatt, Charles W. Frank, and Robert V. Sager. "Incidence of Coronary Heart Disease in a Population Insured for Medical Care." American Journal of Public Health, LIX (1969), 1-101.

Stallones, Reuel A. 'Epidemiology of Cerebrovascular Disease: A Review." Journal of Chronic Diseases, XVIII (1965), 859-72.

U.S. Department of Health, Education, and Welfare. "Guidelines for Coronary Care Units." Public Health Service Publication No. 1824. Washington, D.C., 1968.

Wylie, Charles M. "Death Statistics for Cerebrovascular Disease: A Review of Recent Findings." Stroke, I (1970), 184-93.

Cancer

Bailer, John C., Haitung King, and Marie Joy Mason. Cancer Rates and Risks. Public Health Service Publication No. 547. Washington, D.C.: U.S. Department of Health, Education, and Welfare, 1964.

Chiazze, Leonard, and Antonio Ciacco. "Intracommunity Variation in Cancer Incidence for Pittsburgh." Public Health Reports, LXXXII (1957), 759-70.

Cowdry, E. V. Etiology and Prevention of Cancer in Man. New York: Appleton-Century-Crofts, 1968.

Cutler, Sidney J. "Trends in the Management of Cancer." Cancer Journal for Clinicians, XVIII (1968), 189-204.

Enviro-Med, Inc. "A Study of the Feasibility of the Establishment of a Therapeutic Radiology Center in Peoria, Illinois." La Jolla, Calif., 1969.

Graham, S., H. Levin, and A. H. Lilienfield. "The Socio-Economic Distribution of Cancer of Various Sites in Buffalo, 1948-1952." Cancer, XIII (1960), 80.

Greenburg, Leonard, Franklyn Field, Joseph I. Reed, and Marvin Glasser. "Air Pollution and Cancer Mortality." Archives of Environmental Health, XV (1967), 356-61.

Harris, R. J. C. Cancer. Baltimore: Pelican Books, 1962.

MacDonald, Eleanor J., Dorothy Gaites Wellington, and Patricia F. Wolf. "Regional Patterns in Mortality from Cancer in the United States." Cancer, XX (1967), 617-22.

Mannilla, L., S. Moles, and P. Rentchnick. New Trends in the Treatment of Cancer. New York, 1967.

Miller, R. W. "Environmental Agents in Cancer." Yale Journal of Biology and Medicine, XXXVII (1965), 487-500.

National Cancer Institute. Cancer Mortality Trends in the United States, 1930 to 1955. Public Health Service Monograph No. 6. Washington, D. C.: U. S. Department of Health, Education, and Welfare, 1961.

Patno, Mary Ellen. "Geographic Study of Cancer Prevalence Within an Urban Population." Public Health Reports, LXIX (1954), 705-15.

Regional Medical Programs. "A Prospect for Radiation Therapy in the United States." Final Subcommittee Report, October 24, 1968, 32 pp.

Schultz, Milford D. "Radiation Therapy in the Clinical Management of Cancer." Cancer, XIX (1969), 18-26.

Shimkin, Michael B. "Distribution of Cancer in the United States." Archives of Environmental Health, XVI (1968), 503-12.

________. Science and Cancer. Public Health Service Publication No. 1162. Washington, D. C.: U. S. Department of Health, Education, and Welfare, 1964.

Stein, J. J. "Some Observations on the Logistics of Radiation Therapy for Cancer in the U. S." Cancer, XIX (1969), 96-97.

Characteristics of the Hospital Supply

Berry, Ralph E. "Returns to Scale in the Production of Hospital Services." Health Services Research (Summer, 1967), pp. 123-39.

Carr, W. John, and Paul J. Feldstein. "The Relationship of Cost to Hospital Size." Inquiry, IV (1967), 45-65.

Hefty, Thomas R. "Returns to Scale in Hospitals: A Critical Review of Recent Research." Health Services Research (Winter, 1969), pp. 123-39.

Hospital Planning Council for Metropolitan Chicago. "Utilization of Short-Term General and Special Hospitals in the Chicago Metropolitan Area: Calendar Year 1968." Report No. 9. Chicago, 1969.

________. "Survey of Unusual and Highly Specialized Services in Hospitals." Research Report No. 10. Chicago, 1969.

Long, Millard F., and Paul J. Feldstein. "The Economics of Hospital Systems: Peak Loads and Regional Management." American Economic Review, LVII (1968), 119-29.

Morrill, Richard L. "Hierarchy of Hospital Services: Classification of Hospitals." Chicago Regional Hospital Study, Working Paper No. I. 8, 1966.

________. "Historical Development of the Chicago Hospital System." Chicago Regional Hospital Study, Working Paper No. I. 2, 1966.

________. "Relationship Between Transportation and Hospital Location and Utilization." Chicago Regional Hospital Study, Working Paper No. I. 14, 1967.

Morrill, Richard L., and Robert Earickson. "Hospital Service Areas: Changes in Service Patterns Between 1961 and 1965." Chicago Regional Hospital Study, 1966.

________. "Hospital Service Areas: Distance of Hospital from Patient Home." Chicago Regional Hospital Study, Working Paper No. I.5, 1966.

________. "Hospital Service Areas: General Patterns of Hospital Use." Chicago Regional Hospital Study, Working Paper No. I.3, 1966.

State of Illinois. "The Illinois Hospital Survey and Plan." Illinois Department of Public Health, 1947.

Vise, Pierre de. "Hospital Study Districts for Metropolitan Chicago." Technical Report No. 2. Chicago: Hospital Planning Council for Metropolitan Chicago, 1966.

Methodology

Anderson, Odin W., and Joanna Kravits. Health Services in the Chicago Area: A Framework for Use of Data. Research Monograph No. 26. Chicago: Center for Health Administration Studies, 1968.

Blalock, Hubert M. Theory Construction. Englewood Cliffs, N.J.: Prentice-Hall, Inc., 1969.

Duncan, Otis Dudley. "Path Analysis: Sociological Examples." The American Journal of Sociology, LXXII (1966), 1-16.

Earickson, Robert. The Spatial Behavior of Hospital Patients: A Behavioral Approach to Spatial Interaction in Metropolitan Chicago. Department of Geography Research Paper No. 124. Chicago: University of Chicago, 1970.

Harbaugh, John W., and Daniel F. Merriam. Computer Applications in Stratigraphic Analysis. New York: John Wiley & Sons., Inc., 1968. Pp. 61-100.

Hopps, Howard C. "Computer-Produced Distribution Maps of Disease." Annals of the New York Academy of Sciences, Vol. CLXI (1969).

Hopps, Howard C., and Roger Cuffey. "Cause/Effect Relationships in Disease." International Pathology, X (1969), 23-25.

Li, C. C. Population Genetics. Chicago: University of Chicago Press, 1955. Chap. XII.

Lowry, Ira S. "A Short Course in Model Building." Spatial Analysis: A Reader in Statistical Geography. Edited by Brian J. L. Berry and Duane F. Marble. Englewood Cliffs, N.J.: Prentice-Hall, Inc., 1968. Pp. 53-67.

May, Jacques M. The Ecology of Human Disease. New York: M.D. Publications, 1958.

________. Studies in Disease Ecology. New York: Hofner Publishing Company, 1961.

Morrill, Richard L., and Robert Earickson. "Locational Efficiency of Chicago Hospitals: An Experimental Model." Health Services Research (Summer, 1969).

Mosley, James W. "Transmission of Viral Diseases by Drinking Water." Transmission of Viruses by the Water Route. Edited by Gerald Berd. New York: Interscience Publishers, 1967.

President's Commission on Heart Disease, Cancer, and Stroke. Report to the President: A National Program to Conquer Heart Disease, Cancer, and Stroke. 2 vols. Washington, D. C., 1964.

Pyle, Gerald F. "Some Aspects of Urban Medical Geography." Unpublished Master's dissertation, Department of Geography, University of Chicago, 1968.

Pyle, Gerald F., and Susan M. Davies. "Morbidity and Mortality: Sources of Data and Methods of Analysis." Chicago Regional Hospital Study, Working Paper No. VI. 2. Chicago: Hospital Planning Council for Metropolitan Chicago.

Pyle, Gerald F., and Philip H. Rees "Problems of Modeling Disease Patterns in Urban Areas: The Chicago Example." Economic Geography. Forthcoming.

Regional Medical Programs. Proceedings: Conference Workshop on Regional Medical Programs. 2 vols. Washington, D. C.: U. S. Department of Health, Education, and Welfare, 1968.

Rosenburg, Charles. The Cholera Years. Chicago: University of Chicago Press, 1962.

Schroeder, Henry A. "Relations Between Hardness of Water and Death Rates from Certain Diseases in the United States." Journal of Chronic Diseases, XII (1960), 586-91.

Snow, John, B. W. Richardson, and Wade Hampton Frost. Snow on Cholera. New York: The Commonwealth Fund, 1936.

Stamp, L. Dudley. Some Aspects of Medical Geography. London: Oxford University Press, 1964.

Stewart, William H. "Report on Regional Medical Programs to the President and Congress." Washington, D. C.: U. S. Department of Health, Education, and Welfare, Public Health Service, 1967.

U. S. Department of Health, Education, and Welfare. "Guidelines, Regional Medical Programs." Washington, D. C., 1968.

Vise, Pierre de. Slum Medicine: Chicago's Apartheid Health System. Chicago: University of Chicago Community and Family Study Center, 1969.

Vise, Pierre de, and Siim Soot. "Chicago in the 60's and 70's: A Study of the Chicago Area's Changing Population, 1960-1970, and a Forecast of Population Changes for Municipalities and Counties, 1970-1995." Chicago Regional Hospital Study, Working Paper No. V. 2, 1970.

Wright, Sewall. "The Method of Path Coefficients." Annals of Mathematical Statistics, V (1934), 161-215.

________. "Path Coefficients and Path Regressions: Alternative or Complementary Concepts." Biometrics, XVI (1960), 189-202.

THE UNIVERSITY OF CHICAGO

DEPARTMENT OF GEOGRAPHY

RESEARCH PAPERS (Lithographed, 6×9 Inches)

(*Available from Department of Geography, 5828 S. University Ave. The University of Chicago, Chicago, Illinois 60637. Price: $4.50 each; by series subscription, $4.00 each.*)

*1. GROSS, HERBERT HENRY. *Educational Land Use in the River Forest–Oak Park Community (Illinois)*
*2. EISEN, EDNA E. *Educational Land Use in Lake County, Ohio*
*3. WEIGEND, GUIDO GUSTAV. *The Cultural Pattern of South Tyrol (Italy)*
*4. NELSON, HOWARD JOSEPH. *The Livelihood Structure of Des Moines, Iowa*
*5. MATTHEWS, JAMES SWINTON. *Expressions of Urbanism in the Sequent Occupance of Northeastern Ohio*
*6. GINSBURG, NORTON SYDNEY. *Japanese Prewar Trade and Shipping in the Oriental Triangle*
*7. KEMLER, JOHN H. *The Struggle for Wolfram in the Iberian Peninsula, June, 1942—June, 1944: A Study in Political and Economic Geography in Wartime*
*8. PHILBRICK, ALLEN K. *The Geography of Education in the Winnetka and Bridgeport Communities of Metropolitan Chicago*
*9. BRADLEY, VIRGINIA. *Functional Patterns in the Guadalupe Counties of the Edwards Plateau*
*10. HARRIS, CHAUNCY D., and FELLMANN, JEROME DONALD. *A Union List of Geographical Serials*
*11. DE MEIRLEIR, MARCEL J. *Manufactural Occupance in the West Central Area of Chicago*
*12. FELLMANN, JEROME DONALD. *Truck Transportation Patterns of Chicago*
*13. HOTCHKISS, WESLEY AKIN. *Areal Pattern of Religious Institutions in Cincinnati*
*14. HARPER, ROBERT ALEXANDER. *Recreational Occupance of the Moraine Lake Region of Northeastern Illinois and Southeastern Wisconsin*
*15. WHEELER, JESSE HARRISON, JR. *Land Use in Greenbrier County, West Virginia*
*16. MCGAUGH, MAURICE EDRON. *The Settlement of the Saginaw Basin*
*17. WATTERSON, ARTHUR WELDON. *Economy and Land Use Patterns of McLean County, Illinois*
*18. HORBALY, WILLIAM. *Agricultural Conditions in Czechoslovakia, 1950*
*19. GUEST, BUDDY ROSS. *Resource Use and Associated Problems in the Upper Cimarron Area*
*20. SORENSEN, CLARENCE WOODROW. *The Internal Structure of the Springfield, Illinois, Urbanized Area*
*21. MUNGER, EDWIN S. *Relational Patterns of Kampala, Uganda*
*22. KHALAF, JASSIM M. *The Water Resources of the Lower Colorado River Basin*
*23. GULICK, LUTHER H. *Rural Occupance in Utuado and Jayuya Municipios, Puerto Rico*
*24. TAAFFE, EDWARD JAMES. *The Air Passenger Hinterland of Chicago*
*25. KRAUSE, ANNEMARIE ELISABETH. *Mennonite Settlement in the Paraguayan Chaco*
*26. HAMMING, EDWARD. *The Port of Milwaukee*
*27. CRAMER, ROBERT ELI. *Manufacturing Structure of the Cicero District, Metropolitan Chicago*
*28. PIERSON, WILLIAM H. *The Geography of the Bellingham Lowland, Washington*
*29. WHITE, GILBERT F. *Human Adjustment to Floods: A Geographical Approach to the Flood Problem in the United States*
30. OSBORN, DAVID G. *Geographical Features of the Automation of Industry* 1953. 120 pp.
*31. THOMAN, RICHARD S. *The Changing Occupance Pattern of the Tri-State Area, Missouri, Kansas, and Oklahoma*
*32. ERICKSEN, SHELDON D. *Occupance in the Upper Deschutes Basin, Oregon*
*33. KENYON, JAMES B. *The Industrialization of the Skokie Area*
*34. PHILLIPS, PAUL GROUNDS. *The Hashemite Kingdom of Jordan: Prolegomena to a Technical Assistance Program*
*35. CARMIN, ROBERT LEIGHTON. *Anápolis, Brazil: Regional Capital of an Agricultural Frontier*
*36. GOLD, ROBERT N. *Manufacturing Structure and Pattern of the South Bend–Mishawaka Area*
*37. SISCO, PAUL HARDEMAN. *The Retail Function of Memphis*
*38. VAN DONGEN, IRENE S. *The British East African Transport Complex*
*39. FRIEDMANN, JOHN R. P. *The Spatial Structure of Economic Development in the Tennessee Valley*
*40. GROTEWOLD, ANDREAS. *Regional Changes in Corn Production in the United States from 1909 to 1949*
*41. BJORKLUND, E. M. *Focus on Adelaide—Functional Organization of the Adelaide Region, Australia*
*42. FORD, ROBERT N. *A Resource Use Analysis and Evaluation of the Everglades Agricultural Area*
*43. CHRISTENSEN, DAVID E. *Rural Occupance in Transition: Sumter and Lee Counties, Georgia*
*44. GUZMÁN, LOUIS E. *Farming and Farmlands in Panama*

* Out of print.

*45. ZADROZNY, MITCHELL G. *Water Utilization in the Middle Mississippi Valley*
*46. AHMED, G. MUNIR. *Manufacturing Structure and Pattern of Waukegan–North Chicago*
*47. RANDALL, DARRELL. *Factors of Economic Development and the Okovango Delta*
48. BOXER, BARUCH. *Israeli Shipping and Foreign Trade* 1957. 176 pp.
*49. MAYER, HAROLD M. *The Port of Chicago and the St. Lawrence Seaway*
*50. PATTISON, WILLIAM D. *Beginnings of the American Rectangular Land Survey System, 1784–1800* 1957. 2d printing 1963. 260 pp. Available from Ohio Historical Society.
*51. BROWN, ROBERT HAROLD. *Political Areal-Functional Organization: With Special Reference to St. Cloud, Minnesota.*
*52. BEYER, JACQUELYN. *Integration of Grazing and Crop Agriculture: Resources Management Problems in the Uncompahgre Valley Irrigation Project.*
53. ACKERMAN, EDWARD A. *Geography as a Fundamental Research Discipline* 1958. 40 pp. $1.00
*54. AL-KHASHAB, WAFIQ HUSSAIN. *The Water Budget of the Tigris and Euphrates Basin*
55. LARIMORE, ANN EVANS. *The Alien Town: Patterns of Settlement in Busoga, Uganda* 1958. 210 pp.
56. MURPHY, FRANCIS C. *Regulating Flood-Plain Development* 1958. 216 pp.
*57. WHITE, GILBERT F., *et al. Changes in Urban Occupance of Flood Plains in the United States*
*58. COLBY, MARY MC RAE. *The Geographic Structure of Southeastern North Carolina*
*59. MEGEE, MARY CATHERINE. *Monterrey, Mexico: Internal Patterns and External Relations*
60. WEBER, DICKINSON. *A Comparison of Two Oil City Business Centers* (*Odessa-Midland, Texas*) 1958. 256 pp.
61. PLATT, ROBERT S. *Field Study in American Geography* 1959. 408 pp.
62. GINSBURG, NORTON, editor. *Essays on Geography and Economic Development* 1960. 196 pp.
63. HARRIS, CHAUNCY D., and FELLMANN, JEROME D. *International List of Geographical Serials* 1960. 247 pp.
*64. TAAFFE, ROBERT N. *Rail Transportation and the Economic Development of Soviet Central Asia*
*65. SHEAFFER, JOHN R. *Flood Proofing: An Element in a Flood Damage Reduction Program*
*66. RODGERS, ALLAN L. *The Industrial Geography of the Port of Genova*
67. KENYON, JAMES B. *Industrial Localization and Metropolitan Growth: The Paterson-Passaic District.* 1960. 250 pp.
68. GINSBURG, NORTON. *An Atlas of Economic Development* 1961. 119 pp. 14×8½″. Cloth. University of Chicago Press.
69. CHURCH, MARTHA. *Spatial Organization of Electric Power Territories in Massachusetts* 1960. 200 pp.
70. WHITE, GILBERT F., *et al. Papers on Flood Problems* 1961. 234 pp.
71. GILBERT, E. W. *The University Town in England and West Germany* 1961. 79 pp. 4 plates. 30 maps and diagrams.
72. BOXER, BARUCH. *Ocean Shipping in the Evolution of Hong Kong* 1961. 108 pp.
*73. ROBINSON, IRA M. *New Industrial Towns of Canada's Resource Frontier* (Research Paper No. 4, Program of Education and Research in Planning, The University of Chicago.)
74. TROTTER, JOHN E. *State Park System in Illinois* 1962. 152 pp.
75. BURTON, IAN. *Types of Agricultural Occupance of Flood Plains in the United States* 1962. 167 pp.
*76. PRED, ALLAN. *The External Relations of Cities during 'Industrial Revolution'*
77. BARROWS, HARLAN H. *Lectures on the Historical Geography of the United States as Given in 1933* Edited by WILLIAM A. KOELSCH. 1962. 248 pp.
*78. KATES, ROBERT WILLIAM. *Hazard and Choice Perception in Flood Plain Management*
79. HUDSON, JAMES. *Irrigation Water Use in the Utah Valley, Utah* 1962. 249 pp.
*80. ZELINSKY, WILBUR. *A Bibliographic Guide to Population Geography*
*81. DRAINE, EDWIN H. *Import Traffic of Chicago and Its Hinterland*
*82. KOLARS, JOHN F. *Tradition, Season, and Change in a Turkish Village* NAS-NRC Foreign Field Research Program Report No. 15.
*83. WIKKRAMATILEKE, RUDOLPH. *Southeast Ceylon: Trends and Problems in Agricultural Settlement*
84. KANSKY, K. J. *Structure of Transportation Networks: Relationships between Network Geometry and Regional Characteristics* 1963. 155 pp.
*85. BERRY, BRIAN J. L. *Commercial Structure and Commercial Blight*
86. BERRY, BRIAN J. L., and TENNANT, ROBERT J. *Chicago Commercial Reference Handbook* 1963. 278 pp.
*87. BERRY, BRIAN J. L., and HANKINS, THOMAS D. *A Bibliographic Guide to the Economic Regions of the United States*
*88. MARCUS, MELVIN G. *Climate-Glacier Studies in the Juneau Ice Field Region, Alaska*
*89. SMOLE, WILLIAM J. *Owner-Cultivatorship in Middle Chile*
*90. HELVIG, MAGNE. *Chicago's External Truck Movements: Spatial Interaction between the Chicago Area and Its Hinterland*

* Out of print.

91. HILL, A. DAVID. *The Changing Landscape of a Mexican Municipio, Villa Las Rosas, Chiapas* NAS-NRC Foreign Field Research Program Report No. 26. 1964. 121 pp.
92. SIMMONS, JAMES W. *The Changing Pattern of Retail Location* 1964. 202 pp.
93. WHITE, GILBERT F. *Choice of Adjustment to Floods* 1964. 150 pp.
94. MCMANIS, DOUGLAS R. *The Initial Evaluation and Utilization of the Illinois Prairies, 1815–1840* 1964. 109 pp.
95. PERLE, EUGENE D. *The Demand for Transportation: Regional and Commodity Studies in the United States* 1964. 130 pp.
*96. HARRIS, CHAUNCY D. *Annotated World List of Selected Current Geographical Serials in English*
97. BOWDEN, LEONARD W. *Diffusion of the Decision To Irrigate: Simulation of the Spread of a New Resource Management Practice in the Colorado Northern High Plains* 1965. 146 pp.
98. KATES, ROBERT W. *Industrial Flood Losses: Damage Estimation in the Lehigh Valley* 1965. 76 pp.
*99. RODER, WOLF. *The Sabi Valley Irrigation Projects*
100. SEWELL, W. R. DERRICK. *Water Management and Floods in the Fraser River Basin* 1965. 163 pp.
101. RAY, D. MICHAEL. *Market Potential and Economic Shadow: A Quantitative Analysis of Industrial Location in Southern Ontario* 1965. 164 pp.
102. AHMAD, QAZI. *Indian Cities: Characteristics and Correlates* 1965. 184 pp.
103. BARNUM, H. GARDINER. *Market Centers and Hinterlands in Baden-Württemberg* 1966. 172 pp.
104. SIMMONS, JAMES W. *Toronto's Changing Retail Complex* 1966. 126 pp.
105. SEWELL, W. R. DERRICK, *et al. Human Dimensions of Weather Modification* 1966. 423 pp.
106. SAARINEN, THOMAS FREDERICK. *Perception of the Drought Hazard on the Great Plains* 1966. 183 pp.
107. SOLZMAN, DAVID M. *Waterway Industrial Sites: A Chicago Case Study* 1967. 138 pp.
108. KASPERSON, ROGER E. *The Dodecanese: Diversity and Unity in Island Politics* 1967. 184 pp.
109. LOWENTHAL, DAVID, editor. *Environmental Perception and Behavior* 1967. 88 pp.
110. REED, WALLACE E. *Areal Interaction in India: Commodity Flows of the Bengal-Bihar Industrial Area* 1967. 210 pp.
*111. BERRY, BRIAN J. L. *Essays on Commodity Flows and the Spatial Structure of the Indian Economy*
112. BOURNE, LARRY S. *Private Redevelopment of the Central City: Spatial Processes of Structural Change in the City of Toronto* 1967. 199 pp.
113. BRUSH, JOHN E., and GAUTHIER, HOWARD L., JR. *Service Centers and Consumer Trips: Studies on the Philadelphia Metropolitan Fringe* 1968. 182 pp.
114. CLARKSON, JAMES D. *The Cultural Ecology of a Chinese Village, Cameron Highlands, Malaysia* 1968. 174 pp.
115. BURTON, IAN, KATES, ROBERT W., and SNEAD, RODMAN E. *The Human Ecology of Coastal Flood Hazard in Megalopolis* 1968. 196 pp.
*116. MURDIE, ROBERT, *Factorial Ecology of Metropolitan Toronto, 1951–1961*
117. WONG, SHUE TUCK. *Perception of Choice and Factors Affecting Industrial Water Supply Decisions in Northeastern Illinois* 1968. 96 pp.
118. JOHNSON, DOUGLAS. *The Nature of Nomadism: A Comparative Study of Pastoral Migrations in Southwestern Asia and Northern Africa* 1969. 200 pp.
119. DIENES, LESLIE. *Locational Factors and Locational Developments in the Soviet Chemical Industry* 1969. 285 pp.
120. MIHELIC, DUSAN. *The Political Element in the Port Geography of Trieste* 1969. 104 pp.
121. BAUMANN, DUANE. *The Recreational Use of Domestic Water Supply Reservoir: Perception and Choice* 1969. 125 pp.
122. LIND, AULIS O. *Coastal Landforms of Cat Island, Bahamas: A Study of Holocene Accretionary Topography and Sea-Level Change* 1969. 156 pp.
123. WHITNEY, JOSEPH. *China: Area, Administration and Nation Building* 1970. 198 pp.
124. EARICKSON, ROBERT. *The Spatial Behavior of Hospital Patients: A Behavioral Approach to Spatial Interaction in Metropolitan Chicago* 1970. 198 pp.
125. DAY, JOHN CHADWICK. *Managing the Lower Rio Grande: An Experience in International River Development* 1970. 277 pp.
126. MAC IVER, IAN. *Urban Water Supply Alternatives: Perception and Choice in the Grand Basin Ontario* 1970. 178 pp.
127. GOHEEN, PETER G. *Victorian Toronto, 1850 to 1900: Pattern and Process of Growth* 1970. 278 pp.
128. GOOD, CHARLES M. *Rural Markets and Trade in East Africa* 1970. 252 pp.
129. MEYER, DAVID R. *Spatial Variation of Black Urban Households* 1970. 127 pp.
130. GLADFELTER, BRUCE G. *Meseta and Campiña Landforms in Central Spain* 1971. 204 pp.
131. NEILS, ELAINE M. *Reservation to City: Indian Urbanization and Federal Relocation* 1971. 200 pp.
132. MOLINE, NORMAN T. *Mobility and the Small Town, 1900–1930* 1971. 169 pp.

* Out of print.

133. SCHWIND, PAUL J. *Migration and Regional Development in the United States* 1971. 170 pp.
134. PYLE, GERALD F. *Heart Disease, Cancer and Stroke in Chicago* 1971. 292 pp.
135. JOHNSON, JAMES. *Renovated Waste Water* 1971. 155 pp.
136. BUTZER, KARL W. *Recent History of an Ethiopian Delta* 1971.
137. HARRIS, CHAUNCY D. *Annotated World List of Selected Current Geographical Serials in English, French, and German* 3rd edition 1971. 77 pp.
138. HARRIS, CHAUNCY D., and FELLMANN, JEROME D. *International List of Geographical Serials* 2nd edition 1971.